Greek Medical Manuscripts
Diels' Catalogue

Tome 1: Diels' Catalogue with Indices

Medical Traditions

Edited by
Alain Touwaide

Volume 2/1

De Gruyter

Greek Medical Manuscripts
Diels' Catalogue

Tome 1: Diels' Catalogue with Indices

Newly revised and updated by
Alain Touwaide

De Gruyter

ISBN 978-3-11-060064-3
e-ISBN (PDF) 978-3-11-059996-1
ISSN 2567-6938

Library of Congress Control Number: 2020945916

Bibliographic information published by the Deutsche Nationalbibliothek
The Deutsche Nationalbibliothek lists this publication in the Deutsche Nationalbibliografie; detailed bibliographic data are available on the Internet at http://dnb.dnb.de.

Cover image: Collage of illustrations in medical treatises from the 1st to the 16th century CE, from Greece and Rome, to the Arabic World and China.

Printing: CPI books GmbH, Leck

www.degruyter.com

Table of contents

Foreword

The study of Greek manuscripts of medical content has seen a significant, though not exclusive, investigation by Alain Touwaide, whose life of scholar has been entirely devoted to the knowledge and valorization of the medical traditions of the Mediterranean world with a particular reference to the history of ancient and medieval Greek medicine.

The revisions and updates of the catalogues of Greek medical manuscripts compiled in the early 20th century by an équipe of philologists, guided by the distinguished historian of ancient Greek philosophy and medicine Hermann Diels (*Die Handschriften der antiken Ärzte*), are a cornerstone of Touwaide's scientific research on medical manuscripts, the further developments of which already include plans for a detailed catalogue of all surviving witnesses according to the norms of modern catalography.

Four years after his 2016 voluminous *Census of Greek Medical Manuscripts*, the publication of this new and substantial reference work constitutes a further step, complementary to the previous one, of his programme that will ultimately allow for the critical edition of a series of Greek medical texts in a way reminiscent of the *Corpus Medicorum* conceived by Diels over a century ago as the natural outcome of the catalogues of manuscripts that he coordinated.

If Alain Touwaide embarked on an arduous task with his *Census* and the compilation of an updated list of Greek manuscripts with medical contents—many of which were not listed in Diels' early 20th-century catalogues—the completion of a renewed Diels is a no less demanding endeavour. Diels' catalogues, which have been the reference for over a century for any scholar interested in the study of late antique and medieval Greek medicine from any perspective, are known, indeed, to suffer several limitations—besides the incompleteness of their inventory of manuscripts (well highlighted by the numerous complements provided in the *Census*)—that can be traced to the difficulty in identifying manuscripts generated by Diels' use of shelfmarks which have been made obsolete since by changes in the name of libraries or collections, in ownership, or in the location of collections. To further make research laborious, the printing of Diels' original edition is rather unclear.

Alain Touwaide has chosen to exactly reproduce the substance of Diels' work, even though he significantly intervened with great acumen on the structure, citation format, and presentation of the text, to make its contents more immediately usable and its consultation easier. An innovative organization of data in five tomes (in which the reproduction of Diels' original text in a decidedly more readable form is followed by two different methods of accessing the information, by type of contents—in tomes two through four—and by manuscript—in the fifth and final tome) is accompanied by an articulated system of indices designed to combine the need to reproduce Diels' original text *ad litteram* and the scientific imperative to update and standardize the method of referencing the manuscripts, and also to multiply the keys for searching the texts. In this view, Touwaide's decision to split the list of authors and works is revealing as it allows for the identification of texts by both their Greek and Latin title (albeit following the form, which is not always consistent, of the titles in Diels' original version), thus providing a first effort for a future standardization. Equally inspired by a justifiable need for clarity and simplification is the choice of accompanying the index of the original shelfmarks of manuscripts with a list of the English names of the cities and libraries. Finally, the layout of this renewed Diels clearly improves on the original edition, structuring its presentation in a much clearer and more effective way through different levels of indentation.

Those who are acquainted with Alain Touwaide know that only his visionary and tenacious spirit, supported by an unshakable patience and a truly extraordinary work capacity, could have pushed him to embark alone on the revision of the catalogues that Diels conceived and could complete thanks to the collaboration of a team of no fewer than thirty scholars. Touwaide's revision required many long years of meticulous work, with a sheer quantity of doublechecks, corrections, and identifications of new locations and shelfmarks, as well as *in situ* autoptic inspection of many manuscripts and sometimes even of entire collections.

Though constantly making explicit its connection with Diels' original work through its coherent and functional system of cross-references, the present revision of Diels will ultimately make it unnecessary to refer to the old Diels and make it possible, instead, to work only with updated lists of manuscripts. Furthermore, the multiple indices extremely well designed by Touwaide and the cross-referencing they make possible pave the way to a future, highly desirable transfer of data from a printed form to an open database, much of the necessary material of which is contained in the present work, in addition to the new data already provided by the *Census*. It can be expected that such a database will be constantly expanded and updated by integrating the results of the new developments and research that the catalogue that we have here will undoubtedly contribute to, promote, and generate.

The renewed Diels that we have here deserves to be hailed as an invaluable reference for both the niche of scholars scrutinizing Greek medical manuscripts and texts, and the wider circle of the historians of medicine, pharmacy, and ancient and medieval science, in a way that faithfully reflects the cross-disciplinary approach to the study of medical traditions that Alain Touwaide has convincingly advocated for for years in the name of a fruitful alliance of sciences and the humanities.

We now wish that, as a further contribution to the knowledge of the ancient Greek medical tradition, he will publish a much needed catalogue of Greek medical manuscripts and texts, not only those listed in Diels, but also the many new ones of which he has revealed the existence thanks to his unwavering energy, his devotion to research, and the passion for Greek medicine that has constantly distinguished his life.

Marilena Maniaci
Università degli Studi di Cassino e del Lazio meridionale
Rome, August 2, 2020

Introduction

Just over a century has passed since a team of scholars from across Europe, led by German historian of ancient philosophy and science Hermann Diels (1848–1922)[1], compiled the manuscripts containing Greek medical texts and their medieval translations into a catalogue[2]. Following such classical bibliographies as the *Bibliotheca Graeca* by Johann Albert Fabricius (1668–1736)[3] and the several *Bibliothecae* by Albrecht von Haller (1708–1777)[4], *Diels*, as the catalogue became known, was a landmark in classical and medico-historical scholarship[5]. It was not completely

1 For a broad approach to Diels' multifaceted activity, see for example Calder et al. 1999. All works referred to in this introduction are cited in an abbreviated form (author's last name and year of publication). For the full reference, see the bibliography at pp. xxi–xxx.

2 The catalogue was published in two issues in 1905 and 1906, in the proceedings of Berlin Academy of Science, with a supplement in 1908 in the same series (Diels 1905, 1906a, and 1908, respectively). The 1905 and 1906 issues were published together as a volume in 1906 (Diels 1906b) with a slightly different title (*Die Handschriften der antiken Ärzte, Griechische Abteilung*) which implied that a similar programme would have dealt with the Latin manuscripts. The frontmatter of the second issue (1906a), which provided a general presentation of the programme, the list of the collaborators, and the bibliography, is reproduced as the front matter of this volume with the same pagination as in the first publication. All three issues (1905, 1906a, and 1908) were reprinted in 1970 with an introduction by Fridolf Kudlien (1928–2008) (Kudlien 1970). The translations under consideration were those in Syriac, Arabic, Hebrew, and Latin according to the treatises.
All references to the catalogue here and in the present work comprise two elements: the first identifies the issue of the catalogue (I, II, or N [for *Nachtrag* = Supplement]), and the second (in Arabic numerals) provides the number of the page(s) referred to (e.g., I.22 or N.49). A number in Arabic numerals between parentheses after the second element, such as e.g., II.63 (2), indicates the number of mentions of a manuscript on the same page.

3 Fabricius' *Bibliotheca Graeca* was originally published in 14 volumes between 1705 and 1728, with a second edition started as early as 1708 and pursued until 1754, and also a third edition of Volumes 1 and 2 published in 1718 and 1752, respectively. The whole *Bibliotheca* was further published in a revised edition by Gottlieb Christopher Harles (1738–1815) in 12 volumes published between 1790 and 1809, with an *Index* in 1838. Under the general designation *Bibliotheca Graeca*, all volumes have a distinctive title that indicates their respective contents. In the first volume this title makes an explicit reference to manuscripts (… *notitia Scriptorum Veterum Graecorum quorumcunque monumenta integra, aut fragmenta edita exstant: tum plerorumque è MSS. ac deperditis* …). On Fabricius, see Verner 1966.

4 The first of Haller's *Bibliothecae* was the *Bibliotheca botanica* (1771–1772), which included large chapters on ancient physicians (see for example, Dioscorides, vol. 1, pp. 79–87 [page 79 is numbered 97]). It was followed by the *Bibliotheca chirurgica* (1774–1775), the *Bibliotheca anatomica* (1774–1777), and the *Bibliotheca medicinae practicae* (1776–1788).

5 For the history of the search for the manuscripts of Greek medical texts from the Renaissance to Diels, see Touwaide 2009, particularly pp. 456–508.

unprecedented, however. From the late eighteenth century on, several similar compilations were made, indeed, but they relied either on earlier literature or on *in situ* inspection of just some collections by single scholars. These were the bibliographies compiled by Johann Christian Gottlieb Ackermann (1756–1801)[6] and the pioneering search for manuscripts by the German scholar Friedrich Reinhold Dietz (1804–1836) in the 1830s[7], followed shortly after by the exploratory missions of the French historian of medicine Charles Daremberg (1817–1872), mostly in England[8], with a similar collection of material *in loco* at the Bibliothèque nationale in Paris by the Greek ophthalmologist Georges Costomiris (1849–1902)[9]. Diels' enterprise was different in its systematicity and scale, in addition to its organization, its team[10], and its international network[11] which combined in-house bibliographical research[12] and *in-*

6 Ackermann's bibliographies with their lists of manuscripts for Hippocrates, Dioscorides and Galen, were published in Harles' edition of Fabricius' *Bibliotheca Graeca* (vol. 2 [1791], pp. 506–611, 4 [1795], pp. 673–702, and 5 [1796], pp. 377–500, respectively). The lists of Hippocratic and Galenic manuscripts were reproduced in the edition of these authors in Kühn's *Medicorum Graecorum Opera quae exstant* under the title *Historia literaria* (for Hippocrates, see vol. 1 [1825], pp. I–CCVI; for Galen, see vol. 1 [1821]), pp. XIX–CCLXV). Interestingly enough, Diels referred to these two lists. The list of manuscripts for Dioscorides, *De materia medica*, in Kühn's *Medicorum Graecorum Opera quae exstant* (see vol. 1 [1829], pp. XX–XXVI) did not reproduce Ackermann's, but was compiled by the editor of the text, Kurt Sprengel (1766–1833).

7 Dietz traveled through Germany, Italy, Spain, France, and Britain, systematically searching for codices containing Greek medical texts (see Dietz 1832: IX–X; Dietz 1834: 1.IV), principally Hippocrates, but also Oribasius (he was supposed to prepare an edition for the corpus edited by Kühn), Aetius, the commentators on Hippocrates, Ioannes Zacharias Actuarius, Greek chemical works, Soranus, Paul of Aegina, Rufus of Ephesus, Erotianus, Nicander, Theophilus, Symeon Seth, and others (e.g., Severus iatrosophist whose treatise he published [Dietz 1836]).

8 See the reports of his travels in Daremberg 1845, 1848, 1851, and 1852, with a reproduction of the last two in the form of a monograph in 1853.

9 Costomiris published the results of his investigations at the Bibliothèque nationale in a series of five contributions to the *Revue des études grecques* published between 1889 and 1897.

10 The collaborators of the program are listed in the front matter of the 1906 issue and the 1906 reprint (p. X) with some further names in the 1908 supplement (p. 23). Besides the collaborators *in loco* (among whom were Ph.D. candidates) coordinated in collaboration by Diels and Johan Ludwig Heiberg (1854–1928), the team included several German scholars as Joseph Heeg (1881–1916) in Munich, Georg Helmreich (1849–1921) in Ansbach, Johannes Ilberg (1860–1930) in Leipzig, Karl Kalbfleich (1868–1946) in Marburg, Iwan von Müller (1830–1917) at that time in Munich, Paul Schwarz (1867–1938), then in Berlin, and Max Wellmann (1863–1933). Their number was higher, however, as the reading of the catalogues indicates: the annotations that accompany the mention of some manuscripts refer to scholars whose name does not appear in the two lists of collaborators.

11 The list of collaborators includes several individuals from abroad who were librarians or academics with a special interest in the history of ancient medicine and medical literature, including translations. These scholars were the following (in alphabetical order of last name): Hartwig (Henry) Derembourg (1844–1908) in Paris; Eduard Gottlob (1856–1922) in Krems a.

situ examination of entire library collections by local scholars or members of Diels' team in mission abroad[13].

Remarkably enough, the vast collection of data contained in the two issues of Diels' catalogues was assembled in barely four years[14], witnessing an exceptional mobilization of efforts and resources[15]. Although a supplement—presented as the first—was published in 1908, it was not followed by any other. Shortly after, the team lost some of its collaborators in the First World War[16], and the systematic search for the manuscripts of ancient medical texts was no longer pursued. Nevertheless, several

d. Donau; Montague Rhodes James (1862–1936) in Cambridge; Philip Christian Molhuysen (1870–1944) in Leiden; Alessandro Olivieri (1872–1950) in Naples; Adriano Piccolomini (1843–1907) in Cesena; Anton Ritter von Premerstein (1869–1935) in Vienna; Hans Raeder (1859–1969) in Copenhagen; Walter Scott (1855–1925) in Oxford, with a parenthesis in Montreal (1905–1908); Hermann Schöne (1870–1941) in Basel; Rezső Vári (1867–1940) in Budapest, and Eric Otto Windstedt (1880–1955) in Oxford. This list is not exhaustive, however, as other names appear scattered in the catalogues. The different collaborators interacted as the references to collations (see below) indicate.

12 The consulted bibliography (listed in the 1906a issue [pp. XI–XXIII] with a supplement in 1908 [pp. 23–24]) does not account for the full extent of the library resources consulted by the collaborators of the catalogues, which contain scattered references to works not included in the bibliographical lists.

13 One such mission was that of Max Wellmann, who spent 1906–1907 in Italy, where he particularly investigated the collections of the Vatican and the Marciana libraries. As a result, the 1908 supplement contains multiple annotations made on the basis of his personal consultation of manuscripts.

14 To give an idea of the sheer quantity of data presented in the catalogues, suffice it to say that the number of items from Greek manuscripts only amounts to over 14,000. To this we should add the multiple collations of manuscripts made by the collaborators of the programme during *in loco* research stays or on their behalf that are mentioned in the catalogue. Ilberg, for example, collated himself or received collations of most of the Hippocratic writings from manuscripts at the Vatican Library, and in Florence, Venice, Vienna, and Paris, whereas Helmreich concentrated on Galen (in one case at least, he had a collation of all but one manuscript of a Galenic treatise; see I.83–84).

15 For the history of the programme, see Kollesch 1973, 1989, and 1999; and more recently, Nutton 2004.

16 This was the case of Bruno Rappaport (1875–1915), who managed the data of the catalogues in collaboration with Joahnnes Mewald (1880–1964). On this, see Diels' introductory remarks (*Vorbemerkungen*) to the catalogue (Diels 1906a: pp. I–IX), which include the reports by Rappaport (pp. III–VI) and Mewaldt (pp. VI–VIII). On Rappaport, see the obituary by Regling, 1920. Another victim of the First World War was Joseph Heeg. During the compilation of the catalogues, the program lost another of its members, the orientalist Ludwig Nix (1865–1904) who had collected much material about the Arabic translations of Greek medical works.

editions of Greek medical texts were published thanks to the material collected during the compiling of the catalogues[17].

Addenda and *corrigenda* to Diels[18], studies of the manuscripts or tradition of specific medical treatises[19], and the systematic inventory of the manuscripts of texts to be edited, with the analysis of their tradition[20], punctuated the twentieth-century scholarship devoted to the ancient medical literature. After World War II, an

17 The first such edition was that of Philumenus, *De venenatis animalibus*, by Max Wellmann who discovered the text in the manuscript *Vaticanus graecus* 284 during his research stay at the Vatican Library (Wellmann 1908). This edition, which inaugurated the *Corpus Medicorum Graecorum*, brilliantly illustrated the function of the catalogues as a source of firsthand material for the preparation of the critical editions to be published in the *Corpus*. It is probably significant that it was followed in 1914 by the edition of the Arabic translation of a Pseudo-Galenic treatise by Gotthelf Bergsträsser (1886–1933) (Bergsträsser 1914), and the first edition of Galen in the *Corpus* by three collaborators of the programme (Mewaldt et al. 1914). Another Galenic edition, prepared by another group of three collaborators, followed the next year (Diels et al. 1915), together with Celsus by Friedrich Marx (1869–1941) and, the following year, Quintus Serenus Sammonicus by Friedrich Vollmer (1867–1923). After a short interruption due to World War I, no fewer than 15 editions were published between 1921 and 1937, with one edition every year from 1926 on, including (in chronological order of publication) the vast medical encyclopedias of Paul of Aegina (Heiberg 1921–1924), Oribasius (Raeder 1926, and 1928–1933), and Aetius (*partim*; Olivieri, 1935), in addition to the first Hippocratic edition (Heiberg et al., 1927), Soranus (Ilberg, 1927), Galenic commentaries on Hippocratic treatises (Wenkebach 1934 and 1936) and Galenic works (Koch et al. 1923; De Boer 1937). All this attested to the vitality of the *Corpus* and the usefulness of the catalogue.

18 As early as 1916, Giovanni Mercati (1866–1957), then a *scrittore* at the Vatican Library, published some *addenda* (Mercati 1916, 1917a, and 1917b). Corrections like these are scattered throughout twentieth-century scholarly publications related to the Greek medical literature. Most of them can be found in Touwaide 2016, *passim*, together with new ones. Additions and corrections to Diels' lists of manuscripts of the Latin translations of Greek medical texts have been systematically made, though later. Richard Durling (1932–1999) revised Diels' lists of the Galenic Latin manuscripts (Durling 1967 and 1981, completed only recently by Fortuna and Raia 2006; a cumulative catalogue of the Galenic and Pseudo-Galenic Latin texts [including manuscripts] compiled by Stefania Fortuna and her group is now available online in the form of a constant work in progress [*Galeno. Catalogo delle traduzioni latine*]). Pearl Kibre (1902–1985) compiled new lists of the Hippocratic Latin manuscripts in several installments (1975–1982) followed by a publication in the form of a monographic catalogue in 1985. It may be relevant to note here that Durling expanded his search for Latin medical manuscripts by browsing a collection of material similar to Diels, Kristeller's *Iter Italicum* (Durling 1985–1993).

19 An early work of this type is Ilberg 1911 on Soranus, followed shortly after by Diels 1912 on Galen's commentary on Hippocrates *Prorrheticum*, and Helmreich 1913 on Symeon Seth.

20 The best examples are the introductions to the editions published in the *Corpus Medicorum Graecorum* (which became more developed over time). Their template includes a list of manuscripts, their description, and a detailed philological analysis. Although these introductions focus on identifying the manuscript(s) to be used as a source or sources of the editions, they provide relevant data on codicology and book history.

unprecedented increase in the interest in paleography and codicology[21] soon led to a renewed search for, and study of, manuscripts[22], new catalogues[23], and, more recently, computerized databases allowing for the storage and multi-criteria querying of increasingly larger amounts of information[24], in addition to the digitization of the collections of manuscripts of several libraries across the world[25]. In the field of Greek medical manuscripts and texts, this resulted in the rediscovery or, in some cases, in the true discovery of manuscripts[26], new catalogues of medical manuscripts[27], the history

---

21 In the field of Greek codicology and palaeography, and also textual history, this interest was pioneered by such scholars as Joseph Mogenet (1913–1980), Herbert Hunger (1914–2000), Jean Irigoin (1920–2006), and Paul Canart (1927–2017). It subsequently led to an increased institutionalization of these disciplines illustrated, among others, by a series of international conferences started in 1974 (see *Paléographie,* 1977). For a recent esquisse of the history of codicology and paleography during the twentieth century, see, for example, Touwaide 2010.

22 Whereas the type of research by Alphonse Dain (1896–1964), Paul Henry (1906–1984), Alexander Turyn (1900–1981), and Jean Irigoin on technical texts (Dain 1930, 1933, 1946), Plotin (Henry 1938, 1941), the Greek tragics (Turyn 1943, 1952, 1957) and Pindar (Turyn 1932, and Irigoin 1952), respectively, was relatively rare until then in the academic production, it became more common later. For examples of such a line of investigation, see Eleuteri 1981 on a literary text (Musaeus) and Sonderkamp 1987 on a Greek medical treatise (Theophanes Nonnos/Chrysobalantes).

23 The increase in the publication of catalogues of manuscripts can be best measured by comparing the successive editions of the so-called *Richard* (Richard 1948, 1958, and 1964, followed by such a punctual review of new catalogues as Irigoin 1970, and the major updated editions of *Richard* by Olivier 1995 and 2018).

24 One such database is PINAKES currently hosted and maintained by the Section Grecque of the Institut de Recherche et d'Histoire des Textes (IRHT) of the Centre National de la Recherche Scientifique (CNRS), in Paris. It is built on the basis of the earlier research conducted at the Pontifical Institute of Medieval Studies at University of Toronto by Robert E. Sinkewicz, who compiled available printed catalogues of manuscripts and published the resulting data in the form of microfiches (Sinkewicz and Hayes 1989; Sinkewicz 1990 and 1992). In the matter of medical manuscripts and texts, see the database built on Diels accessible online through the website of the Institute for the Preservation of Medical Traditions. A precursor of this type of database was the catalogue of incipits of Latin medical treatises compiled as early as 1937 by Lynn Thorndike (1882–1965) and Pearl Kibre (1937). After a revised edition published in 1963, this catalogue has been complemented by Linda E. Voigts and Patricia D. Kurtz (Voigts and Kurz 2004), and transformed in digital form (first as a CD-Rom and now as a database consultable online on the site of the University of Missouri Kansas City).

25 See, for example, the site *Gallica*, of the Bibliothèque nationale de France, *teca* of the Biblioteca Medicea Laurenziana in Firenze, *DVL-DigiVatLib* of the Vatican Library, *DigitalBodleian*, *Digitised Manuscripts* of the British Library or, to mention just some, *e-codices* for the manuscripts in Swiss collections. Significantly enough, the most recent release of the site of the *Corpus Medicorum Graecorum* includes links to the digital version of the manuscripts of the authors for which critical editions have been published in the *Corpus*.

26 The most spectacular case has been the discovery of the forgotten manuscript Thessaloniki, Vlatadon 14, which contains a Galenic text which had remained unknown thus far. See Pietrobelli, 2010, for example. For other cases, see, for example, Roselli 2009 ([Hippocrates]) or

of collections of such codices[28], an accrued attention to medical illustration[29], studies of the textual tradition of Greek medical texts[30] or genres[31], the medical production of some regions[32], and new critical editions, particularly from the mid-twentieth century onward[33]. This activity, which also generated a forum in the form of a series of conferences launched by Antonio Garzya (1927–2012) in 1990 and regularly held

---

Perilli 2011 (Galen's Hippocratic lexicon), and Chatzopoulou 2014 and Tselikas 2014 about *iatrosofia*.

27 For some catalogues, see Hunger and Kresten as early as 1969 about the series *medici graeci* of the National Library of Austria in Vienna, and, more recently, Bouras-Vallianatos 2015 about the holdings of the Wellcome Library in London, with a short supplement in Bouras-Vallianatos 2020. A different type of catalogue is that of Formentin 1978, about the libraries of a region.

28 See, for example, Formentin 1997 about the medical manuscripts in the collection of the national library in Naples.

29 A pioneering work in this field was MacKinney 1965, which lists the medieval manuscripts known at that time in several languages with medical illustrations, with some descriptive elements. Recently see Bernabò 2010.

30 For the entire tradition of some works, see, for example (in chronological order of publication), Kudlien 1960 (Hippocrates, *De articulis*), Rivier 1962 (Hippocrates, *De morbo sacro*), and Alexanderson 1963 (Hippocrates, *Prognosticon*) and 1967 (Galen, *De crisibus*). Among the studies in subsequent years, one might cite Morani 1981 (Nemesius) or, more recently, Perilli 1999 (Galen's Hippocratic lexicon). Similar work is being done in Latin, for example by Green 1996 and 1997, on *Trotula*. Research was also devoted to some lesser-known physicians such as Mercurius (see the study by Masullo 2006), or to some segments or manuscripts of the tradition of one or more works. This is the case of Wilson 1987, for example, regarding a group of Galenic manuscripts (the codices copied by Ioannikios), and Petit 2006 on a group of manuscripts in relation with a text ([Galen], *Introductio*).

31 For this type of catalogue, see, for example, Ihm 2002 on medical commentaries (with references to the manuscripts), or Karas 1994, and Tselikas 1995 on *iatrosophia* (Byzantine and later).

32 For Southern Italy, for example, see Ieraci Bio 1989.

33 After an interruption provoked by World War II, the *Corpus Medicorum Graecorum* published anew critical editions as early as 1950 with a predilection for Galen, also including, however, Hippocratic treatises, Aretaeus, Rufus of Ephesus, Aetius, and Leo medicus, and, more recently (from 1983 on), Stephanus of Athens and Johannes of Alexandria. In the 1960s, the French *Collection des universités de France* launched a new Hippocrates (see Joly 1978 for the first volume; the programme has been pursued by Jacques Jouanna) and, very recently, a new Galen (see Boudon 2000 for the first volume). All this in addition to editions in series specifically devoted to the history of ancient and medieval/Byzantine medicine as *Studies in Ancient Medicine* (for example, Dickson 1998 on Stephanus, and Zipser 2009 on Johannes archiater) or, more recently, *Medicine in the Medieval Mediterranean* (Bennett 2016 on hospital formularies) and *Textos Médicos – Ediciones Críticas* (Lamagna 2017 on Johannes Actuarius' Greek translation of Avicenna, *De urinis*). See also such volumes as Pritchet 1975 and 1982 (both on Johannes of Alexandria) or Garzya and Masullo 2004 (on Cassius Iatrosophista). To this, one might add editions of *iatrosofia* (for example, Tselikas and Ilioudis 1995 and 1997, or Clark 2011).

since[34], was accompanied by a transformation in the history of science and the history of the book. While the former moved its focus from the *Great Scientists*[35] to the *histoire vécue*[36], the latter shifted from book production[37] to book use, that is, to reading, studying, annotating, sharing, and collecting[38].

Both transformational trends highlighted limitations of Diels' catalogues: they are devoted to authored works with a focus on the major physicians of classical antiquity and of the period that became defined in the meantime as *Late Antiquity*, that is, the period up to the end of the School of Alexandria in the 7th century A.D[39]. With only some exceptions[40], they omit the multiple small, but no less important, anonymous works, notebooks, and other formularies that give witness to the practice of medicine[41], and also many of the physicians of all epochs (but especially the Byzantine ones, also with some exceptions, however[42]) who have not been credited with such a foundational role as Hippocrates and Galen.

---

34 For the proceedings of the first conference, see Garzya 1992. The conference has been fairly consistently held every four years, alternately in Naples and Paris. The many communications presented in each edition dealt with a great many authors and texts, including lesser known physicians and their treatises. The proceedings were first edited by Antonio Garzya, and then by Garzya in collaboration with Jacques Jouanna before being edited by both, along with Véronique Boudon-Millot and Amneris Roselli.

35 As an example of this historiography, see the monumental encyclopedic *Introduction to the History of Science* (1927–1948) of George Sarton (1884–1956).

36 See, for example, Perrin 1988 on the skin (followed by Herida 1998, on skin in the Hippocratic writings), Rey 1993 on pain, or Dumouchel 1995 on emotions. One might also mention here the development of the history of the body, particularly its specific perception and its representation, including its defects (Fischer 1991).

37 The focus on book production might be best identified by the development of codicology, explicitly formalized as a discipline in its own right during this period (see Dain 1949).

38 On this approach, see, for example, the works of Guglielmo Cavallo, particularly Cavallo 1988 about libraries, and Cavallo and Chartier 1995 on reading, with a panoramic presentation of medieval reading culture. On reading Greek medical literature, more specifically, see, for example, Cavallo 1993 or, more recently, Mondrain 2003.

39 On the chonological span of the catalogues (from the 5th century B.C. to the 7th A.D.), see Bruno Rappaport's report in the 1906 issue, p. III.

40 Some of these exceptions might be the *Excerpta* (or *Excerpta varia*) listed for several authors, as well as the pseudepigraphic literature (mostly Hippocratic and Galenic) (see for example the remedies attributed to, or extracted from the works of, Hippocrates [I.48–49] and Galen [I.132–133]), in addition to some *iatrosophia* of the Ottoman period listed mostly under Hippocrates (I.42), Galen (I.123 and N.38) and Meletius (II.64), but also under Erasistratos (II.36) and Magnus (II.59), besides references to *iatrosophic* literature about Iustus (N.56), Logadius (N.56), Lucas (N.56), and Syncellus (N.66).

41 For such works (hospital formularies), see, for example, Bennett, 2016.

42 These exceptions are the following (in alphabetical order of their names as in Diels) with their reference to Diels: Abraham (II.3; N.42), Antonius Pyropulus (II.15; N.45), Beniaminus (II.22;

A *New Diels* is now a desideratum of the scholarly community[43]. While urgently needed, it would require that Greek medical manuscripts be newly catalogued and their texts accurately identified, building on the twentieth-century classical scholarship briefly presented above and indeed, going even further through a renewed *in situ* autoptic analysis of manuscripts and the reading of their many texts[44]. Whereas codicological analysis would allow for a better approximation of the time or period and place of production of the manuscripts (and also of their texts in some cases), reading and precise identification of all their texts would lead to a more complete and accurate knowledge of medical literature and practice from antiquity to the Renaissance, particularly thanks to the treatises of the period posterior to the 7th century and, for all periods, the multiple anonymous texts of all types not considered in Diels' catalogues.

The present work aims to lead the study of Greek medical manuscripts and literature of the classical and post-classical periods in that direction. While it fundamentally reproduces Diels' lists of Greek manuscripts, it reformats them in different, yet complementary, ways and provides new search tools that may be used for at least two purposes: compiling a catalogue of Greek medical manuscripts that will eventually generate the material necessary for a *New Diels*, and investigating the tradition, reception, and intellectual, and scientific history of Greek medical literature and medicine.

N.46), Cassius iatrosophista (II.22; N.46), Chariton (II.23), Constantinus Meliteniota (II.24; N.47), Damascenus (II.25), Eleutherus (II.35), Esdras propheta (II.37–38; N.50–51), Euphemius Siculus (II.38; N.51), Iacobus Psychrestus (II.50), Ioannes Chumnos (II.52), Ioannes Esdra (II.53), Ioannes episcopus Prisdyanesis (II.54; N.55), Ioannes Staphidaces (II.55; N.55), Leo (II.57; N.56), Manuel Comnenus (N.57), Maximus (Planudes?) (II.62; N.57), Neophytus Prodromenus (II.68; N.60), Nicolaus Myrepsus (II.69; N.60), Nicomedes iatrosophista (II.69), Paulus Nicaeensis (II.81; N.63), Perzoe (II.81), Philippus Xerus (N.63), Photius monachus (II.85),Taronitus (II.100; N.67), Theophilus (II.101–106; N.68), Theophylactus Simocata (II.106; N.68), and Ioannes Zacharias Actuarius (II.108–111; N.69).

43 Some *instrumenta studiorum* that might be considered as partial *New Diels* are already available. One of them is the catalogue of the manuscripts of the Latin translations of Hippocrates compiled by Pearl Kibre (above). Other two are the analytical lists of the manuscripts of the Arabic translations of Greek medical literature and original Arabic medical literature compiled by Sezgin 1970 (medicine, pharmacy, and zoology) and 1971 (alchemy, chemistry, botany, and agriculture), and Ullmann 1970 (medicine). One might also add the inventory of illustrated medical manuscripts compiled by MacKinney as early as 1965 (not only Greek and Latin, but also Syriac, Arabic and Turkish, and the roman languages, English, and German). Relevant also, the bibliographical lists compiled by Gerhard Fichtner (1932–2012) for Hippocrates and Galen (first published on demand, with several successive versions from 1985 on, and now available on line on the website of *Corpus Medicorum Graecorum*).

44 For a proposal in that sense, see Touwaide 2018. Whereas a publication upon completion of the research would be highly desirable, a gradual publication of available data in the form of a work in progress on the Internet might be useful, be it for a catalogue of manuscripts or a *New Diels*.

As such, the present work offers a set of new *instrumenta studiorum* for further developments in manuscript studies, the classical, medical and scientific traditions, and medical history.

Each of the five tomes of the present work has a specific content and purpose. The first tome exactly reproduces Diels' lists of Greek medical manuscripts[45], excluding the lists of the manuscripts containing the possible medieval translations of Greek medical texts into Syriac, Arabic, Hebrew, or Latin according to the treatises. It is not a photographic reproduction of Diels' original pages, however. Whereas lists of manuscripts in the original printing of Diels are presented in the form of blocks of continuous texts, they are rearranged here in the form of enumerations that clearly distinguish each item. The bibliography of Diels has been treated in a similar way for the purposes of clarity. The lists of manuscripts and the bibliography comprise most of the first tome, which is complemented by two indices: one of the authors and texts included in Diels, and the other of the manuscripts listed in Diels. For the purposes of easy and direct consultation, both of these indices open the first tome, which aims to not only make Diels available in a handy format, but to facilitate its use in research.

The remaining four tomes differ with regard to substance and purpose. All of them reproduce the contents of the manuscripts as described in Diels, including all annotations about title, *incipit*, *desinit* and lacunae, in addition to possible similarities with other manuscripts, sources, or copies. They proceed by manuscript (instead of by authors and works as in Diels' original publication). Identification of manuscripts exactly reproduces Diels' elements (city, library, and collection as appropriate, followed by shelfmark). The identification of many manuscripts required updating. This is the case for the several items known in Diels through earlier literature without exact identification. It is also the case of the codices destroyed during the two World Wars of the twentieth century, and of those that have changed location after the publication of Diels. Finally, it is also the case for those manuscripts which have received new shelfmarks. For all of these manuscripts, tomes two through five provide supplementary information with their exact identification, their state of preservation and location, or

45 Until a new reprint is published, Diels does not seem to be widely available (in spite of the 1970 reprint). WorldCat lists only 20 copies across the world. Nevertheless, digital copies are available on the Internet with different levels of quality, accuracy, and completeness via such sites as the *Corpus Medicorum Graecorum*, the Royal College of Physicians (RCP) in London, the Medic@ collection of the BIUSanté in Paris, the Digitale Bibliothek of the Münchener DigitalisierungsZentrum of the Bayerische Staatsbibliothek in Munich, and Google. These copies are linked on some other websites such as the Internet Archive, the UK Medical Heritage Library, the Medical Heritage Library, and European Libraries. As mentioned above, a database built on the basis of Diels is available on the website of the Institute for the Preservation of Medical Traditions.

their new shelfmark[46]. Another contribution of these tomes is their index of manuscripts, which includes possible new locations and shelfmarks, thus allowing one to search for manuscripts in two different, yet complementary ways: by their location and shelfmark as in Diels' time or in present time.

Besides these shared features, tomes two through five differ further by their content. Tomes two through four are each devoted to one author or a group of authors: tome two is devoted to Hippocrates, tome three to Galen, and tome four to the authors defined in Diels as *the remaining physicians* (*Die übrigen griechischen Ärzte ausser Galenos und Hippocrates*), that is, all the other authors of classical and late antiquity, with some Byzantine ones as well[47]. These three volumes aim to allow for a general study of the whole manuscript tradition of the textual bodies they are devoted to. Although they still have a limited documentary basis, they compensate for the lack of relevant instruments in currently available literature, and they provide the substance for first reconstructions of the whole tradition of the treatises by (or attributed to) Hippocrates, Galen, and the other Greek physicians considered by Diels.

Tome five goes further in laying down the basis of what will become a general catalogue of Greek medical manuscripts, as it lists the entire contents of all the manuscripts mentioned in Diels. It proceeds as do tomes two through four, by city and library in alphabetical order and, for each library, by collection and shelfmark, with their new locations and identifications as relevant. It also contains all the descriptive annotations about the texts included in Diels. Like tomes two through four, it contains an index of manuscripts that also lists possible new locations and identifications, allowing one to search for manuscripts on the basis of Diels or by their present location and identification.

By reproducing Diels' inventory of, and data on, Greek medical manuscripts, by rearranging them for new investigations, and by providing them with updated identification and new *instrumenta studiorum*, this work aims to not only make Diels newly available in a handy format with updated information and to expand the range of its applications, but to make further strides in the direction of a general catalogue of Greek medical manuscripts. This catalogue, in turn, will lead to the much needed *New Diels* that may be expected to transform the study and understanding of the Greek medical literature and medicine, with their tradition.

46 For these data, see Touwaide, 2016.
47 For these physicians, see note 42.

Bibliography

Ackermann 1791: Johannes Chr. Ackermann, "Caput XXIII De Hippocrate, Medicorum Principe, et Polybo eius Discipulo", in Ioannes Albertus Fabricius, *Bibliotheca Graeca sive Notitia Scriptorum Veterum Graecorum quorumcumque Monumenta Integra aut Fragmenta edita exstant tum plerorumque e MSS. ac deperditis ab auctore recognita*. Editio quarta variorum curis emendatior atque auctior curante Gottlieb Christophoro Harles. Accedunt B. I. A. Fabricii et Christoph. Augusti Heumanni Supplementa inedita, Volumen secundum. Hamburgi: apud Carolum Ernestum Bohn; Lipsiae: Ex Officina Breitkopfia, 1791, pp. 506–611.

Ackermann 1795: Johannes Chr. Ackermann, "Caput III De Dioscoride", in Ioannes Albertus Fabricius, *Bibliotheca Graeca sive Notitia Scriptorum Veterum Graecorum quorumcumque Monumenta Integra aut Fragmenta edita exstant tum plerorumque e MSS. ac deperditis ab auctore recognita*. Editio tertia variorum curis emendatior atque auctior curante Gottlieb Christophoro Harles. Accedunt Christophori Augusti Heumanni Supplementa inedita, Volumen quartum. Hamburgi: apud Carolum Ernestum Bohn; Lipsiae: Ex Officina Breitkopfia et Haertelia, 1795, pp. 673–702.

Ackermann 1796: Johannes Chr. Ackermann, " Caput XIX (olim XVII) Claudius Galenus", in Ioannes Albertus Fabricius, *Bibliotheca Graeca sive Notitia Scriptorum Veterum Graecorum quorumcumque Monumenta Integra aut Fragmenta edita exstant tum plerorumque e MSS. ac deperditis ab auctore recognita*. Editio tertia variorum curis emendatior atque auctior curante Gottlieb Christophoro Harles. Accedunt Christophori Augusti Heumanni Supplementa inedita, Volumen quintum. Hamburgi: apud Carolum Ernestum Bohn; Lipsiae: Ex Officina Breitkopfia et Haertelia, 1796, pp. 377–500.

Ackermann 1821: Johannes Chr. Ackermann, "Historia literaria Claudii Galeni ... ex Jo. Alb. Fabricii Biblioth. Graec. ex ed. Gli. Cph. Harles, vol. V. P. 377–500", in Carolus Gottlob Kühn (ed.), *Claudii Galeni Opera omnia*, Tomus 1 (Medicorum Graecorum Opera quae exstant 1). Leipzig: Carl Cnobloch, 1821, pp. XVII–CCLXV.

Ackermann 1825: Johannes Chr. Ackermann, "Historia literaria Hippocratis ... ex Jo. Alb. Fabricii Biblioth. Graec. ex edit. Gli. Cph. Harles, vol. II. P. 506–511. Desunta et hinc inde aucta et emendata", in Carolus Gottlob Kühn (ed.), *Magni Hippocratis Opera omnia*, Tomus 1 (Medicorum Graecorum Opera quae exstant 21). Leipzig: Carl Cnobloch, 1825, pp. I–CCVI).

Alexanderson 1963: Bengt Alexanderson, *Die Hippokratische Schrift Prognostikon. Überlieferung and Text* (Studia Graeca et Latina Gothoburgensia 17). Göteborg: Acta Universitatis Gothoburgensis, 1963.

Alexanderson 1967: Bengt Alexanderson, *Galenos, Περὶ κρίσεων. Uberlieferung und Text* (Studia Graeca et Latina Gothoburgensia 23). Göteborg: Acta Universitatis Gothoburgensis, 1967.

Bennett 2016: David Bennett, *Medicine and Pharmacy in Byzantine Hospitals. A study of the extant formularies* (Medicine in the Medieval Mediterranean 7). London and New York, NY: Routledge, 2016.

Bersgträsser 1914: Gotthelf Bergsträsser (ed.), *Pseudogaleni in Hippocratis de septimanis* (Corpus Medicorum Graecorum XI 2,1). Lipsiae et Berolini: B.G. Teubner, 1914.

Bernabò 2010: Massimo Bernabò (ed.), *La collezione di testi chirurgici di Niceta. Firenze, Biblioteca Medicea Laurenziana, plut. 74.7. Tradizione medica classica a Bisanzio* (Folia Picta. Manoscritti miniati medievali 2). Roma: Storia e Letteratura, 2010.

Boudon 2000: Véronique Boudon, *Galien*, Tome II: *Exhortation à l'étude de la médecine. Art médical*. Texte établi et traduit (Collection des Universités de France). Paris: Belles Lettres, 2000.

Bouras-Vallianatos 2015: Petros Bouras-Vallianatos, "Greek Manuscripts at the Wellcome Library in London: A Descriptive Catalogue", *Medical History* 59 (2015), pp. 275–326.

Bouras-Vallianatos 2020: Petros Bouras-Vallianatos, "Addenda et Corrigenda to the 'Greek Manuscripts at the Wellcome Library in London: A Descriptive Catalogue', *Medical History* 59 (2015): 275–326", in Petros Bouras-Vallianatos (ed.), *Exploring Greek Manuscripts in the Library at Wellcome Collection in London*. London: Routledge, 2020, pp. 181–182.

Calder et al. 1999: William M. Calder III, and Jaap Mansfeld (eds.), with the participation of Alex Leukart, François Paschould, and Olivier Reverdin, *Hermann Diels (1848–1922) et la science de l'Antiquité. Huit exposés suivis de discussion … Vandoeuvres-Genève, 17–21 août 1998* (Entretiens sur l'Antiquité classique 45). Genève: Fondation Hardt, 1999.

Cavallo 1988: Guglielmo Cavallo, *Le biblioteche nel mondo antico e medievale* (Biblioteca universale Laterza 250). Bari and Roma: Laterza, 1988.

Cavallo 1993: Guglielmo Cavallo, "Libri di medicina: gli usi di un sapere", in Evelyne Patlagean (ed.), *Maladie et société à Byzance* (Collectanea 3). Spoleto: Centro italiano di studi sull'alto medioevo, 1993, pp. 43–56.

Cavallo and Chartier 1995: Guglielmo Cavallo and Roger Chartier (eds), *Storia della lettura nel mondo occidentale* (Storia e Società). Bari and Roma: Laterza, 1995.

Chatzopoulou 2014: Βενετία Χατζοπούλου, "Δύο ἄγνωστα ἰατρικά χειρόγραφα μὲ ἔργα τοῦ Νικολάου Βελισδονίτη", in Παναγιώτης Βλάχος, *Όσιος Ευγένιος ο Αιτωλός και αι Σχολαί των Αγράφων κατά την Τουρκοκρατία. Καρπενήσιον, 7–9 Όκτωβρίου 2011. Πρακτικά*. Αθήνα: Σύνδεσμος "Ευγένιος ο Αιτωλός", 2014, vol. 2, pp. 573–581.

Clark 2011: Patricia A. Clark, *A Cretan Healer's Handbook in the Byzantine Tradition: Text, Translation and Commentary* (Medicine in the Medieval Mediterranean 3). Aldershot, and Burlington, VT: Ashgate, 2011.

Costomiris 1889: Georges A. Costomiris, "Etudes sur les écrits inédits des anciens médecins grecs et ceux dont le texte original est perdu, mais qui existent en latin ou en arabe. Première série: Hippocrate, Cratevas, Aelius Promotus, Galien", *Revue des études grecques* 1 (1889), pp. 343–383.

Costomiris 1890: Georges A. Costomiris, "Etudes sur les écrits inédits des anciens médecins grecs et ceux dont le texte original est perdu, mais qui existent en latin ou en arabe. Deuxième série: L'Anonyme de Daremberg, Métrodora, Aétius", *Revue des études grecques* 3 (1890), pp. 145–179.

Costomiris 1891: Georges A. Costomiris, "Etudes sur les écrits inédits des anciens médecins grecs et ceux dont le texte original est perdu, mais qui existent en latin ou en arabe. Troisième série: Alexandre (Sophiste et Roi), Timothée, Léon le Sophiste, Théophane Nonnos, les Ephodes", *Revue des études grecques* 4 (1891), pp. 97–110.

Costomiris 1892: Georges A. Costomiris, "Études sur les écrits inédits des anciens médecins grecs. Quatrième série: Hippiatriques et auteurs du XIe siècle: Psellus, Siméon Seth, Damnastès", *Revue des études grecques*, 5 (1892), pp. 61–72.

Costomiris 1897: Georges A. Costomiris, "Etudes sur les écrits inédits des anciens médecins grecs et ceux dont le texte original est perdu, mais qui existent en latin ou en arabe. Cinquième série: XIIIe–XIVe siècles, Jean Tzetzès, Nicolas Myrepsus, Jean Actuarius", *Revue des études grecques* 10 (1897), pp. 405–445.

Dain 1930: Alphonse Dain, *Les manuscrits d'Onesandros* (Collection d'études anciennes). Paris: Belles Lettres, 1930.

Dain 1933: Alphonse Dain, *La tradition du texte d'Héron de Byzance* (Collection d'études anciennes). Paris: Belles Lettres, 1933.

Dain 1946: Alphonse Dain, *Histoire du texte d'Élien le Tacticien des origines à la fin du moyen âge* (Collection d'études anciennes). Paris: Belles Lettres, 1946.

Dain 1949: Alphonse Dain, *Les manuscrits*. Paris: Belles Lettes, 1949.

Daremberg 1845: Charles Daremberg, "Rapport adressé à M. le Ministre de l'Instruction Publique par .. chargé d'une mission médico-littéraire en Allemagne" *Journal général de l'Instruction publique* 14, no. 33 (23 avril 1845), pp. 193–196, and no. 34 (26 avril 1845), pp. 198–202 (also printed as a booklet under the same title, in Paris, P. Dupont, 15 avril 1845, 32 p.).

Daremberg 1848: Charles Daremberg, "Résumé d'un voyage médico-littéraire en Angleterre. Lu à l'Académie des inscriptions et belle-lettres, dans la séance du 6 octobre", *Gazette médicale de Paris*, 4 novembre 1848, pp. 3–18.

Daremberg 1851: Charles Daremberg, "Notices et extraites des manuscrits médicaux d'Angleterre", *Archives des Missions scientifiques et littéraires*, 1851,VII, VIII, and IX.

Daremberg 1852: Charles Daremberg, "Notices et extraites des manuscrits médicaux d'Angleterre", *Archives des Missions scientifiques et littéraires* 1852, I.

Daremberg 1853: Charles Daremberg, *Notices et extraits des manuscrits médicaux grecs, latins et français, des principales bibliothèques de l'Europe, I: Manuscrits grecs d'Angleterre suivis d'un fragment de Gilles de Corbeil et de scolies inédites sur Hippocrate*. Paris: Imprimerie impériale, 1853.

De Boer 1937: Wilko De Boer (ed.), *Galeni De propriorum animi cuiuslibet dignotione et curatione. De animi cuiuslibet peccatorum dignotione et curatione. De atra bile* (Corpus Medicorum Graecorum V 4, 1. 1). Lipsiae et Berolini: B. G. Teubner, 1937.

Dickson 1998: Keith Dickson (ed.), *Stephanus the Philosopher and Physician, Commentary on Galen's Therapeutics to Glaucon* (Studies in Ancient Medicine 19). Leiden, Boston, MA, Köln: Brill, 1998.

Diels 1905: Hermann Diels (ed.), *Die Handschriften der antiken Ärzte. I. Teil. Hippokrates und Galenos. Im Auftrage der akademischen Kommission herausgegeben* (Abhandlungen der Königlich Preussischen Akademie der Wissenschaften vom Jahre 1905, Philosophisch-historische Klasse, Abhandlung III). Berlin: Königliche Akademie der Wissenschaften, 1905.

Diels 1906a: Hermann Diels, *Die Handschriften der antiken Ärzte. II. Teil. Die übrigen griechischen Ärzte ausser Hippokrates und Galenos. Im Auftrage der akademischen Kommission herausgegeben von -* (Abhandlungen der Königlich Preussischen Akademie der Wissenschaften vom Jahre 1906, Philosophisch-historische Klasse, Abhandlung I). Berlin: Königliche Akademie der Wissenschaften, 1906.

Diels 1906b: Hermann Diels, *Die Handschriften der antiken Ärzte. Griechische Abteilung. Im Auftrage der akademischen Kommission herausgegeben von - aus den Abhandlungen der Königlich Preussischen Akademie der Wissenschaften der Jahre 1905 und 1906*. Berlin: Königliche Akademie der Wissenschaften, 1906.

Diels 1908: Hermann Diels, *Bericht über den Stand des interakademischen Corpus Medicorum Antiquorum und Erster Nachtrag zu den in den Abhandlungen 1905 und 1906 veröffentlichten Katalogen: Die Handschriften der antiken Ärzte. I. und II. Teil. Zusammengestellt im Namen der Kommission der Königlich Preussischen Akademie der Wissenschaften von -* (Abhandlungen der Königlich Preussischen Akademie der Wissenschaften vom Jahre 1907, Philosophisch-historische Klasse, Abhandlung II). Berlin: Königliche Akademie der Wissenschaften, 1908.

Diels 1912: Hermann Diels, *Die handschriftliche Überlieferung des galenischen Commentars zum Prorrheticum des Hippocrates* (Abhandlungen der Königlich Preussischen Akademie der Wissenschaften vom Jahre 1912, Philosophisch-historische Klasse, Abhandlung I). Berlin: Königliche Akademie der Wissenschaften, 1912.

Diels et al. 1915: Hermann Diels (ed.), *Galeni, In Hippocratis Prorrheticum I commentaria III*; Johannes Mewaldt (ed.), *Galeni, De comate secundum Hippocratem*; Josef Heeg (ed.), *Galeni, In Hippocratis Prognosticum commentaria III* (Corpus Medicorum Graecorum V 9, 2). Lipsiae et Berolini: B. G. Teubneri, 1915.

Dietz 1832: Friedrich Reinhold Dietz, *Galeni de dissectione musculorum et de consuetudine libri. Ad fidem codicum manuscriptorum alterum secundum, primum alterum graece edidit.* Lipsiae: Leopold Voss, 1832.

Dietz 1834: Friedrich Reinhold Dietz, *Apollonii Citiensis, Stephani, Palladii, Theophili, Meletii, Damasci, Ioannis aliorum Scholia in Hippocratem et Galenum e codicibus mss. Vindobonens. Monacens. Florentin. Mediolanens. Escorialens. etc. primum graece edidit*, 2 volumes. Regimontii Prussorum: apud fratres Borntraeger, 1834.

Dietz 1836: Friedrich Reinhold Dietz, *Severi Iatrosophistae De clysteribus liber. Ad Fidem Codicis Manuscripti unici Florentini primum Graece edidit.* Regimontii Prussorum: apud Fratres Borntraeger, 1836.

Dumouchel 1995: Paul Dumouchel, *Emotions. Essai sur le corps et le social* (Collection Les Empêcheurs de penser en rond). Le Plessis-Robinson: Synthélabo, 1995.

Durling 1967: Richard J. Durling, "Corrigenda and addenda to Diels' Galenica. I. Codices Vaticani". *Traditio* 23 (1967), pp. 461–476.

Durling 1981: Richard J. Durling, "Corrigenda and addenda to Diels' Galenica. II. Codices Miscellanei". *Traditio* 37 (1981), pp. 373–381.

Durling 1985–1993: Richard J. Durling, "A Guide to the Medical Manuscripts Mentioned in Kristeller's *Iter Italicum*", *Traditio* 41 (1985), pp. 341–365; 44 (1988), pp. 485–536; 46 (1991), pp. 347–379; 48 (1993), pp. 253–316.

Eleuteri 1981: Paolo Eleuteri, *Storia della tradizione manoscritta di Museo* (Biblioteca di Studi Antichi 30). Pisa: Giardini, 1981.

Fabricius 1705–1728: Jo. Alberti Fabricii, *Bibliotheca Graeca* ... Hamburgi: Sumptu Christiani Lievezeit, Typis Spiringlanis, 1705–1728, 14 volumes (after the general title as above, each volume has a specific subtitle that details its contents).

Fabricius ed. Harles 1790–1838: Gottlieb Christophorus Harles, *Ioannis Alberti Fabricii ... Bibliotheca Graeca sive notitia scriptorum veterum graecorum quorumcunque monumenta integra aut fragmenta edita exstant tum plerorumque e MSS. ac deperditis ab auctore tertium recognita et plurimis locis aucta editio quarta variorum curis emendatior atque auctior ... Accedunt B. I. A. Fabricii et Christoph. Augusti Heumanni supplementa inedita*. Hamburgi: apud Carolum Ernestum Bohn; Lipsiae: ex Officina Breitkoppia, 1790–1838, 13 volumes.

Fichtner 1985a: Gerhard Fichtner, *Corpus Galenicum. Verzeichnis der galenischen und pseudogalenischen Schriften*. Tübingen: the author, 1985.

Fichtner 1985b: Gerhard Fichtner, *Corpus Hippocraticum. Verzeichnis der hippokratischen und pseudohippokratischen Schriften.* Tübingen: the author, 1985.

Fischer 1991: Jean-Louis Fischer, *Monstres. Histoire du corps et de ses défauts*. Paris: Syros Alternatives, 1991.

Formentin 1978: Mariarosa Formentin, *I codici greci di medicina nelle tre Venezie* (Università di Padova, Studi bizantini e neogreci 10). Padova: Liviana editrice, 1978.

Formentin 1997: Maria Rosa Formentin, "Codici greci di medicina nella Biblioteca Nazionale Vittorio Emanuele III di Napoli: le vie di acquisizione", in Sergio Sconocchia and Lucio Toneatto (eds.), in collaboration with Daria Crismani, Michele Faraguna, and Italo Pin, *Lingue tecniche del greco e del latino II. Atti del II Seminario internazionale sulla letteratura scientifica e tecnica greca e latina (Trieste, 4–5 ottobre 1993).* Bologna: Pàtron, 1997, pp. 208–216.

Fortuna and Raia 2006: Stefania Fortuna and Annamaria Raia, "Corrigenda and Addenda to Diels *Galenica* by Richard J. Durling: III. Manuscripts and Editions", *Traditio* 61 (2006), pp. 1–30.

Garzya 1992: Antonio Garzya (ed.), *Tradizione e ecdotica dei testi medici tardo-antichi e bizantini. Atti del Convegno internazionale, Anacapri, 29–31 ottobre 1990* (Collectanea 5). Napoli: D'Auria, 1992.

Garzya and Masullo 2004: Antonio Garzya and Rita Masullo (eds), *I problemi di Cassio Iatrosofista. Testo critico, introduzione, apparato critico, traduzione e note*. Napoli: Accademia Pontaniana, 2004.

Green 1996: Monica H. Green, "A Handlist of the Latin and Vernacular Manuscripts of the So-Called Trotula Texts. Part I: The Latin Manuscripts", *Scriptorium* 50 (1996), pp. 137–175.

Green 1997: Monica H. Green, "A Handlist of the Latin and Vernacular Manuscripts of the So-Called Trotula Texts. Part II: The Vernacular Texts and Latin Re-Writings", *Scriptorium* 51 (1997), pp. 80–104.

Haller 1771–1772: Albrecht von Haller, *Bibliotheca botanica qua scripta ad rem herbariam facientia a rerum initiis recensentur*, 2 volumes. Tiguri: Orell, Gessner, Fuessli, et Socc., 1771–1772.

Haller 1774–1775: Albrecht von Haller, *Bibliotheca chirurgica qua scripta ad artem chirurgicam facientia a rerum initiis recensentur*, 2 volumes. Bernae: Em. Haller; Basileae: Joh. Schweighauser, 1774–1775.

Haller 1774–1777: Albrecht von Haller, *Bibliotheca anatomica qua scripta ad anatomen et physiologiam facientia a rerum initiis recensentur*, 2 volumes. Tiguri: Orell, Gessner, Fuessli, et Socc., 1774–1777.

Haller 1776–1788: Albrecht von Haller, *Bibliotheca medicinae practicae qua scripta ad partem medicinae practicam facientia a rerum initiis ad A. MDCCLXXV recensentur*, 4 volumes. Basileae: Joh. Schweighauser, and Bernae: Em. Haller, 1776–1788.

Heiberg 1921–1924: Johannes L. Heiberg (ed.), *Paulus Aegineta*, 2 volumes (Corpus Medicorum Graecorum IX 1–2). Lipsiae et Berolini: B. G. Teubner, 1921–1924.

Heiberg et al. 1927: Johannes L. Heiberg, Johannes Mewaldt, Ernst Nachmanson, Hermann Schoene (eds), *Hippocratis opera: Indices librorum, Iusiurandum, Lex, De arte, De medico, De decente habitu, Praeceptiones, De prisca medicina, De aere locis aquis, De alimento, De liquidorum usu, De flatibus* (Corpus Medicorum Graecorum I 1). Lipsiae et Berolini: B. G. Teubner, 1927.

Helmreich 1913: Georg Helmreich, *Handschriftliche Studien zu Symeon Seth* (Programm des K. humanistischen Gymnasiums in Ansbach für das Schuljahr 1912/13). Ansbach: C. Brügel & Sohn, 1913.

Henry 1938: Paul Henry, *Études Plotiniennes I. Les Etats du texte de Plotin* (Museum Lessianum, Section Philosophique, no 20). Paris: Desclée de Brouwer et Cie; Bruxelles: L'Edition Universelle, 1938.

Henry 1941: Paul Henry, *Études Plotiniennes II. Les Manuscrits des Ennéades* (Museum Lessianum, Section Philosophique 21). Bruxelles: L'Edition Universelle; Paris: Desclée de Brouwer et Cie, and A. et J. Picard, 1941.

Herida 1998: Magid Herida, *La peau dans les écrits hippocratiques* (Thèse de médecine). Paris: Université Paris 6, 1998.

Hunger and Kresten 1969: Herbert Hunger, and Otto Kresten, *Katalog der griechischen Handschriften der Österreichischen Nationalbibliothek*, Teil 2: *Codices juridici, codices medici* (Museion, Veröffentlichungen der Österreichischen Nationalbibliothek, Neue Folge, Vierte Reihe: Veröffentlichungen der Handschriftensammlung, Erster Band: Katalog der griechischen Handschriften der Österreichischen Nationalbibliothek, Teil 2). Wien: Georg Prachner, 1969.

Ieraci Bio 1989: Anna Maria Ieraci Bio, "La trasmissione della letteratura medica greca nell'Italia meridionale fra X e XV secolo", in Antonio Garzya (ed.), *Contributi alla cultura greca nell'Italia meridionale* (Hellenica et Byzantina Neapolitana 13). Napoli: Bibliopolis, 1989, pp. 133–257.

Ihm 2002: Sibylle Ihm, *Clavis Commentariorum der antiken medizinischen Texte* (Clavis Commentariorum Antiquitatis et Medii Aevi 1). Leiden, Boston and Köln: Brill, 2002.

Ilberg 1911: Johannes Ilberg, *Die Überlieferung der Gynäkologie des Soranos von Ephesos* (Abhandlungen der philologisch-historischen Klasse der Königl. Sächsischen Gesellschaft der Wissenschaften Bd. 28, Abhandlung 2). Leipzig: B. G. Teubner, 1911.

Ilberg 1927: Ioannes Ilberg (ed.), *Soranus* (Corpus Medicorum Graecorum IV). Lipsiae et Berolini: B. G. Teubner, 1927.

Irigoin 1952: Jean Irigoin, *Histoire du Texte de Pindare* (Etudes et Commentaires 13). Paris: Klincksieck, 1952.

Irigoin 1970: Jean Irigoin, "Les manuscrits grecs. I. Quelques catalogues récents", *Revue des études grecques* 83 (1970), pp. 500–529.

Joly 1978: Robert Joly, *Hippocrate. Oeuvres complètes*, Tome XIII: *Les lieux dans l'homme. Du système des glandes. Des fistules. Des hémorrhoïdes. De la vision. Des chairs. De la dentition*. Texte établi et traduit (Collection des Universités de France). Paris: Belles Lettres, 1978.

Karas 1994: Γιάννης Καράς, *Οι επιστήμες στην Τουρκοκρατία. Χειρόγραφα και έντυπα*, Τόμος Γ': Οι επιστήμες της ζώης. Παράρτημα. Έργα γενικόν γνωσέων (Κέντρο Νεοελληνικών Ερευνών, Ἐθνικό Ἵδρυμα Ερευνών 48). Αθήνα: Βιβλιοπωλείον της «Εστίας», 1994.

Kibre 1975–1982: Pearl Kibre, "Hippocrates Latinus. Repertorium of Hippocratic Writings in the Latin Middle Ages", *Traditio* 31 (1975), pp. 99–126; 32 (1976), pp. 257–292; 33 (1977), pp. 253–295; 34 (1978), pp. 193–226; 35 (1979), pp. 273–302; 36 (1980), pp. 347–392; 37 (1981), pp. 267–289; 38 (1982), pp. 165–192.

Kibre 1985: Pearl Kibre, *Hippocrates Latinus. Repertorium of Hippocratic Writings in the Latin Middle Ages*. Revised Edition. New York: Fordham University Press, 1985.

Koch et al. 1923: Konrad Koch (ed.), *Galeni, De sanitate tuenda libri VI*; Georg Helmreich (ed.), *Galeni, De alimentorum facultatibus libri III*; *Galeni, De bonis malisque sucis lber*; Karl Kalbfleisch (ed.), *Galeni, De victu attenuante*; Otto Hartlich (ed.), *Galeni, De ptisana* (Corpus Medicorum Graecorum V 4, 2). Lipsiae et Berolini: B. G. Teubner, 1923.

Kollesch 1973: Jutta Kollesch, "Hermann Diels in seiner Bedeutung für die Geschichte der antiken Medizin", *Philologus* 117 (1973), pp. 278–283.

Kollesch 1989: "Die Erschliessung der antiken medizinischen Texte und ihre Probleme – das *Corpus Medicorum Graecorum et Latinorum*", *Gesnerus* 46 (1989), pp. 195–210.

Kollesch 1999: "Die Organisation und Herausgabe des *Corpus Medicorum Graecorum*: ergänzenden Details aus der Korrespondenz zwischen Hermann Diels und Johannes Mewaldt", in William M. Calder III, and Jaap Mansfeld (eds.), with the participation of Alex Leukart, François Paschould, and Olivier Reverdin, *Hermann Diels (1848–1922) et la science de l'Antiquité. Huit exposés suivis de discussion ... Vandoeuvres-Genève, 17–21 août 1998* (Entretiens sur l'Antiquité classique 45). Genève: Fondation Hardt, 1999, pp. 207–223.

Kudlien 1960: Fridolf Kudlien, *Die handschriftliche Überlieferung des Galenkommentars zu Hippokrates de articulis* (Deutsche Akademie der Wissenschaften zu Berlin, Schriften der Sektion für Altertumswissenschaft 27). Berlin: Akademie Verlag, 1960.

Kudlien 1970: Fridolf Kudlien (ed.), *Hermann Alexander Diels, Die Handschriften der antiken Ärzte. I Hippokrates und Galenos II Die übrigen griechische Ärzte III Nachtrag*. Mit einem Vorwort. Leipzig: Zentralantiquariat der deutschen demokratischen Republik, 1970.

Kühn 1821: Karl Gottlieb Kühn (ed.), *Claudii Galeni Opera omnia*, Tomus I (Medicorum graecorum opera quae exstant 1). Lipsiae: Cnobloch, 1821.

Kühn 1825: Karl Gottlieb Kühn (ed.), *Magni Hippocratis Opera omnia*, Tomus I (Medicorum graecorum opera quae exstant 21). Lipsiae: Cnobloch, 1825.

Lamagna 2017: Mario Lamagna, *Giovanni Attuario, L'eccellente trattato sulle urine di Avicenna*. Introduzione, testo critico, traduzione e note al testo (Serie Textos Médicos – Ediciones Críticas.

Ediciones críticas de la Escuela de traductores de Toledo 21). Cuenca: Ediciones de la Universidad de Castilla-La Mancha, 2017.

MacKinney 1965: Loren MacKinney, *Medical Illustrations in Medieval Manuscripts* (Publications of the Wellcome Historical Medical Library, New Series, V). London: Wellcome Historical Medical Library, 1965.

Marx 1915: Fridericus Marx (ed.), *A. Cornelii Celsi quae supersunt* (Corpus Medicorum Latinorum I). Lipsiae et Berolini: In aedibus B. G. Teubneri, 1915.

Masullo 2006: Rita Masullo, "Sul ΠΕΡΙ ΣΦΥΓΜΩΝ attribuito a Mercurio Monaco", in Véronique Boudon-Millot, Antonio Garzya, Jacques Jouanna, and Amneris Roselli (eds.), *Ecdotica e ricezione dei testi medici greci. Atti del V Convegno Internazionale Napoli, 1–2 ottobre 2004* (Collectanea 24). Napoli: M. D'Auria, 2006, pp. 335–346.

Mewaldt et al. 1914: Johannes Mewaldt (ed.), *Galeni, In Hippocratis De natura hominis commentaria III*; Georg Helmreich (ed.), *Galeni, In Hippocratis De victu acutorum commentaria IV*; Johann Westenberger (ed.), *Galeni, De diaeta Hippocratis in morbis acutis* (Corpus Medicorum Graecorum V 9, 1). Lipsiae et Berolini: B. G. Teubner, 1914.

Mercati 1916: Giovanni Mercati, "Minuzie. – 6–8. Pretesi scritti di Paolo l'Egineta e di Galeno. – 9–11. Pretesi scritti di medicina greca", *Bessarione* 32 (1916), pp. 208–211 (reprinted in Giovanni Mercati, *Opere minori raccolte in occasione del settantesimo natalizio sotto gli auspicii di S. S. Pio XI*, vol. 3 [1907–1916] (Studi e Testi 780. Città del Vaticano: Biblioteca Apostolica Vaticana, 1937, pp. 521–524).

Mercati 1917a: Giovanni Mercati, "Minuzie. – 13–17. Altre correzioni ed aggiunte all'op. Die Handschriften der antiken Aerzte. – 18. Per Aezio", *Bessarione* 38 (1917), pp. 50–55 (reprinted in Giovanni Mercati, *Opere minori raccolte in occasione del settantesimo natalizio sotto gli auspicii di S. S. Pio XI*, vol. 4 [1917–1936] (Studi e Testi 79). Città del Vaticano: Biblioteca Apostolica Vaticana, 1937, pp. 16–21).

Mercati 1917b: Giovanni Mercati, "I. Filippo Xeros Reggino, Giovanni Alessandrino iatrosofista e altri nel codice Vaticano degli Ephodia, and II. Un nuovo capitolo di Sorano e tre nuove ricette superstiziose in Aezio", in Giovanni Mercati, *Notizie varie di antica letteratura medica e di bibliografia* (Studi e Testi 31). Roma: Tipografia Poliglotta Vaticana, 1917, pp. 9–41, and 42–46.

Mondrain 2003: Brigitte Mondrain, "Comment était lu Galien à Byzance dans la première moitié du XVe siècle? Contribution à quelques aspects de l'histoire des textes", in Antonio Garzya and Jacques Jouanna (eds), *Trasmissione e ecdotica dei testi medici greci. Atti del IV Convegno internazionale, Parigi 17–19 maggio 2001* (Collectanea 21). Napoli: D'Auria, 2003, pp. 361–384.

Morani 1981: Moreno Morani, *La tradizione manoscritta del "De natura hominis" di Nemesio* (Scienze filologiche e letteratura 18). Milano: Vita e pensiero, 1981.

Nutton 2004: Vivian Nutton, "Ancient Medicine: From Berlin to Baltimore", in Frank Huisman, and John Harley Warner (eds), *Locating Medical History. The Stories and Their Meanings.* Baltimore, MD, and London: Johns Hopkins University Press, 2004, pp. 115–138.

Olivier 1995: Jean-Marie Olivier, *Répertoire des bibliothèques et des catalogues de manuscrits grecs de Marcel Richard. Troisième édition entièrement refondue* (Corpus Christianorum). Turnhout: Brepols, 1995.

Olivier 2018: Jean-Marie Olivier, *Supplément au répertoire des bibliothèques et des catalogues de manuscrits grecs,* 2 volumes (Corpus Christianorum). Turnhout: Brepols, 2018.

Olivieri 1935: Alessandro Olivieri (ed.), *Aetii Amideni Libri medicinales I–IV* (Corpus Medicorum Graecorum VIII 1). Lipsiae et Berolini: B. G. Teubner, 1935.

***Paléographie* 1977:** *La paléographie grecque et byzantine: actes du colloque international sur la paléographie grecque et byzantine organisé dans le cadre des colloques internationaux du Centre*

National de la recherche scientifique, Paris du 21 au 25 octobre 1974 (Issue 559 of Colloques internationaux du Centre National de la Recherche Scientifique 559). Paris: Editions du CNRS, 1977.

Perilli 1999: Lorenzo Perilli, "La tradizione manoscritta del Glossario ippocratico di Galeno (e l'ordinamento alfabetico delle glosse)", in Antonio Garzya, and Jacques Jouanna (eds.), *I testi medici greci. Tradizione e ecdotica. Atti del III Convegno Internazionale, Napoli 15–18 ottobre 1997.* Napoli: M. D'Auria, 1999, pp. 429–456.

Perilli 2011: Lorenzo Perilli, "Nuovi manoscritti del Glossario Ippocratico di Galeno e considerazioni stemmatiche. *Codex olim Mosquensis, codex Bodleianus Holkhamensis 92*", in Lorenzo Perilli, Christian Brockmann, Klaus-Dietrich Fischer, and Amneris Roselli (eds), *Officina Hippocratica. Beiträge zu Ehren von Anargyros Anastassiou und Dieter Irmer* (Beiträge zur Altertumskunde 289). Berlin and Boston, MA: De Gruyter, 2011, pp. 177–201.

Perrin 1988: Christophe Perrin, *La peau ou la représentation du corps malade: médecines antiques, médecine anatomo-clinique* (Thèse médecine) Nice: Université de Nice, 1988.

Petit 2006: Caroline Petit, "Les manuscrits de Modène et la tradition de l'*Introductio sive medicus* du Pseudo-Galien", in Véronique Boudon-Millot, Antonio Garzya, Jacques Jouanna, and Amneris Roselli (eds), *Ecdotica e ricezione dei testi medici greci. Atti del V Convegno Internazionale, Napoli, 1–2 ottobre 2004* (Collectanea 24). Napoli: M. D'Auria, 2006, pp. 167–185.

Pietrobelli 2010: Antoine Pietrobelli, "Variation autour du Thessalonicensis Vlatadon 14: un manuscrit copié au Xénon du Kral, peu avant la chute de Constantinople", *Revue des études byzantines* 68 (2010), pp. 95–126.

Pritchet 1975: Christopher Dixon Pritchet (ed.), *Iohannis Alexandrini Commentaria in sextum librum Hippocratis Epidemiarum recognovit et adnotatione critica instruxit.* Leiden: Brill, 1975.

Pritchet 1982: Christopher Dixon Pritchet (ed.), *Iohannis Alexandrini Commentaria in librum De sectis Galeni.* Recognovit et adnotatione critica instruxit. Leiden: E. J. Brill, 1982.

Raeder 1926: Ioannes Raeder (ed.), *Oribasii, Synopsis ad Eustathium; Libri ad Eunapium* (Corpus Medicorum Graecorum VI 3). Lipsiae et Berolini: B. G. Teubner, 1926.

Raeder 1928–1933: Ioannes Raeder (ed.), *Oribasii, Collectionum medicarum reliquiae*, 4 volumes (Corpus Medicorum Graecorum VI 1, 1–2; VI 2, 1–2). Lipsiae et Berolini: B. G. Teubner, 1928–1933.

Regling 1920: Kurt Regling, "Bruno Rappaport. Geb. den 4. November 1875, gest. den 20. Juli 1915", *Biographisches Jahrbuch für die Altertumswissenschaft* 40 (1920), pp. 76–83.

Rey 1993: Roselyne Rey, *Histoire de la douleur* (Histoire des sciences). Paris: La Découverte, 1993.

Richard 1948: Marcel Richard, *Répertoire des bibliothèques et des catalogues de nanuscrits grecs* (Publications de l'Institut de recherche et d'histoire des textes 1). Paris: Centre de documentation du Centre National de la Recherche Scientifique, 1948.

Richard 1958: Marcel Richard, *Répertoire des bibliothèques et des catalogues de manuscrits grecs.* Deuxième édition (Centre national de la recherche scientifique, Publications de l'Institut de recherche et d'histoire des textes 1). Paris: Centre national de la recherche scientifique, 1958.

Richard 1964: Marcel Richard, *Répertoire des bibliothèques et des catalogues de manuscrits grecs. Supplément I (1958–1963)* (Documents, études et répertoires publiés par l'Institut de recherche et d'histoire des textes 9). Paris: Éditions du Centre National de la Recherche Scientifique, 1964.

Rivier 1962: André Rivier, *Recherches sur la tradition manuscrite du traité hippocratique "De morbo sacro"* (Travaux publiés sous les auspices de la Société suisse des sciences morales 3). Berne: Francke, 1962.

Roselli 2009: Amneris Roselli, "Due manoscritti medici greci nelle biblioteche di Sofia", *Galenos* 3 (2009), pp. 177–180.

Sarton 1927–1948: George Sarton, *Introduction to the History of Science*, 3 volumes in five tomes. Baltimore: Williams & Wilkins, 1927–1948.

Sezgin 1970: Fuat Sezgin, *Geschichte des arabischen Schrifttums*, Band 3: *Medizin, Pharmazie, Zoologie, Tierheilkunde bis ca. 430 H.* Leiden: E.J.Brill, 1970.

Sezgin 1971: Fuat Sezgin, *Geschichte des arabischen Schrifttums*, Band 4: *Alchimie, Chemie, Botanik, Agrikultur bis ca. 430 H.* Leiden: E.J.Brill, 1971.

Sinkewicz 1990: Robert E. Sinkewicz, *Manuscript Listings for the Authors of Classical and Late Antiquity* (Greek Index Project Series 3). Toronto: Pontifical Institute of Mediaeval Studies, 1990.

Sinkewicz 1992: Robert E. Sinkewicz, *Manuscript Listings for the Authors of the Patristic and Byzantine Periods* (Greek Index Project Series 4). Toronto: Pontifical Institute of Mediaeval Studies, 1992.

Sinkewicz and Hayes 1989: Robert E. Sinkewicz and Walter H. Hayes, *Manuscript Listings for the Authored Works of the Palaeologan Period* (Greek Index Project Series 2). Toronto: Pontifical Institute of Mediaeval Studies, 1989.

Sonderkamp 1987: Joseph A. M. Sonderkamp, *Untersuchung zur Überlieferung der Schriften des Theophanes Chrysobalantes (sog. Theophanes Nonnus)* (Freie Universität Berlin, Byzantinisch-Neogriechisches Seminar, ΠΟΙΚΙΛΑ ΒΥΖΑΝΤΙΝΑ 7). Bonn: Dr. Rudolf Habelt, 1987.

Sprengel 1829: Kurt Sprengel (ed.), *Pedanii Dioscoridis Anazarbei De materia medica ad fidem codicum manuscriptorum, editionis aldinae principis usquequaque neglectae, et interpretum priscroum textum recnesuit, varias addidit lectiones, interpretationem emendavit, commentario illustravit*, Tomus I (Medicorum graecorum opoera quae exstant 1). Lipsiae: Cnobloch, 1829.

Thorndike and Kibre 1937: Lynn Thorndike, and Pearl Kibre, *A Catalogue of Incipits of Mediaeval Scientific Writings in Latin* (Mediaeval Academy of America, Publication 29). Cambridge, MA: Mediaeval Academy of America, 1937.

Thorndike and Kibre 1963: Lynn Thorndike, and Pearl Kibre, *A Catalogue of Incipits of Mediaeval Scientific Writings in Latin*. Revised and augmented edition (Mediaeval Academy of America, Publication 29). Cambridge, MA: Mediaeval Academy of America, 1963.

Touwaide 2009: Alain Touwaide, "Byzantine Medical Manuscripts. Towards a New Catalogue, with a Specimen for an Annotated Checklist of Manuscripts based on an Index of Diels' Catalogue", *Byzantion* 79 (2009), pp. 453–595.

Touwaide 2010: Alain Touwaide, "Codicology and Paleography", in Albrecht Classen (ed.), *Handbook of Medieval Studies. Terms, Methods, Trends*, 3 volumes. Berlin and New York, NY: Walter de Gruyter, 2010, vol. 1, pp. 266–329.

Touwaide 2016: Alain Touwaide, *A Census of Greek Medical Manuscripts. From Byzantium to the Renaissance* (Medicine in the Medieval Mediterranean 6). London and New York, NY: Routledge, 2016.

Touwaide 2018: Alain Touwaide, "Towards a Catalogue of Greek Medical Manuscripts", in Paola Degni, Paolo Eleuteri, and Marilena Maniaci (eds), *Greek Manuscript Cataloguing: Past, Present, and Future* (Bibliologia. Elementa ad librorum studia pertinentia 47). Turnhout: Brepols, 2018, pp. 111–118.

Tselikas 1995: Ἀγαμέμνων Τσελίκας, "Τὰ ἑλληνικὰ γιατροσόφια: μιὰ περιφρονημένη κατηγορία χειρογράφων", in Thanasis Diamantopoulos (ed.), Ιατρικά Βυζάντινα χειρόγραφα. Αθήνα: Δόμος, 1995, pp. 57–69.

Tselikas 2014: Ἀγαμέμνων Τσελίκας, "Δύο συναγωγὲς ἰατρικῶν λέξεων καὶ ἰατρικὲς συνταγὲς ἀπὸ τὸν ἰατροσοφικὸ κώδικα Παναγίου Τάφου 339 τοῦ Πατριαρχείου Ἱρουσολύμων", in *Εύκρατον-Πρακτικά Επιστημονικής Συνάντησης προς τιμήν του κ. Γεωργίου Ν. Αντονακοπούλου ομότιμου καθηγητού της Ιατρικής Σχολής του Πανεπιστημίου Θεσσαλίας. Λάρισσα 10 Μαΐου 2014, Αμφι-*

θέατρο Δημοσίας Κεντρικής Βιβλιοθήκης Λάρισσας «Κωνσταντίνος Κούμας». Λάρισσα: Δημοσίας Κεντρικής Βιβλιοθήκης Λάρισσας «Κωνσταντίνος Κούμας» – Ιατρική Σχολή Πανεπιστημίου Θεσσαλίας, 2014, pp. 107–176.

Tselikas and Ilioudis 1995: Ἀγαμέμνων Τσελίκας, Γιάννης Ἠλιούδης, *Νικολάου Ἱερόπαιδος ἐξ Ἀγράφων, Πραγματεία περὶ Φυσιολογίας καὶ Παθολογίας* (Βιβλιοθήκη Νεωτέρων Ἑλληνῶν Ἰατρῶν 1). Λάρισα: Πανεπιστήμιο Θεσσαλίας, Τμῆμα Ἰατρικῆς, 1995.

Tselikas and Ilioudis 1997: Ἀγαμέμνων Τσελίκας, Γιάννης Ἠλιούδης, *Νικολάου Ἱερόπαιδος ἐξ Ἀγράφων, Ἐκδόσεις μερικαὶ εἰς ἀρχάριον ἰατρόν* (Βιβλιοθήκη Νεωτέρων Ἑλληνῶν Ἰατρῶν 2). Λάρισα: Πανεπιστήμιο Θεσσαλίας, Τμῆμα Ἰατρικῆς, 1997.

Turyn 1932: Aleksander Turyn, *De Codicibus Pindaricis* (Polska Akademja Umiejętności: Archiwum Filologiczne 11). Cracoviae: Academia Polonae Litterarum, 1932.

Turyn 1943: Aleksander Turyn, *The Manuscript Tradition of the Tragedies of Aeschylus*. New York, NY: Polish Institute of Arts and Sciences in America, 1943.

Turyn 1952: Alexander Turyn, *Studies in the Manuscript Tradition of the Tragedies of Sophocles* (Illinois Studies in Language and Literature 36, 1–2.). Urbana, IL: University of Illinois Press, 1952.

Turyn 1957: Alexander Turyn, *The Byzantine Manuscript Tradition of the Tragedies of Euripides* (Illinois Studies in Language and Literature 43). Urbana, IL: University of Illinois Press, 1957.

Ullmann 1970: Manfred Ullmann, *Die Medizin im Islam* (Handbuch der Orientalistik, Erste Abteilung: Der nahe und der mittlere Osten, Ergänzungsband VI, 1. Abschnitt). Leiden and Köln: Brill, 1970.

Verner 1966: Mathilde Verner "Johann Albert Fabricius, Eighteenth-Century Scholar and Bibliographer", *The Papers of the Bibliographical Society of America* 60 (3) (1966), pp. 281–326.

Voigts and Kurtz 2004: Linda Ersham Voigts, and Patricia Deery Kurtz, *Electronic Thorndike Kibre (eTK) and Electronic Voigts Kurtz (eVK)*. CD Rom publication, release 20 August 2004.

Vollmer 1916: Fridericus Vollmer, *Quinti Sereni Liber medicinalis*. Edidit – (Corpus Medicorum Latinorum II 3). Lipsiae et Berolini: B. G. Teubner, 1916.

Wellmann 1908: Max Wellmann (ed.), *Philumeni de venenatis animalibus eorumque remediis ex codice vaticano* primum edidit (Corpus Medicorum Graecorum X 1, 1). Lipsiae et Berolini: B. G. Teubner, 1908.

Wenkebach 1934: Ernst Wenkebach (ed.), *Galeni, In Hippocratis epidemiarum librum I commentarii III*; Franz Pfarr (Germ. transl.), *Galeni, In Hippocratis epidemiarum librum II commentarii V* (Corpus Medicorum Graecorum V 10, 1). Lipsiae et Berolini: B. G. Teubner, 1934.

Wenkebach 1936: Ernst Wenkebach (ed.), *Galeni, In Hippocratis epidemiarum librum IIII commentarii III* (Corpus Medicorum Graecorum V 10, 2. 1). Lipsiae et Berolini: B. G. Teubner, 1936.

Wilson 1987: Nigel G. Wilson, "Aspects of the Transmission of Galen", in Guglielmo Cavallo (ed.), *Le strade del testo* (Studi e commenti 5). Bari: Adriatica Editrice, 1987, pp. 45–64.

Zipser 2009: Barbara Zipser (ed.), *John the Physician's Therapeutics. A Medical Handbook in Vernacular Greek* (Studies in Ancient Medicine 37). Leiden: Brill, 2009.

Acknowledgements

This work is the result of decades of intensive activity in libraries, research centers, universities, and other institutions throughout the world, which have all provided resources, access to collections, expertise and guidance and, most simply, a home. I am pleased to thank all of them and their staff, even though I cannot enumerate them here. In very recent years, the work has benefitted from the active support of De Gruyter, particularly the Senior Editor for Classical Studies Dr. Serena Pirrotta and her team, especially Marco Acquafredda, and De Gruyter computer and technical units in the persons of Anne Hiller and Florian Ruppenstein who have provided much needed assistance. Going slightly back in time, Patricia Kellogg has been an efficient research assistant and Cheyenne Moore has checked the accuracy of my index of Diels against the original. Since its foundation in 2007 the *Institute for the Preservation of Medical Traditions* has hosted the programme. In the very last phase, Marisa Gomez has checked with great linguistic talent the correctness of the introduction to the several parts of the work. More than anyone else, Emanuela Appetiti has accompanied me through multiple peregrinations of all kinds of which this work may give only an imperfect idea. I cannot conclude without remembering Joseph A. M. Sonderkamp with whom I discussed the project of a *New Diels* and a catalogue of Greek medical manuscripts as early as 1983 in Berlin and then in 1987 at Louvain-la-Neuve. We had defined a cooperative programme and had started implementing it when the sinister *Moira* decided shortly after that we would not fully realize it in collaboration.

Indices

Index of Authors and Works

For each author in Diels, this index lists the works for which manuscripts are recorded. It comprises two lists: one with the titles in Greek, and the other with the titles in Latin. In both lists, all the names of author and the titles are provided exactly as they appear in Diels. For the author names, some are in German (e.g., Hippokrates and Galenos) and others are in Latin. For the works, some are not identified by a specific title, but by a generic Latin designation (e.g., *Opera varia*, *Excerpta varia*, or *Excerpta*) or by a reference to an earlier publication. Furthermore, some works do not provide either a Greek title or a Latin translation. Whatever the form, items are listed in alphabetical order and followed by the reference to the part(s) and page number of Diels' lists where they appear, with the following abbreviations: "I" for the first part, devoted to Hippocrates and Galen (published in 1905), "II" for the second part, devoted to all the other physicians (published in 1906), and "N" for the supplement (N for *Nachtrag* = *Supplement*; published in 1908). A reference appearing as II.3, for example, indicates a work mentioned in part II, page 3.

1. Greek titles

2. Latin titles

Index of Manuscripts

This index lists all the manuscripts mentioned in Diels. The identification of the manuscripts exactly reproduces that of Diels, which usually comprises the following three or four elements: city (German form), library (most of the time in the original language, often in an abbreviated form and in all cases in their form in Diels' time), collection (when appropriate), and shelfmark or reference to an earlier work. In some cases, the name of the library is not explicitly mentioned; it can be identified through the list of catalogues in Diels' bibliography where library names appear. All such elements of identification are reproduced here in boldface for purposes of clarity. For example: **Florenz: Laurent. plut. 74, 1**.

For each item in Diels, this index provides the reference to its mention(s) in Diels' lists as described above (p. xxxv) with the following abbreviations: "I" for the first part, devoted to Hippocrates and Galen (published in 1905), "II" for the second part, devoted to all the other physicians (published in 1906), and "N" for the supplement (N for *Nachtrag* = *Supplement*; published in 1908), followed by the page numbers (in Arabic numerals). A reference appearing as II.3, for example, indicates a manuscript mentioned in part II, page 3. In some cases, the page number is followed by a number between parentheses, e.g., II.106 (2). This indicates that the item in reference appears twice on the same page.

A **Table of Concordance** lists the page numbers of Diels (in the left column) with their equivalent in the present volume (in the right column).

This index is preceded by a **Finding Aid** which provides the city and library names in alphabetical order with reference to the present index of manuscripts, and two lists: one with the names as in Diels and the other with their current standard English name.

Table of Concordance

I.3 = 7	I.57 = 90	I.100 = 144	II.4 = 202
I.4 = 8	I.58 = 93	I.101 = 145	II.5 = 203
I.5 = 9	I.59 = 93	I.102 = 147	II.6 = 205
I.8 = 12	I.60 = 95	I.103 = 148	II.7 = 207
I.10 = 13	I.61 = 96	I.104 = 150	II.8 = 209
I.11 = 15	I.63 = 98	I.105 = 151	II.9 = 210
I.12 = 18	I.64 = 98	I.106 = 152	II.10 = 212
I.13 = 21	I.65 = 100	I.107 = 153	II.11 = 213
I.14 = 24	I.66 = 100	I.108 = 155	II.12 = 215
I.17 = 25	I.67 = 101	I.109 = 156	II.13 = 216
I.18 = 25	I.68 = 103	I.110 = 157	II.14 = 216
I.19 = 28	I.69 = 105	I.111 = 159	II.15 = 217
I.20 = 29	I.70 = 105	I.112 = 161	II.16 = 219
I.21 = 32	I.71 = 107	I.113 = 163	II.17 = 219
I.22 = 34	I.72 = 108	I.114 = 165	II.18 = 221
I.23 = 36	I.73 = 110	I.115 = 167	II.19 = 224
I.24 = 39	I.74 = 112	I.116 = 168	II.20 = 225
I.25 = 42	I.75 = 113	I.117 = 169	II.21 = 226
I.26 = 44	I.76 = 114	I.118 = 170	II.22 = 227
I.27 = 46	I.77 = 115	I.119 = 171	II.23 = 229
I.28 = 49	I.78 = 116	I.120 = 173	II.24 = 229
I.29 = 51	I.79 = 118	I.121 = 174	II.25 = 231
I.30 = 54	I.80 = 119	I.122 = 175	II.26 = 232
I.31 = 56	I.81 = 121	I.123 = 176	II.27 = 233
I.32 = 59	I.82 = 122	I.124 = 178	II.28 = 234
I.33 = 61	I.83 = 124	I.125 = 179	II.29 = 235
I.34 = 63	I.84 = 125	I.126 = 181	II.30 = 237
I.35 = 66	I.85 = 126	I.127 = 182	II.31 = 239
I.36 = 68	I.86 = 127	I.128 = 183	II.32 = 239
I.37 = 70	I.87 = 128	I.129 = 184	II.33 = 242
I.38 = 71	I.88 = 129	I.130 = 185	II.34 = 243
I.39 = 73	I.89 = 130	I.131 = 186	II.35 = 245
I.40 = 74	I.90 = 132	I.132 = 187	II.36 = 246
I.41 = 76	I.91 = 133	I.133 = 188	II.37 = 248
I.42 = 78	I.92 = 134	I.134 = 190	II.38 = 249
I.43 = 80	I.93 = 135	I.135 = 191	II.39 = 251
I.44 = 82	I.94 = 136	I.136 = 192	II.40 = 252
I.46 = 83	I.95 = 137	I.148 = 192	II.41 = 254
I.47 = 85	I.96 = 138	I.149 = 193	II.42 = 256
I.48 = 86	I.97 = 141	I.150 = 194	II.43 = 256
I.49 = 87	I.98 = 141	I.151 = 197	II.44 = 258
I.56 = 89	I.99 = 142	II.3 = 201	II.45 = 260

II.47 = 261	II.75 = 294	II.105 = 335	N.42 = 383
II.48 = 261	II.76 = 296	II.106 = 336	N.43 = 384
II.49 = 262	II.77 = 297	II.107 = 337	N.44 = 385
II.50 = 264	II.78 = 299	II.108 = 338	N.45 = 387
II.51 = 265	II.79 = 301	II.109 = 340	N.46 = 388
II.52 = 266	II.80 = 303	II.110 = 342	N.47 = 389
II.53 = 267	II.81 = 305	II.111 = 344	N.48 = 390
II.54 = 268	II.82 = 306	II.112 = 345	N.49 = 391
II.55 = 268	II.83 = 308	II.113 = 349	N.50 = 393
II.56 = 270	II.85 = 308	II.114 = 350	N.51 = 394
II.57 = 270	II.86 = 309	II.115 = 353	N.52 = 396
II.58 = 272	II.87 = 310	N.25 = 359	N.53 = 397
II.59 = 273	II.88 = 311	N.26 = 359	N.54 = 399
II.60 = 274	II.89 = 313	N.27 = 361	N.55 = 400
II.61 = 275	II.90 = 315	N.28 = 362	N.56 = 401
II.62 = 276	II.91 = 316	N.29 = 363	N.57 = 403
II.63 = 277	II.92 = 318	N.29 = 367	N.58 = 404
II.64 = 279	II.93 = 319	N.30 = 367	N.59 = 405
II.65 = 281	II.94 = 321	N.31= 368	N.60 = 407
II.66 = 282	II.95 = 322	N.32 = 370	N.61 = 408
II.67 = 283	II.96 = 323	N.33 = 371	N.62 = 409
II.68 = 286	II.97 = 325	N.34 = 372	N.63 = 411
II.69 = 287	II.98 = 326	N.35 = 373	N.64 = 412
II.70 = 288	II.99 = 327	N.36 = 374	N.65 = 414
II.71 = 290	II.100 = 329	N.37 = 376	N.66 = 416
II.72 = 292	II.101 = 330	N.38 = 377	N.67 = 417
II.73 = 293	II.102 = 332	N.39 = 379	N.68 = 419
II.74 = 293	II.104 = 334	N.41 = 380	N.69 = 420

Finding Aid

City and Library names

1. Names according to Diels

2. Standard English names

Index of Manuscripts

Bibliography

The bibliography in Diels comprises four lists: **(1)** the *Verzeichnis der ausgenutzten Bibliotheken und Bibliothekskataloge* (List of Consulted Libraries and Library Catalogues) included in the front matter (pp. XI–XXIII) of the second issue of the catalogue (1906) and reproduced in the cumulative edition (1906) of the two issues (1905 and 1906) with the same pagination; **(2)** some additional entries to this list in the front matter of the *Nachtrag* (*Supplement*, 1908) (pp. 23–24); and, at the end of the *Nachtrag*, **(3)** a *Verzeichniss gedruckter Anonymi medici graeci* (List of Printed Anonymous Greek Physicians) followed by **(4)** a *Verzeichniss von Nachschlagwerken* (Inventory of Reference Works) (pp. 70–71 and 71–72, respectively). All of these lists are reproduced here with some modifications which are detailed in the introductory notes for each of these bibliographies.

1. Catalogues of Manuscripts

The list of libraries and catalogues below merges the two original lists of Diels (that is, the 1906 and 1908 lists). Furthermore, whereas Diels' bibliography mentions the catalogue(s) of manuscripts in all the languages considered in the lists (Greek, Latin, Arabic, Syriac, and Hebrew), the present bibliography includes only the catalogues of Greek manuscripts.

The format of the resulting list has been slightly modified for purposes of clarity. In the original publication, the bibliographical list includes the full reference of the catalogues under the name of the libraries in each city. As a result, Diels' lists of catalogues by cities are rather dense and do not allow for a general perception of the vast range of works that were consulted to compile the catalogues. The bibliography below proceeds with two separate lists: the first, which lists the catalogues by country, city and library, provides references in an abbreviated form (this is the *Short-reference List*) and the second list (the *Full-reference List*) provides the full references of all catalogues cited in the first list.

The *Short-reference List* proceeds by country identified by its German name, as in Diels. Countries include polities that no longer exist (e.g., *Österreich-Ungarn*, the Austro-Hungarian Empire) and a grouping utilized by Diels (*Türkey und Orient* [Turkey and the East], which corresponds approximately to the Ottoman Empire in the early 20th century). The designations of the countries are those of that time (e.g., *Russland* [Russia]) as is also their extension (portions of modern Greece and the Greek islands do not appear under *Griechenland* [Greece], for example, but under *Türkey und Orient* [Turkey and the East], and such a city as Wroclaw, identified here by its German name *Breslau*, is included in *Deutschland* (Germany) whereas it is in modern-day Poland). Countries, polities, and groupings identified as above are listed here in the alphabetical order of their name whereas in Diels they are listed according to a clockwise movement that proceeds in three concentric circles. The first such circle, which might be identified as *Mediterranean and northwestern European*, goes from Portugal to Italy passing through France and including Belgium, Holland and Switzerland. The second circle, which might be defined as *north-central European*, goes from England to Germany to Austria-Hungary. The third circle, *Scandinavo-Asian* in nature, includes Denmak, Sweden and Russia. This repartition is completed by the region on the East, with Greece, Turkey and the East.

In both Diels and the present list, the section devoted to each country lists the cities alphabetically by name. These names are mostly in German (e.g., *Athen*, *Brüssel*,

Florenz, *Kopenhagen*, *Moskau*, *Venedig*), but sometimes in their original form (e.g., *Bologna*) or a Latinized form (e.g., *Mileae* for Μηλιές). Libraries within each city are designated, both in Diels and the present bibliography, by the German translation of their name (in most cases) or their original name (often in an abbreviated form and, for some of them, in the original Greek alphabet). All city and library names are printed in boldface for purposes of clarity, both in Diels and here.

The short references of catalogues provided in the *Short-reference List* here provide a standardized abbreviated form of the catalogue titles. This abbreviation is made of the author's last name or the title of a work, followed by the year of publication. Titles of works always reflect Diels' usage and might be a title *sensu proprio*, the general title of a series followed by a volume number in such series, or even the title of a journal with the number of the pages where the publication referred to appears.

The *Short-reference List* is followed here by the *Full-reference List*, which reproduces the abbreviated form of the title used in the *Short-reference List* in boldface, immediately followed by the full form of the title according to standard bibliographical practice. Besides providing the key to abbreviations used in the list of catalogues by city and library, this second list allows for a clear vision of the range of catalogues consulted by Diels and his collaborators, something that the original publication does not make possible.

The section devoted to each country opens with the general catalogues as in Diels' original publication. Within each subsection (city and library) items are listed in chronological order of publication.

1. Short-reference List

Allgemeines.

Haenel 1830; Weinberger 1902.

Serapeum I (1840) - XXXI (1870); *Revue des bibliothèques* I (1891) - XIV (1904); *Centralblatt für Bibliothekswesen* I (1884) - XXI (1904).

BELGIEN.

Omont 1884–1885 (= Omont, *Rev. instr. publ.* 1884–1885).

Antwerpen, Stadtbibliothek: Omont 1884–1885: 41–42. **Brüssel, Königl. Bibl.:** Omont 1884–1885: 1–41; Van den Gheyn 1901–1904;

DÄNEMARK.

Kopenhagen, Königl. Bibliothek: Graux 1880: 141–238; **Universitätsbibl.:** Graux 1880: 239–242.

DEUTSCHLAND.

Blau 1886.

Berlin, Königl. Bibl.: Studemund-Cohn 1890; De Boor 1897. **Breslau, Bibl. Korniana:** Henschel 1847. **Bibl. der Maria-Magdalena-Kirche (jetzt Stadtbibliothek):** Henschel 1847. **Stadtbibliothek:** Krantz 1699; Wolf, 1764; Wachler 1828; Neigebauer 1865; *Catalogus Vratislaviensis* 1899. **Universitätsbibliothek:** Schneider 1840/41; Henschel 1847; Neigebauer 1864: 46–48. **Dresden, Königl. Bibl.:** Schnorr v. Carolsfeld 1882–1883. **Erlangen, Universitätsbibliothek:** Irmischer 1852. **Göttingen, Univ.-Bibl.:** Meyer, 1893–1894. **Hamburg, Stadtbibliothek:** *Bibliothecae Uffenbachianae* III 1730; *Catalogus Bibliothecae Loescheri* 1751; Omont 1890: 355–368. *Philologica Hamburgensia* 1905. **Heidelberg, Univ.-Bibl.:** Wilken 1817. **Jena, Universitätsbibl.:** Mylius 1746; *Zentralbl. f. Bibl. Wesen* 19 1902. **Karlsruhe, Großherzogl. Hof- u. Landesbibliothek:** *Die Hdss. der großherzogl.-badischen Hof- u. Landesbibliothek* 1891-1901. **Leipzig, Ratsbibliothek:** Naumann 1838. **Universitätsbibliothek:** Feller 1686; Gardthausen 1898. **München, Hof- und Staatsbibl.:** Hardt 1806–1812. **Tübingen, Univ.-Bibl.:** Keller 1840; 1841; Klüpfel 1843; Schmid 1902, 1903; Nestle 1903. **Wolfenbüttel, Herzogl. Bibl.:** Ebert 1827; v. Heinemann 1884–1888,1890–1903,1903. **Zeitz, Stiftsbibliothek:** Müller 1806–1818; Wegener 1876; Bech 1881.

ENGLAND.

Daremberg 1853.

Cambridge, Gonville and Caius: Smith 1849. **Peterhouse:** James 1899. **St Johns' College:** Cowie 1842–1843. **Trinity College:** Sinker 1891; James 1900–1904. **Universitätsbibliothek:** Daremberg 1853: 164–166; Halliwell 1856–1867. **Cheltenham:** *Catalogus libr. mss. in bibl. Th. Phill.* 1837; Daremberg 1853: 119–156. **Dublin, Trinity College:** Schenkl 1896: 43–69; Abbott 1900. **Holkham, Bibl. des Gr. Leicester:** Roscoe 1815–1828; Foerster 1884. **London, British Museum:** Thompson 1881–1884; *Arundeliani*: (Forshall) 1834; *Burneiani*: (Forshall) 1840; *Harleiani*: (Nares) 1808–1812; *Regii*: Casley 1734; *Index* 1829. *Sloane Mss.*: Ayscough 1782; Scott 1904; *Stowe Mss.*: *Cat. of the Stowe Mss.* 1895–1896. *Additions*: *Index to the Additions 1783–1835* 1849; *List of additions 1836–1897*: *List of Additions 1836–1840* 1843; *Catalogue of Additions 1841–1845* 1850; *Catalogue of Additions 1846–1847* 1864; *Catalogue of Additions 1848–1853* 1868; *Catalogue of Additions 1854–1860* 1875; *Catalogue of Additions 1854–1875* 1877; *Index of the Catalogue of Additions 1854–1875* 1880; *Catalogue of Additions 1876–1881* 1882; *Catalogue of Additions 1882–1887* 1889; *Catalogue of Additions 1888–1893* 1894; *Catalogue of Additions 1894–1899* 1901. *Papyri*: Kenyon 1893–1898. **Lambeth Palace:** Todd 1812. **Medical Society:** Daremberg 1853: 158–164. **Oxford, Bibl. Bodleiana:** *Codd. mss. ... d'Orvilliani* 1806; Black 1845; Coxe 1853; Madan 1895; Daremberg 1853: 14–62, 100–118, 172. **Bibl. aedis Christi:** Kitchin 1867. **Colleg. Mertonense:** Coxe 1852: Part 3. **Colleg. Novum:** Coxe 1852: Part 7.

FRANKREICH.

Catalogue général des mss. des bibl. publiques des départements, 7 Bde. 1849–1885; *Catalogue général des mss. des bibl. publiques de France. Départements*, 43 Bde. 1886–1904; Omont, *Départements* 1886.

Besançon: *Catal. gén. de Fr. Dép. 32* 1897 & *33* 1900. **Carpentras:** *Catal. gén. de Fr. Dép. 34* 1901; *35* 1899; *36* 1902 & 1903. **Lyon, Bibl. de la Ville:** *Catal. gén. de Fr. Dép. 30* 1899 & 1900; *42*, 1904. **Montpellier, Bibliothèque de l'école de médecine:** *Catal. gén. des Dép. 1* 1849. **Orléans:** *Catal. gén. de Fr. Dép. 12* 1889; *42* 1904: 563–649. **Paris, Bibl. Nationale.** [Mellot], *Catalogus codd. mss. bibl. regiae* 1739–1744; Omont 1886–1888, 1898. Neue Erwerbungen: 1888–1892: Omont 1892; 1892–1893: Omont 1894; 1894–1895: Omont 1896; Omont, *Catal. des mss. ... Miller* 1897; 1898–1899: Omont 1900; Omont 1903. **Kleinere Bibliotheken:** Omont 1883. **Bibl. Mazarine:** *Catal. gén. de Fr.* 1885–1895. **Bibliothèque de la faculté de médecine:** Franklin 1864; Omont 1883: 123–124. **Universitäts-Bibliothek:** Chatelain 1892. **Reims:** *Catal. gén. de Fr. Dép. 39*

1904 & 1906. **Rosanbo:** Omont, *Départements* 1886: 67–72. **Sens:** *Catal. gén. de Fr. Dép. 6* 1887: 147–204.

GRIECHENLAND.

Pervanoglu 1868.

Athen, Nationalbibl.: Sakkelion 1892. **Athen, Βιβλ. τῆς Βουλῆς:** Lampros 1905–1907. **Mileae (Griechenland):** Papadopulos-Kerameus 1901.

HOLLAND.

Omont, *Pays-Bas* 1886.

Amsterdam, Universitäts-Bibliothek: Omont, *Pays-Bas* 1886: 195–198; Mendes da Costa 1902. **Leiden, Universitäts-Bibliothek:** *Catalogus librorum ... bibl. publ. universitatis Lugduno-Batav.* 1716; Geel 1852.

ITALIEN.

Tomasini 1639, 1650; Blume 1824–1836, 1834; Vogel 1841–1842; *Statistica del regno d'Italia* 1865; Mazzatinti 1887, 1891–1903; Allen 1890; Ehrhard 1893; *Statistica delle biblioteche* 1893–1894; Martini 1893, 1896, 1902; Bassi 1897–1901; *Biblioteche governative* 1900.

Bologna: Olivieri, Festa 1895; Puntoni 1896/2; **Bibl. Comunale:** Olivieri, Festa 1895: 467–481. **Bibl. Universitaria:** Olivieri, Festa 1895: 387–466; Puntoni 1896/2; *Biblioteche governative* 1900: 275. **Florenz, Bibl. Mediceo Laurentiana:** Bandini 1764–70; Rostagno-Festa 1893; Rostagno 1894, 1898. **Kleinere Bibliotheken:** Vitelli 1894. **Bibl. Marucelliana:** Biagi 1888; Vitelli 1894: 558–562;. **Bibl. Nazionale (= Magliabecchiana):** Vitelli 1894: 543–557. **Bibl. Riccardiana:** Vitelli 1894: 473–542. **Genua:** Ehrhardt 1893. **Bibl. della Congregazione delle Missioni Urbane (mit Bibl. d. Fil. Sauli):** Ehrhardt 1893: 192–218. **Grottaferrata, Klosterbibliothek:** Rocchi 1883. **Mailand, Archivio del Capitolo metropolitano:** Martini 1893: 39–46. **Mailand, Bibliotheca Ambrosiana:** Martini et Bassi 1906. **Bibl. Trivulziana:** Porro 1884; Martini 1893: 373–385. **Messina, Universität:** Blume 1834: 228; Rühl 1889; Fraccaroli 1897; *Biblioteche governative* 1900: 309–323. **Modena, Bibl. Estense:** Puntoni 1896/1. **Neapel, Biblioteca Borbonica:** Cyrillus 1826–1832. **Bibliot. dei Gerolamini:** Martini 1896: 387–415. **Bibl. di S. Giovanni di Carbonara:** Montfaucon 1739: 1.231–233; Fabricius 1796; Capasso 1878: 586–590. **Bibl. Oratoriana:** Mandarini 1897. **Padua:** Tomasini 1639. **S. Antonius:** Minciotti 1842; Iosa 1886. **Bibl. universitaria:** Landi 1902; *Biblioteche governative* 1900: 345–353. **Palermo, Jesuitenkolleg (jetzt Bibl. nazionale):** Blume 1834: 230–

231. **Biblioteca nazionale (mit Bibl. des Jesuitenkollegs):** Martini 1893: 47–138; *Biblioteche governative* 1900: 89–97. **Parma, Bibl. Palatina:** Blume 1834: 234–236; Martini 1893: 149–205; *Biblioteche governative* 1900: 217–223; Modona 1896. **Pistoja, Biblioteca Fabroniana:** Festa 1897: 226–228; Mazzatinti I 1890: 268–277. **Bibl. Forteguerri:** Mazzatinti I 1890: 239–267; Festa 1897: 225. **Ravenna, Biblioteca Classense:** Martin, *Mélanges Graux* 1884; Mazzatinti IV 1894 144–254; V 1895 3–47; **Rom, Bibl. Angelica:** Franchi de' Cavalieri-Muccio 1896; Piccolomini 1898. **Bibl. Barberina:** Blume 1834: 148–155. **Bibl. Casanatensis:** Allen 1890: 45–48; Bancalari 1894. **Bibl. Corsiniana (= Acc. d. Lincei):** Blume 1834: 188–191; Pélissier 1889, 1891; Pierleoni 1901; Gabrieli 1905. **Bibl. St. Peter (Basilicana):** Montfaucon 1739: 1.156–159; Allen 1890: 56; Heiberg 1896. **Bibl. Vallicellana:** Martini 1902. **Bibl. Vaticana:** *Palatini graeci*: Stevenson 1885; *Reg. Sueciae et Pii II*: Stevenson 1888; *Ottoboniani*: Feron et Battaglini. 1893; *Urbinates*: Stornajolo 1895. **Turin, Bibl. Nazionale (Universitaria):** Pasinus 1749; Peyron, 1820; Zuretti 1896; (Cipolla) 1904. **Venedig, Bibl. Nazionale Marciana:** [Zanetti] 1740; Castellani 1895. **Kleinere Bibliotheken:** Tomasini 1650. **Bibl. monasterii St. Michaelis:** Mittarelli 1779. **Verona:** Blume 1824–1836: 1.259–271; Omont 1891. **La capitolare biblioteca:** Giuliari 1875–1876; Omont 1891: 490–495.

ÖSTERREICH-UNGARN.

Goldmann 1881; Huemer 1885, 1887.

Böhmen: Balbini 1780: 1–47. **Budapest, Universitätsbibl.:** Szilágyi 1881–1894. **Raudnitz (Böhmen): Bibl. d. Fürsten Lobkowitz:** Passow 1825: VI. adn.; Dworzak 1843. **Sáros-Patak, Bibl. des reform. Collegiums:** Haenel 1840. **Wien: Jesuitenkollegium:** Gollob 1908.

PORTUGAL.

Graux et Martin 1892: 299–308.

RUSSLAND.

Thraemer 1892; Vater 1843.

Moskau: v. Gebhardt 1898. **Synodalbibl.:** Matthaei 1805. **St. Petersburg: Kaiserl. öffentl. Bibl.:** Muralt 1864. **Warschau, Zamoyskische Majorats-biblithek:** Foerster 1898, 1900.

SCHWEDEN.

Graux et Martin 1889.

Upsala, Universitätsbibl.: Sparfwenfeldt 1706; Svedelius 1806; Graux et Martin 1889: 314–358.

SCHWEIZ.

Omont, *Suisse* 1886; Omont, *Supplément Suisse* 1891; Meier 1887.

Basel, Universitäts-Bibliothek: Montfaucon 1739: 607–615; Haenel 1830: 511–660; Omont, *Suisse* 1886: 386–419; Omont, *Supplément Suisse* 1891:22–24. **Bern, Stadtbibliothek:** Hagen 1875. **Genf, Stadtbibliothek:** Senebier 1779; Omont, *Suisse* 1886: 430–440. **Zürich, Stadtbibliothek:** Weidmann 1841; Omont, *Suisse* 1886: 441–445.

SPANIEN.

Heine, *Serapeum* 7 1846; Heine, *Serapeum* 8 1847; Volger 1858, 1859; Ruelle 1875; Graux 1879; Graux et Martin 1892; Beer 1893

Escurial: Miller 1848. **Madrid, Privatbibliothek des Königs:** Graux et Martin 1892: 55–125. **Nationalbibliothek:** Iriarte 1769; Miller 1886; Omont 1897. **Salamanca, Universitäts-Bibliothek:** Volger, *Philologus* 14 1859; Graux et Martin 1892: 145. **Toledo, Archivo historico = Bibl. Capitolare:** Haenel 1830: 983–999; Ruelle 1875: 506–508; Graux et Martin 1892: 32, 229, 293. **Bibl. del cabillo de la iglesia catedral:** Graux et Martin 1892: 293. **Zaragoza, Bibl. d. Pilar:** Graux et Martin 1892: 207.

TÜRKEI UND ORIENT.

Coxe 1858; Papadopulos-Kerameus 1887.

Athos: Lampros 1895–1900. **Chalke, Bibl. monasterii Deiparae:** Βαρθολομαίου Κουτλουμουσιάνου 1846; Papadopulos-Kerameus 1887: 8; *Byz. Zeitschr.* 2 1893; Papadopulos-Kerameus 1900; Boyens, 1901; *Byz. Zeitschr.* 10 1901;. **Constantinopel:** Weißenborn 1857; *Philolog.* 5 1850: 758–762; Foerster 1877; Codera 1891;. **Bibl. des Sultans:** Mordtmann 1854; Blaß 1888; Foerster, *Philolog.* 42 1884: 167. **Gallipoli, Bibl. d. Kirche d. H. Nikolaus:** Papadopulos-Kerameus 1887: 6–12. **Jerusalem:** Ehrhard 1891–1892; Papadopulos-Kerameus, 1891 ff; Koikylides 1899. **Lesbos, Βιβλ. τῆς τοῦ Λειμῶνος Μονῆς:** Papadopulos-Kerameus, 1886. **(Mitylene), Bibl. d. Gymnasiums:** Papadopulos-Kerameus 1886: 132; 1888: 143. **Patmos:** Guérin 1856: 101–120; Migne 1865; Bidez et Parmentier 1896. **Bibl. des Johannis-Klosters:** Guérin 1856: 101–119.

Rhodope: Βιβλ. τῆς Μονῆς Μπασκόβου: Papageorgios 1887; Papageorgios *Berl. Philol. Woch.* 7 1887. **Smyrna: Βιβλ. τῆς Εὐαγγελικῆς Σχολῆς:** Papadopulos-Kerameus, 1877. **The Greek library at Smyrna:** *The Academy* 1880.

2. Full-reference List

Centralblatt für Bibliothekswesen 1 (1884)–21 (1904).
Revue des bibliothèques 1 (1891)–14 (1904).
Serapeum 1 (1840)–31 (1870).

Abbott 1900: Thomas Kingsmill Abbott, *Catalogue of the manuscripts in the Library of Trinity College, Dublin*. Dublin: Hodges, Figgis, & Co., and London: Longman, Green, & Co., 1900.

Allen 1890: Thomas William Allen, *Notes on Greek Manuscripts in Italian Libraries*. London: David Nutt, 1890.

Ayscough 1782: Samuel Ayscough, *A Catalogue of the Manuscripts preserved in the British Museum hitherto undescribed: consisting of Five Thousand Volumes; includeing the Collections of Sir Hans Sloane, Bart, the Rev. Thomas Birch, D,D, and about Five Hundred Volumes bequeathed, presented, or purchased at various Times. Volume II containing Medicine, Natural History, Voyages, Grammars, &cc, Literary History, Cat. of the mss. pres. in the Brit. Mus. London 1782, Biography, Letters, Poetry, Judicial Astrology, Magic, Miscellaneous, MSS. in Icelandic, and Oriental Languages, with Two Indices*. London: The Author, 1782.

Balbini 1780: Bohuslai Balbini, *Bohemia docta*, Opus posthumus editum, notisque illustratum ab Raphaele Ungar, Pars 3. Pragae: Characteribus Haeredum Rosenmüller per Mathiam Glatz Factorem, 1780.

Bancalari 1894: Francesco Bancalari, "Index codicum graecorum Bibliothecae Casanatensis", *Studi italiani di filologia classica* 2 (1894), pp. 161–207.

Bandini 1764–1770: Angelo Maria Bandini, *Catalogus codicum manuscriptorum Bibliothecae Mediceae Laurentianae ...*, Tomus I–III. Florentiae: Typis Caesareis (Tomus I); Typis Regiis (Tomi II–III), 1764–1770.

Βαρθολομαίου Κουτλουμουσιανοῦ 1846: Βαρθολομαίου Κουτλουμουσιανοῦ, *Ὑπόμνημα ἱστορικὸν Ὑπόμνημα ἱστορικόν περί της κατά την Χάλκην μονής της Θεοτόκου. Ἐκτιθέμενον τὴν φυσικὴν τῆς νήσου θέσιν – Τὴν ἀνέκαθεν οἰκοδομὴν τῆς Μονῆς – Τὰς μετὰ ταῦτα ἀνακαινίσεις – Καὶ ἐπὶ πᾶσι, τὴν μεταῤῥύθμισιν αὐτῆς εἰς Ἑλληνικὸν Φροντιστήριον*. Ἐν Κωναστατινουπόλει: Τυπογραφεῖον 'Αντωνίου Κορομηλά καὶ Πλάτωνος Πασπαλλή, 1846.

Bassi 1897–1901: Domenico Bassi, "Notizie di codici greci nelle biblioteche italiane", *Rivista di filologia e d'istruzione classica* 25 (1897), pp. 265–276; 26 (1898), pp. 118–124; 29 (1901), pp. 77–83.

Bech 1881: Fedor Bech, *Verzeichniss der alten Handschriften und Drucke in der Domherren-Bibliothek zu Zeitz aufgestellt und mit einem Vorworte zur Geschichte der Bibliothek*. Berlin: Weidmannsche Buchhandlung, 1881.

Beer 1893: Rudolf Beer, *Handschriftenschätze Spaniens. Bericht über eine im Auftrage der kaiserlichen Akademie der Wissenschaften in den Jahren 1886–1888* *durchgeführte Forschungsreise* (Sitzungsberichte der philosophisch-historischen Classe der kaiserlichen Akademie der Wissenschaften 128, VIII. Abhandlung; 129, VI. Abhandlung). Wien: Kaiserliche Akademie der Wissenschaften, 1893.

Biagi 1888: Guido Biagi, *Indice del Mare Magnum di Francesco Marucelli* (Ministero della Pubblica Istruzione, Indici e cataloghi 9). Roma: [Ministero della Pubblica Istruzione], 1888.

***Biblioteche governative* 1900**: Ministero della Pubblica Istruzione, *Le Biblioteche Governative Italiane nel MDCCCXCVIII. Notizie storiche, bibliografiche e statistiche*. Roma: Società Editrice Dante Alighieri, 1900.

***Bibliothecae uffenbachianae* III 1730**: *Bibliothecae Uffenbachianeae Universalis Tomus III. Exhibens integrum manuscriptorum tam veterum quam recentium adparatum, quem Z. C. Uffenbach summo studio atque labore conlegit, nunc vero bibliophilis aequo pretio offert*. Francofurti ad Moenum: Jo. Benj. Andreae & Henr. Hort, 1730.

Bidez et Parmentier 1896: Joseph Bidez and Léon Parmentier, "Notes sur quelques manuscrits de Patmos", *Revue de philologie* 20 (1896), pp. 38–40, 116–125.

Black 1845: William Henry Black, *Descriptive, Analytical, and Critical Catalogue of the Manuscripts Bequeathed to the University of Oxford by Elias Ashmole ..., also of Some Additional MSS. Contributed by Kingsley, Lhuyd, Borlase and Others*. Oxford: University Press, 1845.

Blaß 1888: Friedrich Wilhelm Blaß, "Die griechischen und lateinischen Handschriften im Alten Serail zur Konstantinopel"; "Nachtrag", *Hermes. Zeitschrift für classische Philologie* 23 (1888), pp. 219–233, 622–625.

Blau 1886: August Blau, "Verzeichniss der Handschriftenkataloge der deutschen Bibliotheken", *Centralblatt für Bibliothekswesen* 3 (1886), pp. 1–35, 49–108, 160.

Blume 1824–1836: Friedrich Blume, *Iter italicum*, Erster Band. *Archive, Bibliotheken und Inschriften in den Sardinischen und OEsterreichischen Provinzen*; Zweiter Band. *Archive, Bibliotheken und Inschriften in Parma, Modena, Massa, Lucca, Toscana, dem Kirchenstaat und S. Marino*; Dritter Band. *Archive, Bibliotheken und Inschriften in der Stadt Rom*; Vierter und Lezter Band. *Königreich Neapel, nebst Nachträgen und Registern zu allen vier Bänden, und zur Bibliotheca Librorum MSS. Italica*. Berlin und Stetting: In der Nicolaischen Buchhandlung (Bd. 1–2); Halle: Eduard Anton (Bd. 3–4), 1824–1836.

Blume 1834: Friedrich Blume, *Bibliotheca Librorum Manuscriptorum Italica. Indices bibliothecarum Italiae ex schedis Maieri eslingensis, Haenelii lipsiensis, Gottlingii ienensis, Car. Wittii, suisque propriis. In supplementum itineris italici*. Gottingae: impensis Bibliopolii Dietericiani, 1834.

Boyens 1901: Joseph Boyens, "Catalogus codicum hagiographicorum graecorum bibliothecae monasterii Deiparae in Chalce insula", *Analecta Bollandiana* 20 (1901), pp. 45–70.

***Byz. Zeitschr.* 2 1893**: Athanasios Papadopoulos Kerameus, "Handschriftliches zu Ignatios Diakonos", *Byzantinische Zeitschrift* 2 (1893), pp. 126–131.

***Byzant. Zeitschr.* 10 1901**: Eduard Kurz "A. Papadopoulos-Kerameus, Ἡ ἐν τῷ νησίῳ Σωζοπόλεως βασιλικὴ μονὴ Ἰωάννου τοῦ Προδρόμου καὶ ἡ τύχη τῆς βιβλιοθήκης αὐτῆς. Viz.Vrem. 1 (1900) 661–695", *Byzantinische Zeitschrift* 10 (1901), p. 667.

Capasso 1878: Bartolomeo Capasso, "Sulla spogliazione delle biblioteche napolitane nel 1718. Notizie e Documenti.", *Archivio storico per le provincie Napoletane* 3 (1878), pp. 563–594.

Casley 1734: David Casley, *A Catalogue of the Manuscripts of the Kings' Library: An Appendix to the Catalogue of the Cottonian Library Together with an Account of Books burnt or damaged by a late Fire. One Hundred and Fiftly Specimens of the Manner of Writing in different Ages, from the Third to the Fifteenth Century, in Copper-Plates: and some Observations upon MSS, in a Preface*. London: the Author, 1734.

Castellani 1895: Carolus Castellani, *Catalogus codicum graecorum qui in bibliothecam D. Marci Venetiarum inde ab anno MDCCXL ad haec usque tempora inlati sunt*. Venetiis: sumptibus Ferd. Ongania et F. M. Visentini fratrum, 1895.

***Cat. of the Stowe Mss.* 1895–1896**: *Catalogue of the Stowe Manuscripts in the British Museum*, volume 1: *Text*; volume 2: *Index*. London: British Museum, 1895–1896.

***Catal. gén. de Fr.* 1885–1895**: Auguste Molinier, *Catalogue des manuscrits de la Bibliothèque Mazarine* (Catalogue général des manuscrits des bibliothèques publiques de France), 4 volumes. Paris: Librairie Plon, E. Plon, Nourrit et Cie, 1885–1895.

***Catal. gén. de Fr. Dép. 6* 1887**: Auguste Molinier, *Catalogue général des manuscrits des bibliothèques publiques de France,* Départements, Tome VI: *Auxerre ... Sens ...* Paris: Librairie Plon, E. Plon, Nourrit et Cie, 1887.

***Catal. gén. de Fr. Dép. 12* 1889**: Charles Cuissard, *Catalogue général des manuscrits des bibliothèques publiques de France, Départements*, Tome XII: *Orléans*. Paris: Librairie Plon, E. Plon, Nourrit et Cie, 1889.

***Catal. gén. de Fr. Dép. 30* 1899**: Auguste Molinier et Félix Desvernay, *Catalogue général des manuscrits des Bibliothèques publiques de France*, Départements, Tome XXX: *Lyon*. Première partie. Paris: Librairie Plon, E. Plon, Nourrit et Cie, 1899.

***Catal. gén. de Fr. Dép. 30* 1900**: Auguste Molinier et Félix Desvernay, *Catalogue général des manuscrits des Bibliothèques publiques de France*, Départements, Tome XXX: *Lyon*. Seconde partie. Paris: Librairie Plon, E. Plon, Nourrit et Cie, 1900.

***Catal. gén. de Fr. Dép. 32* 1897**: Auguste Castan, *Catalogue général des manuscrits des bibliothèques publiques de France*, Départements, Tome XXXII: *Besançon*. Tome I. Paris: Librairie Plon, E. Plon, Nourrit et Cie, 1897.

***Catal. gén. de Fr. Dép. 33* 1900**: Auguste Castan, *Catalogue général des manuscrits des bibliothèques publiques de France*, Départements, Tome XXXIII: *Besançon*, Tome II. Première partie. Paris: Librairie Plon, E. Plon, Nourrit et Cie, 1900.

***Catal. gén. de Fr. Dép. 34* 1901**: Léopold Duhamel, *Catalogue général des manuscrits des bibliothèques publiques de France, Départements*, Tome XXXIV: *Carpentras*, Tome I. Paris: Librairie Plon, Plon-Nourrit et Cie, 1901.

***Catal. gén. de Fr. Dép. 35* 1899**: Léopold Duhamel et Joseph Liabastres, *Catalogue général des manuscrits des bibliothèques publiques de France, Départements*, Tome XXXV: *Carpentras*, Tome II. Paris: Librairie Plon, E. Plon, Nourrit et Cie, 1899.

***Catal. gén. de Fr. Dép. 36* 1902**: Joseph Liabastres, *Catalogue général des manuscrits des bibliothèques publiques de France, Départements*, Tome XXXVI: *Carpentras*, Tome III. Première partie. Paris: Librairie Plon, Plon-Nourrit et Cie, 1902.

***Catal. gén. de Fr. Dép. 36* 1903**: Léon-Honoré Labande, *Catalogue général des manuscrits des bibliothèques publiques de France, Départements*, Tome XXXVI: *Carpentras*, Tome III. Deuxième partie. Paris: Librairie Plon, Plon-Nourrit et Cie, 1903.

***Catal. gén. de Fr. Dép. 39* 1904**: Henri Loriquet, *Catalogue général des manuscrits des Bibliothèques publiques de France*, Départements, Tome XXXIX: *Reims*, Tome II. Première partie. Paris: Librairie Plon, Plon-Nourrit et Cie, 1904.

***Catal. gén. de Fr. Dép. 39* 1906**: Henri Loriquet, *Catalogue général des manuscrits des Bibliothèques publiques de France*, Départements, Tome XXXIX: *Reims*, Tome II. Deuxième partie. Paris: Librairie Plon, Plon-Nourrit et Cie, 1904.

***Catal. gén. de Fr. Dép. 42* 1904**: Félix Desvernay, *Catalogue général des manuscrits des bibliothèques publiques de France,* Départements, Tome XLII, Supplément, Tome III: *Lyon, Orléans*. Paris: Librairie Plon, Plon-Nourrit et Cie, 1904.

***Catal. gén. des Dép. 1* 1849**: Guillaume Libri, "Catalogue des manuscrits de la Bibliothèque de l'Ecole de médecine de Montpellier", in Félix Raviasson et Guillaume Libri, *Catalogue général des manuscrits des bibliothèques publiques des départements*, Tome I: *Autun, Laon, Montpellier, Albi*. Paris: Imprimerie nationale, 1849, pp. 279–477.

***Catalogue général des mss. des bibl. publiques de France. Départements.* 43 Bde. 1886–1904**: *Catalogue général des manuscrits des bibliothèques publiques de France, Départements 1–43*. Paris: Librarie Plon, E. Plon, Plon-Nourrit et Cie, 1886–1897 (= 1–32); Librairie Plon, Plon-Nourrit et Cie, 1900–1904 (= 33–43).

***Catalogue général des mss. des bibl. publiques des départements.* 7 Bde. 1849–1885**: *Catalogue général des manuscrits des bibliothèques publiques des départements publié sous les auspices du Ministre de l'Instruction publique* (tomes 1–2, 4–7) *du Ministre d'Etat* (tome 3), 7 tomes. Paris: Imprimerie nationale (tomes 1, 4–7); Imprimerie Impériale (tomes 2–3), 1849–1885.

***Catalogue of Additions 1841–1845* 1850**: *Catalogue of Additions to the Manuscripts in the British Museum in the Years 1841–1845*. London: British Museum, 1850.

***Catalogue of Additions 1846–1847* 1864**: *Catalogue of Additions to the Manuscripts in the British Museum in the Years 1846–1847*. London: British Museum, 1864.

***Catalogue of Additions 1848–1853* 1868**: *Catalogue of Additions to the Manuscripts in the British Museum in the Years 1848–1853*. London: British Museum, 1868.

***Catalogue of Additions 1854–1860* 1875**: *Catalogue of Additions to the Manuscripts in the British Museum in the Years 1854–1860*. London: British Museum, 1875.

***Catalogue of Additions 1854–1875* 1877**: *Catalogue of Additions to the Manuscripts in the British Museum in the Years 1854–1875*, volume II. London: British Museum, 1877.

***Catalogue of Additions 1876–1881* 1882**: *Catalogue of Additions to the Manuscripts in the British Museum in the Years 1876–1881*. London: British Museum, 1882.

***Catalogue of Additions 1882–1887* 1889**: *Catalogue of Additions to the Manuscripts in the British Museum in the Years 1882–1887*. London: British Museum, 1889.

***Catalogue of Additions 1888–1893* 1894**: *Catalogue of Additions to the Manuscripts in the British Museum in the Years 1888–1893*. London: British Museum, 1894.

***Catalogue of Additions 1894–1899* 1901**: *Catalogue of Additions to the Manuscripts in the British Museum in the Years 1894–1899*, Part I: Descriptions; Part II: Index. 2 volumes. London: British Museum, 1901.

***Catalogus Bibliothecae Loescheri* 1751**: *Catalogus Bibliothecae viri summi D. Valentini Ernesti Loescheri Theologi Saxoni, cuius pars I continens bibliothecam theologicam hastae publicae subiicietur D. VII. seqq. jan 1750 horis a meridie consuetis, in aedibus viduae B. Hermanni Poligraphi*. Dresdae et Lipsiae: apud Harpeterum, 1751.

***Catalogus librorum … bibl. publ. universitatis Lugduno-Batav.* 1716**: Wolferdius Senguerdius, Jacobus Gronovius, and Johannes Heyman, *Catalogus librorum tam impressorum quam manuscriptorum bibliothecae publicae universitatis lugduno-batavae* … Lugduni apud Batavos: Sumptibus Petri van der Aa, 1716.

***Catalogus libr. mss in bibl. Th. Phill.* 1837**: *Catalogus librorum manuscriptorum in bibliotheca D. Thomae Phillipps Bart. A.D. 1837*. [Middle Hill]: Impressus typis Medio-Montanis, 1837.

***Catalogus Vratislaviensis* 1889:** *Catalogus codicum graecorum qui in Bibliotheca Urbica Vratislaviensi adservantur a philologis vratislaviensibus compositus. Civitatis vratislaviensis sumptibus impressus. Accedit Appendix qua Gymnasii regii Fridericiani codices graeci describuntur.* Vratislavae: Apud Guilelmum Koebnerum, 1889.

Chatelain 1892: Emile Chatelain, *Catalogue des manuscrits de la bibliothèque de l'université*. Paris: Honoré Champion, 1892.

(Cipolla) 1904: Ettore Stampini, Gaetano De Sanctis, Carlo Cipolla, Carlo Frati, "Inventario dei Codici superstiti greci e latini antichi della Biblioteca nazionale di Torino", *Rivista di filologia e d'istruzione classica* 32 (1904), pp. 385–542.

Codera 1891: Francisco Codera y Zaidin, "Informes. I. Catálogos de bibliotecas de Constantinopla", *Boletín de la Real Academia de la Historia* 18 (1891), pp. 297–303.

***Codd. mss. ... D'Orvilliani* 1806**: [Thomas Gaisford], *Codices manuscripti, et impressi cum notis manuscriptis, olim d'Orvilliani, qui in Bibliotheca Bodleiana apud Oxonienses adservantur*. Oxonii: E Typographeo Clarendoniano, 1806.

Cowie 1842–1843: Benjamin Morgan Cowie, *A descriptive catalogue of the manuscripts and scarce books in the library of St. John's College*, 2 volumes (Publications of the Cambridge Antiquarian Society 6). Cambridge: J. & J. J. Deighton, and T. Stevenson, and London: John W. Parker, 1842–1843.

Coxe 1852: Henry O. Coxe, *Catalogus Codicum MSS. qui in Collegiis Aulisque Oxoniensibus hodie adservantur*, 2 volumes. Oxonii: E Typographo Academico, 1852.

Coxe 1853: Henry O. Coxe, *Catalogi Codicum Manuscriptorum Bibliothecae Bodleianae Pars Prima Recensionem Codicum Graecorum Continens*. Oxonii: E Typographo Academico, 1853.

Coxe 1858: Henry O. Coxe, *Report to Her Majesty's Government, on the Greek Manuscripts yet Remaining in Libraries of the Levant*. London: George E. Eyre and William Spottiswoode, 1858.

Cyrillus 1826–1832: Salvator Cyrillus, *Codices Graeci MSS. Regiae Bibliothecae Borbonicae descripti, atque illustrati*, Tomus I. Qui complectitur bibliothecam sacram. Tomus II. Neapoli: Ex Regia Typographia, 1826–1832.

Daremberg 1853: Charles Daremberg, *Notices et extraits des manuscrits médicaux grecs, latins et français des principales bibliothèques de l'Europe*. Ire partie. *Manuscrits grecs d'Angleterre suivis d'un fragment inédit de Gilles de Corbeil et de scolies inédites sur Hippocrate*. Paris: Imprimerie Impériale, 1853.

De Boor 1897: Carl de Boor, *Verzeichniss der griechischen Handschriften der Königlichen Bibliothek zu Berlin*, II. Berlin: A. Asher & Co, 1897.

***Die Hdss. der großherzogl.-badischen Hof- u. Landesbibliothek in Karlsruhe* 1891–1901 (actually 1891–1896)**: *Die Handschriften der grossherzoglich-badischen Hof- und Landesbibliothek in Karlsruhe*. Wilhelm Brambach, *I. Geschichte* *und Bestand der Sammlung*; Wilhelm Brambach, *II. Orientalische Handschriften;* Alfred Holder, *III. Die durlacher und rastatter Handschriften*; Wilhelm Brambach, *IV. Die karlsruher Handschriften*. Karlsruhe: Ch. Th. Gross, 1891–1896.

Dworzak 1843: Dworzak, "Merkwürdigkeiten der Fürstlich von Lobkowitzischen Schlossbibliothek zu Raudnitz an der Elbe in Böhmen", *Serapeum – Zeitschrift für Bibliothekwissenschaft, Handschriftenkunde und ältere Litteratur* 4 (1843) p. 1–11.

Ebert 1827: Friedrich Adolf Ebert, *Bibliothecae Guelferbytanae codices graeci et latini classici*. Lipsiae: apud Steinackerum et Harknochium, 1827.

Ehrhard 1891–1892: Albert Ehrhard, "Die griechische Patriarchal-Bibliothek von Jerusalem. Ein Beitrag zur griechischen Palaeographie", *Römische Quartalschrift für christliche Alterthumskunde und für Kirchengeschichte* 5 (1891), pp. 217–265, 329–331, 383–384; 6 (1892), pp. 339–365.

Ehrhard 1893: Albert Ehrhard, "Zur Catalogisirung der kleineren Bestände griechischer Handschriften in Italien (I. Genova]", *Zentralblatt für Bibliothekswesen* 10 (1893), pp. 189–218.

Fabricius 1796: Gaetano d'Ancora, "Codices graeci MSS. qui adservantur Neapoli in Bibliotheca Augustinensium S. Iohannis ad Carbonariam", in Jo. Alberti Fabricii, *Bibliotheca graeca sive notitia scriptorum veterum graecorum quorumcumque monumenta integra aut fragmenta edita exstant tum plerorumque e mss. ac deperditis ab auctore recognita*. Editio tertia variorum curis emendatior atque auctor curante Gottlieb Christophoro Harles. Accedunt Christophori Augusti Heumanni Supplementa inedita, Volumen quintum. Hamburgi: apud Carolum Ernestum Bohn, Lipsiae: Ex Officina Breitkopfia et Haertelia, 1796, pp. 796–800.

Feller 1686: L. Joachim Feller, *Catalogus codicum manuscriptorum Bibliothecae Paulinae in Academia Lipsiensi*. Lipsiae: Joh. Frid. Gleditsch, 1686.

Feron et Battaglini 1893: Ernest Feron et Fabio Battaglini, *Codices manuscripti graeci Ottoboniani Bibliothecae Vaticanae descripti*. Romae: Ex Typographeo Vaticano, 1893.

Festa 1897: Nicola Festa, "Indice de' codici greci di Lucca e di Pistoia", *Studi italiani di filologia classica* 5 (1897), pp. 221–230.

Foerster 1877: Richard Foerster, *De antiquitatibus et libris manuscriptis constantinopolitanis commentatio*. Rostochii: Formis Academicis Adlerianis, 1877.

Foerster 1884: Richard Foerster, "Mittheilungen aus handschriften. 1. Handschriften in Holkham", *Philologus. Zeitschrift fur das klassische Alterthum* 42 (1884), pp. 158–167.

Foerster 1898: Richard Foerster, "Zur Handschriftenkunde und Geschichte der Philologie. V. Eine griechische Handschrift in Russisch-Polen und das Anthologion des Orion", *Rheinisches Museum für Philologie* Neue Folge 53 (1898), pp. 547–574.

Foerster 1900: Richard Foerster, "Zur Handschriftenkunde und Geschichte der Philologie. VI. Handschriften der Zamoyski'schen Bibliothek", *Rheinisches Museum für Philologie* Neue Folge 55 (1900), pp. 435–459.

Foerster *Philolog.* 42 1884 167: Richard Foerster, "Eine handschrift des Serail", *Philologus. Zeitschrift fur das klassische Alterthum* 42 (1884), p. 167.

(Forshall) 1834: [Josiah Forshall], *Catalogue of the Manuscripts in the British Museum*, New Series, Volume I, Part I. *The Arundel Manuscripts*. London: British Museum, 1834.

(Forshall) 1840: [Josiah Forshall], *Catalogue of the Manuscripts in the British Museum*, New Series, Volume I, Part II. *The Burney Manuscripts*. London: British Museum, 1840.

Fraccaroli 1897: Giuseppe Fraccaroli, "Dei codici greci del Monastero del SS. Salvatore che si conservano nella biblioteca universitaria di Messina", *Studi italiani di filologia classica* 5 (1897), pp. 329–336, 487–514.

Franchi de' Cavalieri-Muccio 1896: Pio Franchi de' Cavalieri e Giorgio Muccio, "Index codicum graecorum Bibliothecae Angelicae", *Studi italiani di filologia classica* 4 (1896), pp. 33–184.

Franklin 1864: Alfred Franklin, *Recherches sur la bibliothèque de la Faculté de médecine de Paris d'après des documents entièrement inédits suivies d'une notice sur les manuscrits qui y sont conservés*. Paris, 1864: Auguste Aubry.

Gabrieli 1905: Giuseppe Gabrieli, "Il «Zad al musafir» di ibn Al Gazzar in un ms. greco corsiniano (ΕΦΟΔΙΑ ΤΟΥ ΑΠΟΔΗΜΟΥΝΤΟΣ)", *Rendiconti della Reale Accademia dei Lincei, Classe di scienze morali, storiche e filologiche*, Serie Quinta, 14 (1905), pp. 29–50.

Gardthausen 1898: Viktor Gardthausen, *Katalog der griechischen Handschriften der Universitäts-Bibliothek zu Leipzig* (Catalogus codicum manuscriptorum Bibliothecae Universitatis Lipsiensis III – Katalog der Handschriften der Universitätsbibliothek zu Leipzig. III Die griechischen Handschriften). Leipzig: O. Harrassowitz, 1898.

Geel 1852: Jacob Geel, *Catalogus librorum manuscriptorum qui inde ab anno 1741 bibliothecae Lugduno Batavae accesserunt*. Lugduni Batavorum: E.J. Brill, 1852.

Giuliari 1875–1876: G. B. Carlo Giuliari, "La capitolare biblioteca di Verona", *Archivio Veneto* 10 (1875) pp. 239–271; 11 (1876) pp. 51–74; 12 (1876) pp. 56–79, 274–293.

Goldmann 1881: Arthur Goldmann, "Verzeichniss der österreich-ungarischen Handschriftenkataloge", *Centralblatt für Bibliothekswesen* 5 (1881), pp. 1–37, 55–73.

Gollob 1908: Eduard Gollob, *Medizinische griechische Handschriften des Jesuitenkollegiums in Wien (XIII. Lainz)* (Sitzungsberichte der Philosophisch-historischen Klasse der Kaiserlichen Akademie der Wissenschaften in Wien, 158. Band, 5. Abhandlung). Wien: Alfred Hölder, 1908.

Graux 1879: Charles Graux, "Rapport sur une mission en Espagne", *Archives des Missions scientifiques et littéraires, choix de rapports et instruction. Choix de rapports et instructions publié sous les auspices du Ministère de l'instruction publique et des beaux-arts,* 3e série, tome 5 (1879), pp. 111–136.

Graux 1880: Charles Graux. "Notices sommaires des manuscrits de la Grande Bibliothèque Royale de Copenhague", *Archives des missions scientifiques et littéraires. Choix de rapports et instructions publié sous les auspices du Ministère de l'instruction publique et des beaux-arts*, 3e série, tome 6 (1880), pp. 133–242.

Graux et Martin 1889: Charles Graux, "Notices sommaires des manuscrits grecs de Suède mises en ordre et complétées par Albert Martin", *Archives des Missions scientifiques et littéraires, choix de rapports et instructions. Choix de rapports et instructions publié sous les auspices du Ministère de l'instruction publique et des beaux-arts*, 3e série, tome 15 (1889), pp. 293–370.

Graux et Martin 1892: Charles Graux and Albert Martin (ed.), "Rapport sur une mission en Espagne et en Portugal. Notices sommaires des manuscrits grecs d'Espagne et de Portugal", *Nouvelles Archives des Missions scientifiques et littéraires. Choix de rapports et instructions publié sous les auspices du Ministère de l'instruction publique et des beaux-arts* 2 (1892), pp. 1–322.

Guérin 1856: Victor Guérin, *Description de l'île de Patmos et de l'île de Samos*. Paris: Auguste Durand, 1856.

Haenel 1830: Gustav Haenel, *Catalogi librorum manuscriptorum, qui in bibliothecis Galliae, Helvetiae, Belgii, Britanniae M., Hispaniae, Lusitaniae asservantur, nunc primum editi*. Lipsiae: I. C. Hinrichs, 1830.

Haenel 1840: Gustav Haenel, "Ungedruckte Handschriften-Kataloge, II. Manuscripta B. Collegii Ref. S. Patak", *Neue Jahrbücher für Philologie und Paedagogik oder Kritische Bibliothek für das Schuhl- und Unterrichtswesen* 6. Supplementband (1840), pp. 423–424.

Hagen 1875: Hermannus Hagen, *Catalogus codicum bernensium (Bibliotheca Bongarsiana)*. Bernae: B. F. Haller, 1875 (first published as *Pars prior* in 1874).

Halliwell 1856–1867: Charles Hardwick and Henry Richards Luard (eds), *A Catalogue of the Manuscripts preserved in the Library of the University of Cambridge*, 5 volumes. Cambridge: University Press, 1856–1867.

Hardt 1806–1812: Ignaz Hardt, *Catalogus Codicum Manuscriptorum Graecorum Bibliothecae Regiae Bavaricae*, 5 volumes. Monachii: Typis I. E. Seidelii Solisbacensis, 1806–1812.

Heiberg 1896: Johannes Ludwig Heiberg, "Biblioteksnotizen. IV. Ein Inventar des Archivio di S. Pietro", *Philologus. Zeitschrift fur das klassische Alterthum* 55 (1896), pp. 742–746.

Heine, *Serapeum* 7 1846: Gustav Heine, "Briefliche Mittheilung des Dr. G. Heine aus Berlin an Hofrath Hänel in Leipzig über spanische und portugiesische

Bibliotheken", *Serapeum-Zeitschrift für Bibliothekwissenschaft, Handschriftenkunde und ältere Litteratur* 7 (1846), pp. 193–204.

Heine, *Serapeum* 8 1847: Gustav Heine, "Zweiter Bericht des Dr. G. Heine in Berlin über seine litterarische Reise in Spanien gerichtet an Hofrath und Prof. Dr. Gustav Hänel und von letzterem mitgetheilt"; "Dritter Bericht des Dr. G. Heine in Berlin über seine litterarische Reise in Spanien, gerichtet an Hofrath und Prof. Dr. Gustav Hänel und von letzterem mitgetheilt", *Serapeum-Zeitschrift für Bibliothekwissenschaft, Handschriftenkunde und ältere Litteratur* 8 (1847), pp. 81–95, 103–105.

Henschel 1847: Augustus Guilelmus Eduardus Theodorus Henschel, *Catalogus codicum medii aevi medicorum ac physicorum qui manuscripti in bibliothecis vratislaviensibus asservantur.* Particula I. *Praemissa sunt de bibliothecarum vratislaviensium codicibus manuscriptis medii aevi medicis ac physicis observationes generales.* Particula II. *Inest synopsis chronologica scriptorum medii aevi medicorum ac physicorum quae codicibus bibliothecarum vratislaviensium continentur.* Vratislaviae: Eduardus Trewendt, [1847].

Huemer 1885: Johannes Huemer, "Aus alten Bücherverzeichnissen. (Ein Beitrag zur lateinischen Literaturkunde.)", *Wiener Studien – Zeitschrift für classische Philologie* 7 (1885), pp. 325–336.

Huemer 1887: Johannes Huemer, "Iter Austriacum I.", *Wiener Studien – Zeitschrift für classische Philologie* 9 (1887), pp. 51–93.

***Index* 1829**: [Frederick Augusta Barnard], *Bibliothecae regiae catalogus*, Tomus quintus: Londini: Guilelmus Nicol, 1829.

***Index of the Catalogue of Additions 1854–1875* 1880**: *Index of the Catalogue of Additions to the Manuscripts in the British Museum in the Years 1854–1875.* London: British Museum, 1880.

***Index to the Additions 1783–1835* 1849:** *Index to the Additional Manuscripts, with those of the Egerton Collection, preserved in the British Museum, and acquired in the years 1783–1835.* London: British Museum, 1849.

Iosa 1886: Antonio Maria Iosa, *I codici manoscritti della Biblioteca Antoniana di Padova descritti ed illustrati*. Padova: Tipografia del Seminario, 1886.

Iriarte 1769: Joannes Iriarte, *Regiae Bibliothecae Matritensis Codices Graeci MSS.* Volumen prius. Matriti: E Typografia Antonii Perez de Soto, 1769.

Irmischer 1852: Johann Conrad Irmischer, *Handschriften-Katalog der Königlichen Universitätsbibliothek zu Erlangen*. Frankfurt a. M. und Erlangen: der Verfasser, 1852.

James 1899: Montague Rhodes James, *A Descriptive Catalogue of the Manuscripts in the Library of Peterhouse*, with an Essay on the History of the Library by John Willis Clark. Cambridge: University Press, 1899.

James 1900–1904: Montague Rhodes James, *The Western Manuscripts in the Library of Trinity College Cambridge. A Descriptive Catalogue*, Volume I containing an account of the manuscripts standing in class B; Volume II containing an account of the manuscripts standing in class R; Volume III containing an account of the manuscripts standing in class O; Volume IV containing plates, addenda, corrigenda and index. Cambridge: University Press, 1900–1904.

Keller 1840, 1841: Adalbert Keller, "Die Handschriften der königlichen Universitätsbibliothek in Tübingen", *Serapeum-Zeitschrift für Bibliothekwissenschaft, Handschriftenkunde und ältere Litteratur* 1 (1840), pp. 124–128, 139–144, 203–206; 2 (1841), pp. 358–368.

Kenyon 1893–1898: Frederic G. Kenyon, *Greek Papyri in the British Museum. Catalogue with Texts*, 2 volumes. London: British Museum, 1893–1898.

Kitchin 1867: George William Kitchin, *Catalogus codicum MSS. qui in Bibliotheca Aedis Christi apud Oxonienses adservantur*. Oxonii: E Typographo Clarendoniano, 1867.

Klüpfel 1843: Karl Klüpfel, "Die Handschriften der königlichen Universitätsbibliothek in Tübingen", *Serapeum-Zeitschrift für Bibliothekwissenschaft, Handschriftenkunde und ältere Litteratur* 4 (1843), pp. 184–190, 205–208.

Koikylides 1899: Κλεόπα Μ. Κοικυλίδου, *Κατάλοιπα χειρογράφων ἱεροσολυμιτικῆς βιβλιοθήκης (Χειρόγραφα ἑλληνικὰ κείμενα ἐν τῇ μικρᾷ βιβλιοθήκῃ τοῦ μοναστηρίου Ἀβρααμίου. Συλλόγη χειρογράφων τοῦ Σεβασμιωτάτου Ἀρχιεπισκόπου Ἰορδάνου Κ. κ. Ἐπιφανίου. Ἐπιστολαι τοῦ Ἀδριανουπολεως Νεοφυτου καὶ Λαρισσης Διονυσίου)*. Ἐν Ἱεροσολύμοις: Ἐκ τοῦ Τυπογραφείου τοῦ Ἱεροῦ Κοινοῦ τοῦ Π. Τάφου, 1899.

Krantz 1699: Gottlob Krantz, *Memorabilia Bibliothecae Publicae Elisabetanae Wratislaviensis, a Fundatore Celeberrimo Rehdigerianae dictae* ... Wratislavae: apud Johannem Georgium Steck, 1699.

Lampros 1895–1900: Spyridon P. Lampros, *Catalogue of the Greek Manuscripts on Mount Athos*, 2 volumes. Cambridge: University Press, 1895–1900.

Lampros 1905–1907: Σπυρίδων Π. Λάμπρος, "Κατάλογος τῶν κωδίκων τῶν ἐν Ἀθήναις βιβλιοθηκῶν πλὴν τῆς Ἐθνικῆς. Α'. Κώδικες τῆς Βιβλιοθήκης τῆς Βουλῆς", *Νέος Ἑλληνομνήμων* 2 (1905), pp. 226–235, 357–364, 490–500; 3 (1906), pp. 113–121, 243–248, 447–473; 4 (1907), pp. 105–112, 225–236, 368–374, 476–483.

Landi 1902: Carolus Landi, "Codices graeci bybliothecae Universitatis patavinae", *Studi italiani di filologia classica* 10 (1902), pp. 18–20, 430–432.

***List of Additions 1836–1840* 1843**: *List of Additions to the Manuscripts in the British Museum in the years 1836–1840*. London: British Museum, 1843.

Madan 1895: Falconer Madan, *A Summary Catalogue of Western Manuscripts in the Bodleian Library at Oxford which have not hitherto been catalogued in the quarto series with references to the Oriental and other manuscripts*, volume 3 (Collections received during the 18th Century). Oxford: Clarendon Press, 1895.

Mandarini 1897: Enrico Mandarini, *I codici manoscritti della Biblioteca Oratoriana di Napoli illustrati*. Napoli and Roma: Andrea e Salvatore Festa, 1897.

Martin, *Mélanges Graux* 1884: Albert Martin, "Notice sur les manuscrits grecs de la bibliothèque Classense à Ravenne", *Mélanges Graux. Recueil de travaux d'érudition classique dédié à la mémoire de Charles Graux* ... Paris: Ernest Thorin, 1884, pp. 553–556.

Martini 1893: Emidio Martini, *Catalogo di manoscritti greci esistenti nelle biblioteche italiane*, volume 1, Parte 1. Milano: Ulrico Hoepli, 1893.

Martini 1896: Emidio Martini, *Catalogo di manoscritti greci esistenti nelle biblioteche italiane*, volume 1, Parte 2. Milano: Ulrico Hoepli, 1896.

Martini 1902: Emidio Martini, *Catalogo di manoscritti greci esistenti nelle biblioteche italiane*. Volume 2: *Catalogus codicum Graecorum qui in Bibliotheca Vallicellana Romae adservantur*. Milano: Ulrico Hoepli, 1902.

Martini et Bassi 1906: Aemidius Martini et Dominicus Bassi, *Catalogus codicum graecorum Bibliothecae Ambrosianae*. Digesserunt –, 2 volumes. Mediolani: Impensis U. Hoepli, 1906.

Matthaei 1805: Christian Friderich de Matthaei, *Accurata codicum graecorum MSS. bibliothecarum mosquensium Sanctissimae Synodi notitia et recensio* ..., Tomus secundus. Lipsiae: Ex Libraria Joachimica, 1805.

Mazzatinti 1887, 1891–1903: Giuseppe Mazzatinti, *Inventari dei manoscritti delle biblioteche d'Italia*. Volume I, fascicolo 1: Torino: Ermanno Loescher, 1887; volumi I–XI: Forlì: Luigi Bordandini, 1891–1901; volume XII: Forlì: Tipografia Sociale (Successori Bordandini), 1902–1903.

Mazzatinti I 1890 239–267: Ernesto Gori e Agostino Zanelli, "Pistoia, Biblioteca Forteguerri", in Giuseppe Mazzatinti, *Inventari dei manoscritti delle biblioteche d'Italia*, 1. Forlì: Luigi Bordandini, 1890, pp. 239–267.

Mazzatinti I 1890 268–277: Agostino Zanelli, "Pistoia, Biblioteca Fabroniana", in Giuseppe Mazzatinti, *Inventari dei manoscritti delle biblioteche d'Italia*, 1. Forlì: Luigi Bordandini, 1890, pp. 268–277.

Mazzatinti IV 1894 144–254; V 1895 3–47: Silvio Bernicoli, "Ravenna, Biblioteca Classense", in Giuseppe Mazzatinti, *Inventari dei manoscritti delle biblioteche d'Italia*, IV, pp. 144–254; V, pp. 3–47. Forlì: Luigi Bordandini, 1894, 1895.

Meier 1887: P. Gabriel Meier, "Verzeichniss der Handschriftenkataloge der schweizerischen Bibliotheken", *Centralblatt für Bibliothekswesen* 4 (1887), pp. 1–19.

[Mellot], *Catalogus codd. mss. bibl. regiae* 1739–1744: *Catalogus Codicum Manuscriptorum Bibliothecae Regiae*. Tomus primus – Tomus quartus. Parisiis: E Typographia Regia, 1739–1744.

Mendes da Costa 1902: Maurits Benjamin Mendes da Costa, *Bibliotheek der Universiteit van Amsterdam, Catalogus der Handschriften*. II. *De Handschriften der Stedelijke Bibliotheke met de latere aanwinsten. Vooral eenige mededeelingen over de geschiedenis van de bibliotheek en hare handschriftenversameling, door den Bibliothecaris Combertus Pieter Burger*. Amsterdam: J. H. de Bussy, 1902.

Meyer 1893–1894: Wilhelm Meyer, *Die Handschriften in Göttingen*, Bd. 1: *Universitätsbibliothek. Philologie, Literärgeschichte, Philosophie, Jurisprudenz*; Bd. 2: *Universitätsbibliothek. Geschichte, Karten, Naturwissenschaften, Theologie, Handschriften aus Lüneburg*; Bd. 3: *Universitätsbibliothek. Nachlässe von Gelehrten, Orientalische Handschriften. Handschriften im Besitz von Instituten und Behörden. Register zu Band 1 – 3* (Verzeichniss der Handschriften im preußischen Staate 1, Hannover, 1–3). Berlin: Bath, 1893–1894.

Migne 1865: Jacques Paul Migne, "Circa annum MCCCLV Catalogus librorum Monasterii insulae Patmi saeculo XIV. Πίναξ τῶν ἐν τῇ σεβασμίᾳ μονῇ τῆς νήσου Πάτμου ἀξιολογωτέρων εὑρισκομένων βιβλίων", in Jacques Paul Migne, *Patrologiae cursus completus, seu bibliotheca universalis, integra, uniformis, commoda, oeconomica, omnium SS. Patrum, Doctorum Scriptorumque Ecclesiasticorum, sive latinorum, sive graecorum* ... Series graeca posterior ... Patrologiae graecae tomus 149: Nicephorus Gregoras, Georgius Lapitha, Theodorus Meliteniota. [Parisiis]: apud J.-P. Migne, 1865, cols 1047–1052.

Miller 1848: Emmanuel Miller, *Catalogue des mss. grecs de la bibliothèque de l'Escurial*. Paris: Imprimerie nationale, 1848.

Miller 1886: Emmanuel Miller, "Bibliothèque royale de Madrid. Catalogue des manuscrits grecs (Supplément au catalogue d'Iriarte)", *Notices et extraits des manuscrits de la Bibliothèque nationale et autres bibliothèques* 31.2 (1886), pp. 1–116.

Minciotti 1842: Luigi Minciotti, *Catalogo dei codici manoscritti esistenti nella biblioteca di Sant' Antonio di Padova con brevissimi cenni biografici degli autori*. Padova: La Minerva, 1842.

Mittarelli 1779: Johannis-Benedicti Mittarelli, *Bibliotheca codicum manuscriptorum Monasterii S. Michaelis Venetiarum prope Murianum una cum Appendice librorum impressorum seculi XV. Opus posthumum*. Venetiis: Ex Typographia Femtiana, Sumptibus Praefati Monasterii, 1779.

Modona 1896: Leonello Modona, "La reale biblioteca di Parma", *Rivista delle Biblioteche e degli Archivi* 6 (1896), pp. 161–168.

Montfaucon 1739: Bernardus De Montfaucon, *Bibliotheca Bibliothecarum Manuscriptorum Nova, Ubi, quae innumeris pene manuscriptorum bibliothecis continentur, ad quodvis litteraturae genus spectantia et notatu digna, describuntur et indicantur* ..., 2 tomi, Parisiis: Apud Briasson, 1739.

Mordtmann 1854: Andreas David Mordtmann, "Verzeichniss der handschriften in der bibliothek sr. maj. des sultans". *Philologus. Zeitschrift fur das klassische Alterthum* 9 (1854), pp. 582–584.

Müller 1806–1818: Christian Gottfried Müller, *Notitia et Recensio Codicum Mss. qui in bibliotheca episcopatus Numburgo-Cizensis asservantur*, particulae 1–8 ... Lipsiae: Ex officina Breitkopfio-Haertelia (particulae 1–4); ex Officina Vogeliana (particulae 5–8), 1806–1818.

Muralt 1864: Eduard von Muralt, *Catalogue des manuscrits grecs de la Bibliothèque impériale publique*, volume 1. St.-Pétersbourg: Imprimerie de l'Académie impériale des sciences, 1864.

Mylius 1746: Iohannes Christophus Mylius, *Memorabilia Bibliothecae Academicae Ienensis sive Designatio codicum manuscriptorum in illa bibliotheca et librorum impressorum, plerumque rariorum concinnata potissimum ad usus suorum in collegiis litterariis auditorum*. Ienae et Weissenfelsae: apud Ioh. Christoph. Croekerum, 1746.

(Nares) 1808–1812: Robert Nares, *A Catalogue of the Harleian Manuscripts in the British Museum with Indexes of Persons, Places, and Matters*, 4 volumes. [London] [G. Eyre and A. Strahan], 1808–1812.

Naumann 1838: Aemilius Guilelmus Robertus Naumann, *Catalogus librorum manuscriptorum qui in Bibliotheca senatoria Civitatis Lipsiensis asservantur ...* Grimae: sumptus fecit Julius Mauritius Gebhardt, 1838.

Neigebauer 1864: Johann Ferdinand Neigebauer, "Die königliche und Universitäts-Bibliothek zu Breslau", *Neuer Anzeiger fur Bibliographie und Bibliothekswissenschaft* 1864, pp. 7–9, 41–51.

Neigebauer 1865: Johann Ferdinand Neigebauer, "Die Stadtbibliothek in Breslau", *Neuer Anzeiger fur Bibliographie und Bibliothekswissenschaft* 1865, pp. 246–253, 293–296.

Nestle 1903: Eberhard Nestle, "Zum Verzeichnis der griechischen Handschriften der K. Universitätsbibliothek in Tübingen", *Centralblatt für Bibliothekswesen* 20 (1903), pp. 277–278.

Olivieri, Festa 1895: Alessandro Olivieri, and Nicola Festa, "Indice dei codici greci delle biblioteche Universitaria e Comunale di Bologna", *Studi italiani di Filologia classica* 3 (1895), pp. 385–495.

Omont 1883: Henri Auguste Omont, "Inventaire sommaire des manuscrits grecs conservés dans les bibliothèques publiques de Paris autres que la Bibliothèque nationale", *Bulletin de la Société de l'Histoire de Paris et de l'Île-de-France* 10 (1883), pp. 118–125.

Omont 1885: Henri Auguste Omont, *Catalogue des manuscrits grecs de la Bibliothèque royale de Bruxelles et des autres bibliothèques publiques de Belgique*. Gand: Imprimerie Eug. Vanderhaeghen, and Paris: Alph. Picard, 1885.

Omont 1886–1888: Henri Auguste Omont, *Inventaire sommaire des manuscrits grecs de la Bibliothèque nationale et des autres bibliothèques de Paris et des Départements*, 3 volumes. Paris: Ernest Leroux, 1886–1888.

Omont 1890: Henri Auguste Omont, "Notes sur les manuscrits grecs des villes hanséatiques Hambourg, Brême et Lübeck", *Centralblatt für Bibliothekswesen* 7 (1890), pp. 351–377.

Omont 1891: Henri Auguste Omont, "Les manuscrits grecs de la Bibliothèque Capitulaire et de la Bibliothèque Communale de Vérone", *Centralblatt für Bibliothekswesen* 8 (1891), pp. 489–497.

Omont 1892: Henri Auguste Omont, "Nouvelles acquisitions du département des manuscrits de la Bibliothèque nationale pendant l'année 1891–1892", *Bibliothèque de l'école des chartes* 53 (1892), pp. 333–382.

Omont 1894: Henri Auguste Omont, "Nouvelles acquisitions du département des manuscrits de la Bibliothèque nationale pendant les années 1892–1893", *Bibliothèque de l'école des chartes* 55 (1894), pp. 61–114, 241–258.

Omont 1896: Henri Auguste Omont, "Nouvelles acquisitions du département des manuscrits de la Bibliothèque nationale pendant les années 1894–1895", *Bibliothèque de l'école des chartes* 57 (1896), pp. 161–196; 339–372.

Omont 1897: Henri Auguste Omont, "Complément du catalogue des manuscrits grecs de la Bibliothèque royale de Madrid", *Revue des bibliothèques* 7 (1897), pp. 149–154.

Omont 1898: Henri Auguste Omont, *Inventaire sommaire des manuscrits grecs de la Bibliothèque nationale et des autres bibliothèques de Paris et des Départements. Table alphabétique*. Paris: Ernest Leroux, 1898.

Omont 1900: Henri Auguste Omont, *Nouvelles acquisitions du Départment des Manuscrits pendant l'année 1898–1899*. Paris: E. Leroux, 1900.

Omont 1903: Henri Auguste Omont, "Mnauscrits de la bibliothèque de Sir Thomas Phillipps récemment acquis pour la Bibliothèque nationale", *Revue des bibliothèques* 13 (1903), pp. 189–206.

Omont, *Catal. des mss. ... Miller* 1897: Henri Auguste Omont, *Catalogue des manuscrits grecs, latins, français et espagnols et des portulans recueillis par feu Emmanuel Miller*. Paris: Ernest Leroux, 1897.

Omont, *Départements* 1886: Henri Auguste Omont, *Catalogue des manuscrits grecs des départements*. Paris: Librarie Plon, E. Plon, Nourrit et Cie, 1886.

Omont, *Pays-Bas* 1886: Henri Auguste Omont, "Catalogue des manuscrits grecs des bibliothèques publiques des Pays-Bas (Leyde exceptée)", *Centralblatt für Bibliothekswesen* 4 (1886), pp. 185–214.

Omont, *Rev. instr. publ.* 1884–1885: Henri Auguste Omont, "Catalogue des manuscrits grecs de la Bibliothèque royale de Bruxelles et des autres bibliothèques publiques de Belgique", *Revue de l'Instruction Publique (supérieure et moyenne) en Belgique* 27 (1884), pp. 311–319, 374–383; 28 (1885), pp. 6–21, 82–89, 168–181.

Omont, *Suisse* 1886: Henri Auguste Omont, "Catalogue des manuscrits grecs des Bibliothèques de Suisse: Bâle, Einsiedeln, Genève, St Gall, Schaffouse et Zürich", *Centralblatt für Bibliothekswesen* 3 (1886), pp. 385–452.

Omont, *Supplément Suisse* 1891: Henri Auguste Omont, "Supplément au Catalogue des manuscrits grecs des Bibliothèques de Suisse", *Centralblatt für Bibliothekswesen* 8 (1891), pp. 22–26.

Papadopulos 1877: Ἀθανάσιος Παπαδόπουλος Κεραμεύς, *Κατάλογος τῶν χειρογράφων τῆς ἐν Σμύρνῃ βιβλιοθήκαις τῆς Εὐαγγελικῆς Σχολῆς μετὰ παραρτήματος περιέχοντος καί τινα ἀνέκδοτα* (Μουσεῖον καὶ Βιβλιοθηκὴ τῆς Εὐαγγελικῆς Σχολῆς). Σμύρνη: Ὑπογράφειον ὁ «Τύπος», 1877.

Papadopulos-Kerameus 1886: Ἀθανάσιος Παπαδόπουλος Κεραμεύς, "Κατάλογος τῶν ἐν ταῖς βιβλιοθήκαις τῆς νήσου Λέσβου ἑλληνικῶν χειρογράφων", *Σύγγραμμα Περιοδικόν – Ὁ ἐν Κωνσταντινουπόλει Ἑλληνικὸς Φιλολογικὸς Σύλλογος*, *Παράρτημα τοῦ ΙΖ΄ τόμου*, 1886, pp. 85–140.

Papadopulos-Kerameus 1887: Ἀθανάσιος Παπαδόπουλος-Κεραμεύς, "Ἔκθεσις παλαιογρα-φικῶν καὶ φιλολογικῶν ἐρευνῶν ἐν Θράκῃ καὶ Μακεδονίᾳ κατὰ τὸ ἔτος διὰ τὴν «Μαυρογορδάτειον Βιβλιοθήκην» ", *Ἀρχαιολογικὴ Ἐπιτροπή* (Σύγγραμμα Περιοδικόν – Ὁ ἐν Κωνσταντινουπόλει Ἑλληνικὸς Φιλολογικὸς Σύλλογος, Παράρτημα τοῦ ΙΖ΄). Κωνσταντινουπόλει: Ε.Φ.Σ.-Τύποις Σ. Ι. Βουτυρά 1887, pp. 3–64 (the *Supplement* [Παράρτημα] contains two title pages; both are exactly identical, except the year of publication: one [the second] is dated to 1886 and the other [the first] to 1887).

Papadopulos-Kerameus 1888: Ἀθανάσιος Παπαδόπουλος Κεραμεύς, "Κατάλογος τῶν ἐν ταῖς βιβλιοθήκαις τῆς νήσου Λέσβου ἑλληνικῶν χειρογράφων", *Σύγγραμμα Περιοδικόν – Ὁ ἐν Κωνσταντινουπόλει Ἑλληνικὸς Φιλολογικὸς Σύλλογος*, *Παράρτημα τοῦ ΙΗ΄ τόμου*, 1888, pp. 141–212.

Papadopulos-Kerameus, *Ἱεροσολυμιτικὴ Βιβλιοθήκη* 1891 ff: Ἀθανάσιος Παπαδόπουλος-Κεραμεύς, *Ἱεροσολυμιτικὴ βιβλιοθήκη ἤτοι Κατάλογος τῶν ἐν ταῖς βιβλιοθήκαις τοῦ ἁγιωτάτου ἀποστολικοῦ τε καὶ ὀρθοδόξου πατριαρχικοῦ θρόνου τῶν Ἱεροσολύμων καὶ πάσης Παλαιστίνης ἀποκειμένων κωδίκων συνταχθεῖσα μὲν καὶ φωτοτυπικοῖς κοσμηθεῖσα πίναξιν*, 4 τόμοι. Πετρουπόλει: Β. Κιρσπάουμ, 1891–1899.

Papadopulos-Kerameus 1900: Ἀθανάσιος Ι. Παπαδόπουλος-Κεραμεύς, "Ἡ ἐν τῷ νησίῳ Σωζοπόλεως βασιλικὴ μονὴ Ἰωάννου τοῦ Προδρόμου καὶ ἡ τύχη τῆς βιβλιοθήκης αὐτῆς", *Vizantijskij Vremenik* 7 (1900), pp. 661–695.

Papadopulos-Kerameus 1901: Ἀθανάσιος Παπαδόπουλος-Κεραμεύς, "Κατάλογος τῶν ἑλληνικῶν κωδίκων τῆς ἐν Μηλέαις βιβλιοθήκης", *Ἐπετηρὶς τοῦ Φιλολογικοῦ Συλλόγου Παρνασσοῦ* 5 (1901), pp. 20–74.

Papageorgios 1887: Πέτρος Ν. Παπαγεώργιος, "Παλαιογραφικὴ ἐκδρομὴ εἰς τὴν μονὴν Μπατσκόβου", *Ἡμερολόγιον τῆς Ἀνατολῆς Φιλολογικὸν καὶ Ἐπιστημονικόν* 6 (1887), pp. 115–120.

Papageorgios *Berl. Philol. Woch.* 7 1887: Peter N. Papageorgios, " Ἡμερολόγιον τῆς Ἀνατολικῆς φιλολογικὸν καὶ ἐπιστημονικὸν τοῦ ἔτους 1887 ὑπὸ Ἀθ. Παλαιολόγου, Konstantinopel, Pallamari. S. η' 224. 4 fr.", *Berliner Philologische Wochenschrift* 7 (1887), cols. 821–823.

Pasinus 1749: Iosephus Pasinus, Antonius Rivautella, and Franciscus Berta, *Codices manuscripti Bibliothecae Regii Taurinensis Athenaei Per Linguas digesti, & binas in partes distributi, in quarum Prima Hebraei, & Graeci, in altera Latini, Italici,*

& Gallici. Recensuerunt, & animadversionibus illustrarunt. Taurini: Ex Typographia Regia, 1749.

Passow 1825: Franciscus Passow, *Dionysii Orbis Terrarum Descriptio. Recensuit et adnotatione critica instruxit. Accessit tabula geographica lapidi inscripta*. Lipsiae: B.G. Teubner, 1825.

Pélissier 1889: Léon G. Pélissier, "Un inventaire des manuscrits de la Bibliothèque de Corsini à Rome dressé par la Porte du Theil", *Mélanges d'archéologie et d'histoire de l'École de Rome* 9 (1889), pp. 389–429.

Pélissier 1891: Léon G. Pélissier, "Inventaire sommaire de soixante-deux manuscrits de la Bibliothèque Corsini (Rome)", *Centralblatt für Bibliothekswesen* 8 (1891), pp. 176–202, 297–324.

Pervanoglu 1868: Johannes Pervanoglu, "Griechenlands neueste handschriftliche Forschungen", *Neue Jahrbücher für Philologie und Paedagogik* 98 (1868), pp. 466–470.

Peyron 1820: Amedeus Peyron, *Notitia librorum manu typisve descriptorum qui donante ab. Thoma Valperga-Calusio V. Cl. illati sunt in Reg. Taurinensis Athenaei Bibliothecam bliographica et critica descriptione illustravit anecdota passim inseruit*. Lipsiae: Impensis Ioa. Aug. Gottl. Weigelii, 1820.

***Philolog.* 5 1850 758–62**: Friedrich Wilhelm Schneidewin, "Handschriften in Konstantinopel", *Philologus. Zeitschrift fur das klassische Alterthum* 5 (1850), pp. 758–760.

***Philologica Hamburgensia* 1905**: Robert Münzel (ed.), *Philologica Hamburgensia für die Mitglieder der 48. Versammlung deutscher Philologen und Schulmänner ausgestellt von der Stadtbibliothek zu Hamburg*. Hamburg: Lütcke und Wulff, 1905.

Piccolomini 1898: Aeneas Piccolomini, "Index codicum graecorum Bibliothecae Angelicae ad praefationem additamenta", *Studi italiani di filologia classica* 6 (1898), pp. 167–184.

Pierleoni 1901: Gino Pierleoni, "Index codicum graecorum qui Romae in Bybliotheca Corsiniana nunc Lynceorum adservantur", *Studi italiani di filologia classica* 9 (1901), pp. 467–478.

Porro 1884: Giulio Porro, *Catalogo dei codici manoscritti della Trivulziana* (Biblioteca storica, Reale Deputazione di Storia patria 2). Torino: Fratelli Bocca (Stamperia Reale), 1884.

Puntoni 1896/1: Vittorio Puntoni, "Indice dei codici greci della Biblioteca Estense di Modena", *Studi italiani di filologia classica* 4 (1896), pp. 379–536.

Puntoni 1896/2: Vittorio Puntoni, "Indicis codicum graecorum Bononiensium ab Al. Oliverio compositi supplementum", *Studi italiani di filologia classica* 4 (1896), pp. 365–378.

Rocchi 1883: Antonius Rocchi, *Codices cryptenses seu Abbatiae Cryptae Ferratae in Tusculano digesti et illustrati*. Romae: Ex Typographia Pacis, Philippi Cuggiani, 1883.

Roscoe 1815–1828: William Roscoe, *Catalogue of manuscripts in the library at Holkham in the County of Norfolk, belonging to Thomas William Coke, Esq., M.P.* Compiled and arranged by William Roscoe; collated and enlarged by Frederic Madden, 8 volumes, 1815–1828.

Rostagno 1894: Enrico Rostagno, "Codici greci Laurenziani meno noti", *Studi italiani di filologia classica* 2 (1894), p. 154.

Rostagno 1898: Enrico Rostagno, "Indicis codicum graecorum bybliothecae Laurentianae supplementum", *Studi italiani di filologia classica* 6 (1898), pp. 129–166.

Rostagno–Festa 1893: Enrico Rostagno e Nicola Festa, "Indice dei codici greci Laurenziani non compresi nel catalogo del Bandini", *Studi italiani di filologia classica* 1 (1893), pp. 129–232.

Ruelle 1875: Charles Emile Ruelle, "Rapports sur une mission littéraire et philologique en Espagne", *Archives des missions scientifiques et littéraires. Choix de rapports et instructions publié sous les auspices du Ministère de l'instruction publique et des beaux-arts*, 3e série, tome 2 (1875), pp. 497–627.

Rühl 1889: Franz Rühl, "Bemerkungen über einige Bibliotheken von Sicilien", *Philologus. Zeitschrift fur das klassische Alterthum* N. F. 1 = 47 (1889), pp. 577–588.

Sakkelion 1892: Ἰωάννης Σακκελίων καὶ Ἀλκιβιάδης Σακκελίων, *Κατάλογος τῶν χειρογράφων τῆς Ἐθνικῆς Βιβλιοθήκης τῆς Ἑλλάδος*. Ἀθῆναι: Ἐκ τοῦ Ἐθνικοῦ Τυπογραφείου καὶ Λιθογραφείου, 1892.

Schenkl 1896: Heinrich Schenkl, *Bibliotheca patrum latinorum Britannica. VII* (Sitzungsberichte der kaiserlichen Akademie der Wissenschaften, Philosophish-historische Classe 133 [1895], Abhandlung 7). Wien: Kaiserliche Akademie der Wissenschaften, 1896.

Schmid 1902: Wilhelm Schmid, *Verzeichnis der griechischen Handschriften der königlichen Universitätsbibliothek zu Tübingen*. Tübingen: Buchdruckerei von G. Schnürlen, 1902.

Schmid 1903: Wilhelm Schmid, "Zum Verzeichnis der Tübinger griechischen Handschriften", *Centralblatt für Bibliothekswesen* 20 (1903), pp. 462–464.

Schneider 1840/41: Karl Ernst Christoph Schneider, "Descriptio duorum codicum MSS. Galeni libros latinam in linguam translatos continentium", in *Index lectionum in Universitate Litterarum Vratislaviensi per hiemem Anni MDCCCXL. a Die XIX M. Octobris instituendarum*. Vratislavae: Universitas Literarum Vratislaviensis, 1840/41, pp. 1–14.

Schnorr v. Carolsfeld 1882–1883: Franz Schnorr von Carolsfeld, *Katalog der Handschriften der Königl. öffentlichen Bibliothek zu Dresden*. Im Auftrage der Generaldirection der königlichen Sammlungen für Kunst und Wissenschaft bearbeitet von –. Erster Band. (enthaltend die Abtheilungen A–D und F–H). Zweiter Band. (enthaltend die Abteilungen J–M). Leipzig: Druck und Verlag von B. G. Teubner, 1882–1883.

Scott 1904: Edward J. L. Scott, *Index to the Sloane manuscripts in the British Museum*. London: British Museum, 1904.

Senebier 1779: Jean Senebier, *Catalogue raisonné des manuscrits conservés dans la Bibliothèque de la Ville et République de Genève*. Genève: Barthelemy Chirol, 1779.

Sinker 1891: Robert Sinker, *The Library of Trinity College, Cambridge*. Cambridge: Deighton, Bell and Co., and London: George Bell and Sons, 1891.

Smith 1849: John James Smith, *A Catalogue of the Manuscripts in the Library of Gonville and Caius College, Cambridge*. Cambridge: J. Deighton, and Macmillan & Co.; London: John W. Parker; Oxford: J. Parker, 1849.

Sparfwenfeldt 1706: Ioan. Gabr. Sparvenfeldius, *Catalogus centuriae librorum rarissimorum manuscript. Et partim impressorum, Arabicorum, Persicorum, Turcicorum, Graecorum, Latinorum, etc. Qua anno MDCCV Bibliothecam Publicam Academiae Upsalensis auxit et exornavit Vir illustris et generosissimus* ... Upsaliae: Typis Joh. Henr. Werneri, 1706.

***Statistica del regno d'Italia* 1865**: *Statistica del regno d'Italia. Biblioteche. Anno 1863*. Firenze: Tipografia dei successori Le Monnier, 1865.

***Statistica delle biblioteche* 1893–1894**: Ministero di Agricoltura, Industria e Commercio (Direzione generale della statistica), *Statistica delle biblioteche*. Parte I. *Biblioteche dello stato, delle provincie, dei comuni ed altri enti morali aggiuntevi alcune biblioteche private accessibili agli studiosi, tra le più importanti per numero di volumi o per rarità di collezioni*. Volume I. *Piemonte, Liguria, Lombardia, Veneto ed Emilia;* Volume II. *Toscana, Marche, Umbria, Roma, Abruzzi e Molise, Campania, Puglie, Basilicata, Calabria, Sicilia e Sardegna*. Roma: Tipografia nazionale di G. Bertero, 1893–1894.

Stevenson 1885: Henry Stevenson, *Codices manuscripti Palatini graeci Bibliothecae Vaticanae descripti*. Romae: Ex Typographeo Vaticano, 1885.

Stevenson 1888: Henry Stevenson, *Bibliothecae Apostolicae Vaticanae ... Codices Reginae Suecorum et Pii PP. II graeci*. Romae: Ex Typographeo Vaticano, 1888.

Stornajolo 1895: Cosimo Stornajolo, *Codices urbinates graeci Bibliothecae Vaticanae descripti ... Accedit Index vetus Bibliothecae urbinatis nunc primum editus*. Romae: Ex Typographeo Vaticano, 1895.

Studemund–Cohn 1890: Wilhelm Studemund und Leopold Cohn, *Codices ex Bibliotheca Meermanniana Phillippici Graeci nunc Berolinenses* (Verzeichniss der griechischen Handschriften der königlichen Bibliothek zu Berlin 1). Berolini: A. Asher & Co, 1890.

Svedelius 1806: Pehr Fabian Aurivillius, *Notitia codicum manuscriptorum Græcorum biblioth. acad. Upsaliensis. Quam consensu ampliss. fac. phil. Ups. præside Petro Fabiano Aurivillio ... pro gradu philosophico publico examini subjicit Petrus Gustavus Svedelius, Dalekarlus. In audit. Gust. maj. d. VI. Junii MDCCCVI* ... Upsaliæ: typis Edmannianis, [1806].

Szilágyi 1881–1894: Sándor Szilágyi, *Catalogus manuscriptorum Bibliothecae Regiae Scientiarum Universitatis Budapestinensis*, 3 volumes. Budapestini: Typis Typographiae Universitatis Regiae Scientiarum, 1881–1894.

***The Academy* 1880**: Greville John Chester, "The Greek Library at Smyrna", *The Academy – A Weekly Review of Literature Science, and Arts* 17 (January–June 1880), p. 178.

Thompson 1881–1884: [Edward Maunde Thompson, and George F. Warner], *Catalogue of Ancient Manuscripts in the British Museum*, 2 volumes. London: British Museum, 1881–1884.

Thraemer 1892: Eduard Thrämer, "Auf der Suche nach der Bibliothek Iwans des Schrecklichen", *Allgemeine Zeitung, Beilage*, 1892, Heft 1, pp. 4–7; Heft 2, pp. 1–4; Heft 3, pp. 3–5.

Todd 1812: Henry John Todd, *A catalogue of the archiepiscopal manuscripts in the library at Lambeth Palace. With an account of the archiepiscopal registers and other records there preserved*. London: Law and Gilbert, 1812.

Tomasini 1639: Iacobus Philippus Tomasini, *Bibliothecae patavinae manuscriptae publicae et privatae*. Utini: Typis Nicolai Schiratti, 1639.

Tomasini 1650: Iacobus Philippus Tomasini, *Bibliothecae venetae manuscriptae publicae et privatae*. Utini: Typis Nicolai Schiratti, 1650.

Van den Gheyn 1901–1904: Joseph Van den Gheyn, *Catalogue des manuscrits de la Bibliothèque Royale de Belgique*, vol. 1: *Écriture sainte et liturgie*; vol. 2: *Patrologie*; vol. 3: *Théologie*; vol. 4: *Jurisprudence et philosophie*, Brussels: Lambertin, 1901–1904.

Vater 1843: Friedrich Vater, "Zur Kunde griechischer Handschriften in Russland", *Neue Jahrbücher für Philologie und Paedagogik oder Kritische Bibliothek für das Schul- und Unterrichtswesen* 9. Supplementband (1843), pp. 5–49.

Vitelli 1894: Girolamo Vitelli, "Indice de' codici greci Riccardiani, Magliabechiani e Marucelliani", *Studi italiani di filologia classica* 2 (1894), pp. 471–570.

Vogel 1841–1842: Ernst Vogel, "Ueber einige frühere italienische Bibliotheken", *Serapeum – Zeitschrift für Bibliothekswissenschaft, Handschriftenkunde und ältere Literatur* 2 (1841), pp. 24–32, 41–46, 52–59, 72–79, 318–319, 321–330; 3 (1842), pp. 140–144.

Volger 1858: Ernst Volger, "Mittheilungen aus handschriften", *Philologus. Zeitschrift für das klassische Alterthum* 13 (1858), pp. 192–195.

Volger 1859: Ernst Volger, "Mittheilungen aus Spanien", *Philologus. Zeitschrift für das klassische Alterthum* 14 (1859), pp. 161–168.

Volger, *Philologus* 14 1859: Ernst Volger, "Mittheilungen aus Spanien. 23. Verzeichniss der classischen HSS. der Universitätsbibliothek von Salamanca", *Philologus. Zeitschrift für das klassische Alterthum* 14 (1859), pp. 373–379.

v. Gebhardt 1898: Oscar von Gebhardt, "Christian Friedrich Matthaei und seine Sammlung griechischer Handschriften. II. Zur Orientierung über die Moskauer Bibliotheken", *Centralblatt für Bibliothekswesen* 15 (1898), pp. 393–420.

v. Heinemann 1884–1888: Otto von Heinemann, *Die Handschriften der Herzoglichen Bibliothek zu Wolfenbüttel*. Erste Abteilung. *Die Helmstedter Handschriften*, 3 volumes. Wolfenbüttel: Druck und Verlag Julius Zwissler, 1884–1888.

v. Heinemann 1890–1903: Otto von Heinemann, *Die Handschriften der Herzoglichen Bibliothek zu Wolfenbüttel*. Zweite Abteilung. *Die Augusteischen Handschriften*. 5 volumes. Wolfenbüttel: Julius Zwissler, 1890–1903.

v. Heinemann 1903: Otto von Heinemann, *Die Handschriften der Herzoglichen Bibliothek zu Wolfenbüttel*. Dritte Abteilung. *Die Weissenburger Handschriften*. Wolfenbüttel: Julius Zwissler, 1903.

Wachler 1828: Albrecht W. J. Wachler, *Thomas Rhediger und seine Büchersammlung in Breslau. Ein biographisch-literärischer Versuch*. Breslau: Grüson,1828.

Wegener 1876: Philipp Wegener, "Verzeichnis der auf der Zeitzer Stiftsbibliothek befindlichen Handschriften", *Programm des Königlichen Stifts-Gymnasiums in Zeitz* ... (Programm 206). Zeitz: 1876, pp. 1–22.

Weidmann 1841: Franz Weidmann, "Verzeichniss der im Jahre 1712 nach Zürich abgeführten und nicht zurückgegebenen sanctgallischen Handschriften", in Weidmann, *Geschichte der Bibliothek von St. Gallen seit ihrer Gründung um das Jahr 830 bis auf 1841. Aus den Quellen bearbeitet auf die Tausendjährige Jubelfeier*. St. Gallen: Scheitlin und Zollikofer, 1841, pp. 423–441.

Weinberger 1902: Wilhelm Weinberger, *Catalogus catalogorum. Verzeichnis der Bibliotheken, die ältere Handschriften lateinischer Kirchenschriftsteller enthalten im Auftrage cer Kaiserlichen Akademie der Wissenschaften in Wien zusammengestellt*. Prag: F. Tempsky; Wien: F. Tempsky; Leipzig: G. Freitag, 1902.

Weißenborn 1857: Hermann Johann Christian Weißenborn, "Die Bibliotheken zu Constantinopel und deren alte Handschriften", *Neue Jahrbücher für Philologie und Paedagogik* 76 (1857) pp. 201–203.

Wilken 1817: Friedrich Wilken, *Geschichte der Bildung, Beraubung und Vernichtung der alten Heidelbergischen Büchersammlungen: ein Beytrag zur Literärgeschichte vornehmlich des funfzehnten und sechszehnten Jahrhunderts ; nebst einem meist beschreibenden Verzeichniß der im Jahr 1816 von dem Papst Pius VII. der Universität Heidelberg zurückgegebenen Handschriften und einigen Schriftproben*. Heidelberg: August Oswald's Universitäts-Buchhandlung, 1817.

Wolf 1764: Johann David Wolf, *Compendiaria Bibliothecae Neapolitanae Vratislaviensis ad Aedem S. Bernardini servatae descriptio* ... Bregae: Gottfr. Boerner, 1764.

[Zanetti] 1740: Anton Maria Zanetti and Antonio Bongiovanni, *Graeca D. Marci Bibliotheca codicum manuscriptorum per titulos digesta* ... Venetiis: apud Simonem Occhi, 1740.

***Zentralbl. f. Bibl. Wesen* 19 1902**: Karl Konrad Müller, “Besichtigung der Universitätsbibliothek und ihrer Cimelien mit einleintenden Worten des Direktors”; “Die Ausstellung auf der Universitätsbibliothek in Jena gelegentlich der Bibliothekarversammlung (S. 384) umfasste von Hss.”, *Centralblatt für Bibliothekswesen* 19 (1902), pp. 380–384, 428–429.
Zuretti 1896: Carlo Oreste Zuretti, “Indice de’ mss. greci torinesi non contenuti nel catalogo del Pasini”, *Studi italiani di Filologia classica* 4 (1896), pp. 201–223.

2. Editions of Anonymous Greek Medical Texts

This bibliography of printed anonymous Greek medical texts provides references to the edition of ca. fifty anonymous texts found in manuscripts and papyri. Although it is not comprehensive, in a certain way it complements the lists of manuscripts by authors and texts which make up the substance of Diels.

Though not explicitly divided into two parts, this bibliography comprises two sections: texts in manuscripts and texts in papyri (in this order). These two parts are clearly distinguished here. In both, items are identified as they are in Diels, by the title of the text (in many cases in Greek) or by another type of title (from an edition or from the scholarly tradition). These titles are exactly reproduced here in boldface for purposes of clarity. They are listed in alphabetical order and followed by the reference to the edition(s) listed in Diels. Whereas in Diels, these references are mostly in an abbreviated form, they are fully expanded here, and formatted according to standard bibliographical practice. In several cases, more than one edition is mentioned in Diels. All are listed here in chronological order. In some cases, such different editions are distinguished in Diels by textual characteristics (e.g., the *incipit* of the text). All these distinctive elements are exactly reproduced here.

In some cases, new elements of identification of the works referred to are added here (for instance, the exact pages where the edition of the text can be read).

1. Texts from manuscripts

Anonymi metrologici: Friedrich Hultsch, *Metrologicorum scriptorum reliquiae*, collegit, recensuit, partim nunc primum edidit –, volumen I. Lipsiae: B.G. Teubner, 1864.

Carmen de viribus herbarum: Moritz Haupt, *Index lectionum quae auspiciis Regis augustissimi Guilelmi Imperatoris germanici in universitate litterarum Frideria Guilelma per semestre hibernum a. d. XVI. m. octobris A. MDCCCLXXIII usque ad d. XXII. m. martii MDCCCLXXIV habentur*. Berolini: Formis Academicis (G. Vogt), 1873–1874. *Inc.*: Carmen graecum de viribus herbarum quod dicitur ...

Vgl. Mauricius Hauptius, *Opuscula*, volumen secundum: *Prooemia indicibus lectionum praefixa*. Lipsiae: Salomon Hirzelius, 1876, pp. 475–489: "Index Lectionum Hibernarum 1873". *Inc.*: Carmen Graecum de viribus herbarum ...

Georg Kaibel, "Sententiarum Liber Quintus", *Hermes. Zeitschrift für classische Philologie* 25 (1890), pp. 97–112 (see section VII, pp. 103–109).

See also Ποίημα περὶ βοτανῶν (e cod. Vindob.) (below).

Fragmentum medicum (aus cod. bibl. Lips. 175 f. 17): Conrad Bursian, "Fragmentum medicum Graecum", in *Index scholarum publice et privatim in Universitate Litterarum Ienensi inde a Die XX M. Octobris A. MDCCCLXXXIII usque ad Diem XXI M. Martii A. MDCCCLXXIIII habendarum*. Ienae: Officina Neuenhahni, 1873, pp. 3–14.

Laterculi medicorum graecorum: *bei* Otto Kröhnert, *Canonesne poetarum, scriptorum artificum per antiquitatem fuerunt*? Dissertatio inauguralis philologa quam consensu et auctoritate amplissimi philosophorum ordinis in Alma Litterarum Universitate albertina Regimontana ad summos in philosophia honores rite capessendos die XXVIII. mensis Iunii. a. MDCCCXCVII ... Regimonti Prussorum: Officina Leopoldiana, 1897, esp. pp. 54–63.

Laterculi medicorum graecorum et latinorum (cod. Laur. lat. 73, 1): *bei* Max Wellmann, "Zur Geschichte der Medizin im Alterthum" *Hermes. Zeitschrift für classische Philologie* 35 (1900), pp. 349–384 (see especially pp. 367–382, section VI about the text on ff. 142v–143r of the manuscript).

Διάγνωσις περὶ τῶν ὀξέων καὶ χρονίων νοσημάτων: siehe H. Diels, *Die Handschriften der antiken Ärzte* II, p. 48 s. v. Herodotus.

Εἰσαγωγὴ ἀνατομική: Petrus Lauremberg, *Ἀνωνύμου εἰσαγωγὴ ἀνατομική, Anonymi philosophi antiquiss: Isagoge Anatomica*. Nunc primùm è suâ Bibliotheca edidit, & vertit –. Hamburgi: Paulus Langius, 1616.

edd. Daniel Wilhelm Triller et Johannes Stephanus Bernard, *Anonymi Introductio Anatomica Gr. et Lat. Item Hypatus De partibus corporis, Gr. et Lat.* cum notis –. *Accedunt Figurae Anatomicae cum explicatione Graeca, nunc primum ex Codice MS. Bibliothecae Leidensis editae*. Lugduni Batavorum: Philippus Bonk, 1744, pp. 1–141.

Vgl. Wilhelm Schmidt, *De Anonymi Laurembergiani introductione anatomica*. Dissertatio inauguralis quam ad summos in philosophia honores impetrandos consensu et auctoritate amplissimi philosophorum ordinis in Alma Litterarum Universitate Friderica Guilelma Berolinensi scripsit –. Berolini: Noske Bornensis, 1905.

Ἐκ τοῦ Φυσιολόγου περὶ φύσεως καὶ εἴδους ζῴων καὶ ἑρπετῶν καὶ ἡ ἀναγωγὴ τῶν ἀνθρώπων ὡς ἔχει: Charles Gidel et Emile Legrand, "Etude sur un poëme grec inédit intitulé Ο ΦΥΣΙΟΛΟΓΟΣ", *Annuaire de l'association pour l'encouragement des études grecques* 7 (1873), pp. 188–296 (edition of the Greek text by Legrand, pp. 225–286).

Vgl. Karl Krumbacher, *Geschichte der byzantinischen Litteratur von Justinian bis zum Ende des oströmischen Reiches (527–1453)*, 2. Auflage, bearbeitet unter Mitwirkung von Albert Ehrhard und Heinrich Gelzer. München: C. H. Beck'sche Verlagsbuchhandlung, 1897, pp. 874–877.

Ἑρμηνεία περὶ τῶν στοιχείων τοῦ ἀνθρώπου: Julius Ludwig Ideler, *Physici et Medici graeci minores. Congessit, ad fidem codd. MSS. praesertim eorum, quos beatus Dinzius contulerat, veterumque editionum partim emendavit partim nunc prima vice edidit, commentatiis criticis indicibusque tan rerum quam verborum instruxit*, 2 volumes. Berolini: G. Reimer, 1841–1842, vol. 1, pp. 301–302.

Ἑρμηνεία πρόχειρος ὀνομάτων βοτανῶν καὶ ἑτέρων εἰδῶν ἰατρικῶν ἀπὸ διαφόρων βιβλίων συλλεγεῖσα κατὰ ἀλφάβητον: Jean-François Boissonade, *ΑΝΕΚΔΟΤΑ. Anecdota graeca e codicibus regiis* descripsit annotatione illustravit, vol. II. Parisiis: In Regio Typographeo, 1830, pp. 394–408.

Ὀνόματα τῶν ἀνατομικῶν ἐργαλείων:

Friedrich Reinhold Dietz, *Severi sophistae de clysteribus liber ad fidem cod. manuscripti unici Florentini primum graece editus*. Regimontii Prussorum: apud fratres Borntraeger, 1836, pp. 46–48.

Hermann Schoene, "Zwei Listen chirurgische Instrumente", *Hermes. Zeitschrift für classische Philologie* 38 (1903), pp. 280–284.

Περὶ γεννήσεως ἀνθρώπου καὶ γονῆς: Julius Ludwig Ideler, *Physici et Medici graeci minores. Congessit, ad fidem codd. MSS. praesertim eorum, quos beatus Dinzius contulerat, veterumque editionum partim emendavit partim nunc prima vice edidit, commentatiis criticis indicibusque tan rerum quam verborum instruxit*, 2 volumes. Berolini: G. Reimer, 1841–1842, vol. 1, pp. 294–296.

Περὶ διαίτης: Julius Ludwig Ideler, *Physici et Medici graeci minores. Congessit, ad fidem codd. MSS. praesertim eorum, quos beatus Dinzius contulerat, veterumque editionum partim emendavit partim nunc prima vice edidit, commentatiis criticis indicibusque tan rerum quam verborum instruxit*, 2 volumes. Berolini: G. Reimer, 1841–1842, vol. 2, pp. 194–198.

Περὶ λυκανθρωπίας: Julius Ludwig Ideler, *Physici et Medici graeci minores. Congessit, ad fidem codd. MSS. praesertim eorum, quos beatus Dinzius contulerat, veterumque editionum partim emendavit partim nunc prima vice edidit, commentatiis criticis indicibusque tan rerum quam verborum instruxit*, 2 volumes. Berolini: G. Reimer, 1841–1842, vol. 2, p. 282.

Περὶ οὔρων ἐκ συρικοῦ βιβλίου: Julius Ludwig Ideler, *Physici et Medici graeci minores. Congessit, ad fidem codd. MSS. praesertim eorum, quos beatus Dinzius contulerat, veterumque editionum partim emendavit partim nunc prima vice edidit, commentatiis criticis indicibusque tan rerum quam verborum instruxit*, 2 volumes. Berolini: G. Reimer, 1841–1842, vol. 2, pp. 303–304.

Περὶ οὔρων ἐν πυρετοῖς: Julius Ludwig Ideler, *Physici et Medici graeci minores. Congessit, ad fidem codd. MSS. praesertim eorum, quos beatus Dinzius contulerat, veterumque editionum partim emendavit partim nunc prima vice edidit, commentatiis criticis indicibusque tan rerum quam verborum instruxit*, 2 volumes. Berolini: G. Reimer, 1841–1842, vol. 2, pp. 323–327.

Περὶ ὀφθαλμῶν (Alexander Trall.?): Theodor Puschmann, *Nachträge zu Alexander Trallianus. Fragmente aus Philumenus und Philagrius, nebst einer Bisher noch ungedruckten Abhandlung über Augenkrankheiten.* Nach den Handschriften herausgegeben und ins Deutsche übersetzt (Berliner Studien für classische Philologie und Archaeologie 5. Band, 2. Heft). Berlin: S. Calvary & Co., 1886, pp. 130–179.

Vgl. Georg Helmreich, "Zum Anonymus Περὶ ὀφθαλμῶν", *Philologus. Zeitschrift für das klassische Alterthum* 51 (N.F. 5) (1892), p. 746.

Περὶ παθῶν: Richard Schneider, *Excerpta περὶ παθῶν* (Beigabe zu den Jahresbericht des Königlichen Gymnasiums zu Duisburge 1895, Programm Nummer 446). Leipzig: B. G. Teubner, 1895.

Περὶ σφυγμῶν: Julius Ludwig Ideler, *Physici et Medici graeci minores. Congessit, ad fidem codd. MSS. praesertim eorum, quos beatus Dinzius contulerat, veterumque editionum partim emendavit partim nunc prima vice edidit, commentatiis criticis indicibusque tan rerum quam verborum instruxit*, 2 volumes. Berolini: G. Reimer, 1841–1842, vol. 2, p. 317.

Περὶ τῆς τοῦ κόσμου κατασκευῆς τοῦ ἀνθρώπου: Julius Ludwig Ideler, *Physici et Medici graeci minores. Congessit, ad fidem codd. MSS. praesertim eorum, quos beatus Dinzius contulerat, veterumque editionum partim emendavit partim nunc prima vice edidit, commentatiis criticis indicibusque tan rerum quam verborum instruxit*, 2 volumes. Berolini: G. Reimer, 1841–1842, vol. 1, pp. 303–304.

Περὶ τροφῶν: Franciscus Zacharias Ermerins, "Incerti auctoris tractatus de cibis, e libro de medicina ad Costantinum Pogonatum", in Idem, *Anecdota medica graeca*. Lugduni Batavorum: Luchtmans, 1840, pp. 223–275 (actual Greek title: Ἐξ ἰατρικῆς βίβλου πρὸς Κωνστάντινον Βασιλέα τῶν Πωγανατῶν, Περὶ τροφῶν σύνταγμα).

Περὶ τῶν δώδεκα μηνῶν τοῦ ἐνιαυτοῦ, ὁποίαις δεῖ χρῆσθαι τροφαῖς ἐν ἑκάστῳ αὐτῶν καὶ ἀπὸ ποίων ἀπέχεσθαι:

Jean-François Boissonade, *ΑΝΕΚΔΟΤΑ. Anecdota graeca e codicibus regiis* descripsit annotatione illustravit, vol. III. Parisiis: In Regio Typographeo, 1830, pp. 409–421.

Julius Ludwig Ideler, *Physici et Medici graeci minores. Congessit, ad fidem codd. MSS. praesertim eorum, quos beatus Dinzius contulerat, veterumque editionum partim emendavit partim nunc prima vice edidit, commentatiis criticis indicibusque tan rerum quam verborum instruxit*, 2 volumes. Berolini: G. Reimer, 1841–1842, vol. 2, pp. 423–429.

Περὶ ὑδροφοβίας:

ed. James Sims, *De hydrophobia. Graece et latine.* Interprete –. [Arnhem: W. Troost, 1791].

Reproduction of Sims' edition and translation (originally published in the *Memoirs of the Medical Society of London* 2 [1789], pp. 2–9 under the title "Of the Hydrophobia, from a Greek manuscript, in the possession James Sims ... with a translation by the fame") by Jo. Steph. Bernard, with Sims' Greek and Latin text pp. 1–10, and Bernard's commentary pp. 11–31.

Christianus Gothfr. Gruner, *Ioannis Stephani Bernard Reliquiae medico-criticae* edidit –. Ienae: [s.n.], 1795. See pp. 54–116 (reproduction of the work above, originally printed in a limited number of copies).

Περὶ χροιᾶς αἵματος τοῦ ἀπὸ φλεβοτομίας ἐκ τῆς ἰατρικῆς τῶν Περσῶν:

Christian Godofredus Gruner, "Anonymi fragmentum de venae sectione", in *Ordinis medici in Universitate Litteraria Ienensi H. T. Decanus D. Christ. Godofred. Gruner … sollemnia inauguralia viri praenobilissimi atque experientissimi Frederici Hoffmann … A. D. XVIIII. August. MDCCLXXX. indicit*. Ienae: Litteris Fickelscherrii, 1780, pp. 3–13.

Julius Ludwig Ideler, *Physici et Medici graeci minores. Congessit, ad fidem codd. MSS. praesertim eorum, quos beatus Dinzius contulerat, veterumque editionum partim emendavit partim nunc prima vice edidit, commentatiis criticis indicibusque tan rerum quam verborum instruxit*, 2 volumes. Berolini: G. Reimer, 1841–1842, vol. 1, p. 293.

Περὶ χυμῶν, βρωμάτων καὶ πομάτων: Julius Ludwig Ideler, *Physici et Medici graeci minores. Congessit, ad fidem codd. MSS. praesertim eorum, quos beatus Dinzius contulerat, veterumque editionum partim emendavit partim nunc prima vice edidit, commentatiis criticis indicibusque tan rerum quam verborum instruxit*, 2 volumes. Berolini: G. Reimer, 1841–1842, vol. 2, pp. 257–281.

Ποίημα περὶ βοτανῶν (e cod. Vindob.): Ludwig Choulant und Julius Sillig, *Una cum Walafridi Strabonis Othonis Cremonensis et Ioannis Folcz Carminibus similis argumenti quae secundum codices manuscriptos et veteres editiones recensuit, supplevit et adnotatione critica instruxit L. C. Accedit anonymi carmen graecum de herbis quod e codice vindobonensi auxit et cum Goddfredi Hermanni suisque emendationibus edidit J. S.* Lipsiae: Leopoldi Vossii, 1832, pp. 195–216.

Στίχοι τῶν ιβ′ μηνῶν (e cod. Paris. 2286. f. 124):

Jean-François Boissonade, "Traité alimentaire du médecin Hérophile extrait de deux manuscrits de la bibliothèque du roi", *Notices et Extraits des manuscrits de la bibliothèque du roi et autres bibliothèques* 11 (1827), seconde partie, pp. 178–273.

Julius Ludwig Ideler, *Physici et Medici graeci minores. Congessit, ad fidem codd. MSS. praesertim eorum, quos beatus Dinzius contulerat, veterumque editionum partim emendavit partim nunc prima vice edidit, commentatiis criticis indicibus-*

que tan rerum quam verborum instruxit, 2 volumes. Berolini: G. Reimer, 1841–1842, vol. 1, pp. 421–422.

Στοῖχοι τῶν δώδεκα μηνῶν: Julius Ludwig Ideler, *Physici et Medici graeci minores. Congessit, ad fidem codd. MSS. praesertim eorum, quos beatus Dinzius contulerat, veterumque editionum partim emendavit partim nunc prima vice edidit, commentatiis criticis indicibusque tan rerum quam verborum instruxit,* 2 volumes. Berolini: G. Reimer, 1841–1842, vol. 1, pp. 299–300.

Σύνοψις ἀκριβεστάτη περὶ οὔρων ἑρμηνευθεῖσα ἐκ τῆς ἰατρικῆς τέχνης τῶν Περσῶν: Julius Ludwig Ideler, *Physici et Medici graeci minores. Congessit, ad fidem codd. MSS. praesertim eorum, quos beatus Dinzius contulerat, veterumque editionum partim emendavit partim nunc prima vice edidit, commentatiis criticis indicibusque tan rerum quam verborum instruxit*, 2 volumes. Berolini: G. Reimer, 1841–1842, vol. 2, pp. 305–306.

Σύνοψις περὶ οὔρων: Julius Ludwig Ideler, *Physici et Medici graeci minores. Congessit, ad fidem codd. MSS. praesertim eorum, quos beatus Dinzius contulerat, veterumque editionum partim emendavit partim nunc prima vice edidit, commentatiis criticis indicibusque tan rerum quam verborum instruxit*, 2 volumes. Berolini: G. Reimer, 1841–1842, vol. 2, pp. 307–316.

2. Texts from papyri

A medical papyrus fragment: Edgar Johnson Goodspeed, "A Medical Papyrus Fragment", *American Journal of Philology* 24 (1903), pp. 327–329.

Anonymi Londinensis ex Aristotelis Iatricis Menoniis et aliis medicis eclogae: Hermann Diels, *Anonymi Londinensis ex Aristotelis Iatricis Menoniis et aliis medicis eclogae* (Supplementum Aristotelicum voluminis III pars 1). Berolini: G. Reimer, 1893.

Papyri Argentoratenses graecae (Remedia oculorum. De febribus): Karl Kalbfleisch, *Papyri Argentoratenses graecae* editae (*Ad Scholas quae in has Universitate Rostochiensi per semestre aestivum inde a D. XV M. Aprilis usque a D.XV M. Augusti Z. MDCCCI habebuntur invitant Rector et Concilium*). Rostochii: Typis academicis Adlerianis, 1901, pp. 3–12.

Papyrus Berolinensis 7763. 9776 (Medicinische Recepte): ed. Hermann Schoene, in Karl Kalbfleisch und Hermann Schöne (herausgegeben von –), *Berliner Klassikertexte*, Heft III, *Griechische Papyri medizinischen und naturwissenschaftlichen Inhalts*. Berlin: Weidmannsche Buchhandlung, 1905, pp. 32–33, 33–34.

Papyrus Berolinensis 9015 (Lehre der empirischen Ärzte): ed. Hermann Schoene, in Karl Kalbfleisch und Hermann Schöne (herausgegeben von –), *Berliner Klassikertexte*, Heft III, *Griechische Papyri medizinischen und naturwissenschaftlichen Inhalts*. Berlin: Weidmannsche Buchhandlung, 1905, pp. 29–30.

Papyrus Berolinensis 9095 (Behandlung einer Verstopfung): ed. Karl Kalbfleisch, in Karl Kalbfleisch und Hermann Schöne (herausgegeben von –), *Berliner Klassikertexte*, Heft III, *Griechische Papyri medizinischen und naturwissenschaftlichen Inhalts*. Berlin: Weidmannsche Buchhandlung, 1905, pp. 19–21.

Papyrus Berolinensis 9764 (Medizinischer Unterricht): ed. Hermann Schoene, in Karl Kalbfleisch und Hermann Schöne (herausgegeben von –), *Berliner Klassikertexte*, Heft III, *Griechische Papyri medizinischen und naturwissenschaftlichen Inhalts*. Berlin: Weidmannsche Buchhandlung, 1905, pp. 22–26.

Papyrus Berolinensis 9765 (Gewinnung und Reinigung von Rindstalg): ed. Hermann Schoene, in Karl Kalbfleisch und Hermann Schöne (herausgegeben von –), *Berliner Klassikertexte*, Heft III, *Griechische Papyri medizinischen und naturwissenschaftlichen Inhalts*. Berlin: Weidmannsche Buchhandlung, 1905, pp. 30–31.

Papyrus Berolinensis 9770 A. B (Aus einer anatomisch-physiologischen Schrift): ed. Karl Kalbfleisch, in Karl Kalbfleisch und Hermann Schöne (herausgegeben von –), *Berliner Klassikertexte*, Heft III, *Griechische Papyri medizinischen und naturwissenschaftlichen Inhalts*. Berlin: Weidmannsche Buchhandlung, 1905, pp. 10–19.

Papyrus Cairensis Cattaui (Chirurgisches Fragment, wahrscheinlich Heliodorus):

ed. Jules Nicole, "Fragment d'un Traité de Chirurgie", *Archiv für Papyrusforschung und verwandte Gebiete* 4 (1908), pp. 269–271.

Johannes Ilberg, "Kommentar", *ibidem*, pp. 271–283.

Papyrus Cairensis Musei 10160: Edgar Johnson Goodspeed, "Greek Papyri from the Cairo Museum together with Papyri of Roman Egypt from American Collections", *Decennial Publications of the University of Chicago* 5 (1902), pp. 1–78; see pp. 6–7 for papyrus Cairo Museum 10160.

Papyrus Genevensis 111 (»Un questionnaire de chirurgie«): Jules Nicole, "Un questionnaire de chirurgie", *Archiv für Papyrusforschung und verwandte Gebiete* 2 (1903) pp. 1–3.

Papyrus Golenischtschew; saec. III (Gynaekologische Fragment): Albert Bäckström, "Fragment einer medizinischen Schrift", *Archiv für Papyrusforschung und verwandte Gebiete* 3 (1906), pp. 158–162.

Papyri graecae Musei Britannici et Musei Berolinensis (De maxilla reponenda. De excrementis. De ponderibus et mensuris): Karl Kalbfleisch, "Papyri Graecae Musei Britannici et Musei Berolinensis", in *Ad Scholas quae in hac Universitate Rostochiensi per semestre aestivum inde a D. XV M. Aprilis usque a D. XV M. Augusti A. MDCCCII habebuntur* invitant Rector et Concilium. Rostochii: Typis academicis Adlerianis, 1902. pp. 3–14.

De maxilla reponenda: see pp. 3–8; De excrementis: see pp. 8–9 (same as Papyrus Berolinensis 9095 above); De ponderibus et mensuris: see pp. 11–14.

Papyrus Magica: Frederic George Kenyon, *Greek Papyri in the British Museum. Catalogue, with texts*. London: British Museum, 1893.

Reference is made to pp. 89 ff. This is a part of the description of papyrus CXXI described pp. 83–115. At pp. 89–90, Kenyon reproduces, and comments on, the text of ll. 168–185, which contain, according to him (see p. 89, note ad ll. 168–185), "A number of recipes for various purposes, not magical".

Papyrus Oxyrhynchus, nr. 234 (Recepte): Bernard P. Grenfell and Arthurs S. Hunt, *The Oxyrhynchus Papyri*, Part II. Edited with translations and notes (Egypt Exploration Fund, Graeco-Roman Branch). London: Egypt Exploration Fund, and Kegan Paul, Trench, Trübner & Co., 1899, pp. 134–136.

Vgl. Alessandro Olivieri, "Papiro medicinale (Pap. di Oxyrhynchus Vol. 2°, 135–6)", *Bolletino di filologia classica* 8 (1901–1902), pp. 229–237.

Vgl. Wilhelm Crönert "Adnotamenta in papyros Musei Britannici graecas maximam partem lexicographica", *Classical Review* 17 (1903) pp. 26–27.

Vgl. Wilhelm Crönert, "Sprachliches zu griechischen Ärzten, eine Untersuchung über den Verfasser des griechischen Papyrus Lond. Nr. 155", *Archiv für Papyrusforschung und verwandte Gebiete* 2 (1903), pp. 475–482.

Περὶ μέτρων: edd. Bernard P. Grenfell and Arthurs S. Hunt, *The Oxyrhynchus Papyri*, Part IV. Edited with translations and notes (Egypt Exploration Fund, Graeco-Roman Branch). London: Egypt Exploration Fund, and Kegan Paul, Trench, Trübner & Co., 1904, pp. 116–121.

3. Reference Works

The list of reference works provided at the end of the 1908 *Nachtrag* (*Supplement*) provides over 40 titles referenced in a summary form. It is reproduced below with the full references of cited works formatted according to current standard bibliographical practices. For purposes of clarity, full references are introduced by a short reference in boldface, utilizing the last name of the author(s) and the year of publication of the work. The full reference follows in regular typeface.

Listed works range from the classical *Elenchus medicorum veterum* compiled by Johann Albert Fabricius (1668–1736) and published in 1726 or the *Bibliothecae* (*botanica*, *chirurgica*, *anatomica* and *medicinae practicae*) by Albrecht von Haller (1708–1777) published between 1771 and 1788, to the more recent inventoires and descriptions of Greek medical manuscripts by Georges Costomiris (1849–1902), the revised edition (then in the making) of *Paulys Realencyclopädie der classischen Altertumswissenschaft* or the recent *Hanbuch der Geschichte der Medizin* edited by Max Neuburger (1868–1955) and Julius Pagel (1851–1912). The works are mostly in German, with some in French and few in English, besides earlier works in Latin. While they reflect the intellectual tradition of which Diels' catalogues were the heirs, they also integrate the new medical history in the making at that time, with a broad range of disciplines: neurology, ophthalmology, obstetrics, surgery, epidemiology, venereology, and surgery, in addition to pharmacy, botany and materia medica, and also medical education and hospital.

André-Pontier 1900: Léon-Charles André-Pontier, *Histoire de la pharmacie. Origines, Moyen Age, Temps Modernes*. Paris: Octave Doin, 1900.

Berendes 1891: Julius Berendes, *Die Pharmazie bei den alten Culturvölkern. Historisch-kritische Studien*, 2 Bände. Halle: Tausch & Grosse 1891.

Choulant 1841: Ludwig Choulant, *Handbuch der Bücherkunde für die ältere Medicin zur Kenntniss der griechischen, lateinischen und arabischen Schriften im ärztlichen Fache und zur bibliographischen Unterscheidung ihrer verschiedenen Ausgaben, Uebersetzungen und Erläuterungen*, 2. Auflage. Leipzig: Leopold Voss, 1841.

Choulant 1842: Ludwig Choulant, *Bibliotheca medico-historica sive catalogus librorum historicorum de re medica et scientia naturali systematicus*. Lipsiae: Gul. Engelmann, 1842.

Costomiris 1889: Georges A. Costomiris, "Etudes sur les écrits inédits des anciens médecins grecs et ceux dont le texte original est perdu, mais qui existent en latin ou en arabe. Première série: Hippocrate, Crateuas, Aelius Promotus, Galien", *Revue des études grecques* 2 (1889), pp. 343–383.

Costomiris 1890: Georges A. Costomiris, "Etudes sur les écrits inédits des anciens médecins grecs. Deuxième série: L'Anonyme de Daremberg, Métrodora, Aétius", *Revue des études grecques* 3 (1890), pp. 145–179.

Costomiris 1891: Georges A. Costomiris, "Etudes sur les écrits inédits des anciens médecins grecs. Troisième série: Alexandre (Sophiste et Roi), Timothée, Léon le Sophiste, Théophane Nonnos, les Ephodes", *Revue des études grecques* 4 (1891), pp. 97–110.

Costomiris 1892: Georges A. Costomiris, "Etudes sur les écrits inédits des anciens médecins grecs. Quatrième série: Hippiatriques et auteurs du XIe siècle: Psellus, Siméon Seth, Damnastès", *Revue des études grecques* 5 (1892), pp. 61–72.

Costomiris 1897: Georges A. Costomiris, "Etudes sur les écrits inédits des anciens médecins grecs. Cinquième série: XIIIe–XIVe siècles, Jean Tzetzès, Nicolas Myrepsus, Jean Actuarius", *Revue des études grecques* 10 (1897), pp. 405–445.

Espérandieu 1894: Emile Espérandieu, *Recueil de cachets d'oculistes romains*. Paris: Ernest Leroux, 1893 (not 1894).

Fabricius 1726: Johannes Albertus Fabricius, "Elenchus medicorum veterum, praecipue eorum uorum scripta desiderantur, vel de quibus mentio in priscis monumentis occurrit" in: Idem, *Bibliotheca graeca*, volumen XIII, *quo continetur elenchus medicorum veterum, et notitia collectionum ac scriptorum graecorum junctim editorum, liturgicorumque. Accedunt Anonymi Hoescheliani definitiones, latina versione donatae: Sententiae variorum et secundi philosophi, emendatae ex MS. nuncupationes ecclesiasticae quibus utuntur in suo litterarum commercio Graeci recentiores. Theophili Corydalei expositio rhetorices, &c.* Hamburgi: Theodorus Christophorus Felginer, 1726, pp. 15–456.

Gurlt 1898: Ernst Julius Gurlt, *Geschichte der Chirurgie und hihrer Ausübung. Volkschirurgie, Alterthum, Mittelalter, Renaissance*, Erster Band. Berlin: August Hirschwald, 1898.

Haeser 1875: Heinrich Haeser, *Lehrbuch der Geschichte der Medicin und der epidemischen Krankheiten*. Erster Band: *Geschichte der Medicin im Alterthum und Mittelalter*, 3. Bearbeitung. Jena: Hermann Dufft, 1875.

Hahn 1897: Lucien Hahn, *Essai de bibliographie médicale. Etude analytique des principaux répertoires bibliographiques concernant les sciences médicales; de leur utilité dans les recherches scientifiques*. Paris: G. Steinheil, 1897.

Hirsch 1893: August Hirsch, *Geschichte der medicinischen Wissenschaften in Deutschland* (Geschichte der Wissenschaften in Deutschland, Neuere Zeit. 22). München und Leipzig: Druck und Verlag R. Oldenbourg, 1893.

Hirschberg 1899: Julius Hirschberg, *Geschichte der Augenheilkunde im Alterthum* (Handbuch der gesamten Augenheilkunde, 2. Auflage, 12. Band, Kapitel XXIII. *Geschichte der Augenheilkunde*, Erstes Buch). Berlin: Springer, 1899.

Hoffmann 1838–1845: Samuel Friedrich Wilhelm Hoffmann, *Lexicon bibliographicum. Sive Index editionum et interpretationum scriptorium graecorum tum sacrorum tum profanorum*, zweite umgearbeitete, verbesserte und fortgesetzte Ausgabe, 3 Bände. Leipzig: A. F. Böhme, 1838–1845 (the 2nd edition [1845] referred to here is titled *Bibliographisches Lexicon der gesamten Literatur der Griechen*).

Index-Catalogue: *Index-Catalogue of the library of the Surgeon-generals Office, United States Army. Authors and Subjects*, 16 Bde. Washington: Government Printing Office, 1880–1895; Second Series, 1896 ff.

Kühn 1826–1837: Carolus Gottlob Kühn, *Additamenta ad elenchum medicorum veterum, a Io. A. Fabricio in biblioth. graec. vol. XIII, p. 17–456 exhibitum*, I–XXX. Lipsiae: Universitas Literarum Lipsiensis, 1826–1837.

Kühn 1829–1830: Carolus Gottlob Kuehn, *Index medicorum oculariorum inter Graecos Romanosque*. I–XI. Lipsiae: Universitas Literarum, 1829–1830.

Kühn 1830–1832: Carolus Gottlob Kuehn, *Additamenta ad indicem medicorum arabicorum a J. A. Fabricio in bibl. Grec. Vol. XIII. exhibitum*. Manip. I–IX. Lipsiae: Universitas Literarum Lipsiensis, 1830–1832.

Magnus 1901: Hugo Magnus, *Die Augenheilkunde der Alten*. Breslau: J.U. Kern, 1901.

Meyer 1854 ff.: Ernst H. F. Meyer, *Geschichte der Botanik*. 4 Bände. Königsberg: Gebrüder Bornträger, 1854–1857.

Neuburger–Pagel 1902: Max Neuburger und Julius Pagel (herausgegeben von –), *Handbuch der Geschichte der Medizin*, Erster Band. Jena: Gustav Fischer, 1902.

Oehler 1906–1907: Johann Oehler, *Epigraphische Beiträge zur Geschichte des Ärztestandes* (Jahres-Bericht des k. k. Maximilians –Gymnasiums in Wien. Für das Schuljahr 1906/1907). Wien: Selbstverlag des Gymnasiums, 1907, pp. 3–25.

Pagel 1898: Julius Pagel, *Historisch-Medicinische Bibliographie für die Jahre 1875–1896* (*Geschichte der Medizin*, Zweite Theile, II). Berlin: S. Karger, 1898.

Pauly 1872: Alphonse Pauly, *Bibliographie des sciences médicales*. 1er fascicule. Paris: Tross, 1872.

Pauly–Wissowa 1894 ff: Georg Wissowa (herausgegeben von –), *Paulys Realencyclopädie der classischen Altertumswissenschaft*, Neue Bearbeitung. Stuttgart: J. B. Metzlersche Verlagsbuchhandlung, 1894 ff.

Petit 1887: Louis Henri Petit, *Essais de bibliographie médicale. Conseils aux étudiants sur les recherches bibliographiques, la manière de faire sa thèse, de ranger sa bibliothèque, etc.* Paris: G. Masson, 1887.

Pohl 1905: Rudolfus Pohl, *De graecorum medicis publicis* (Dissertatio inauguralis Berolinensis). Berolini: Georgius Reimer, 1905.

Puschmann 1889: Theodor Puschmann, *Geschichte des medizinischen Unterrichts von den ältesten Zeiten bis zur Gegenwart*. Leipzig: Veit & Comp., 1889.

Reinach 1904: Salomon Reinach, “Medicus”, in Charles Daremberg, Edmond Saglio et Edmond Pottier, *Dictionnaire des antiquités grecques et romaines d’après les textes et les monuments contenant l’explication des termes qui se rapportent aux mœurs, aux institutions, à la religion, aux arts, aux sciences, au costume, au mobilier, à la guerre, à la marine, aux métiers, aux monnaies, poids et mesures, etc., etc. et en général à la vie publique et privée des anciens.* Tome troisième, Deuxième partie (L–M). Paris: Librarie Hachette, 1904, pp. 1669–1700.

Rosenbaum 1842: Julius Rosenbaum, *Additamenta ad Lud. Choulanti bibliothecam medico-historicam*. Halis Saxonum: Jo. Fr. Lippert, 1842.

Rosenbaum 1847: Julius Rosenbaum, *Additamenta ad Lud. Choulanti bibliothecam medico-historicam. Specimen secundum.* Halis Saxonum: C. A. Schwetschke et filius, 1847.

Rosenbaum 1882: Julius Rosenbaum, *Geschichte der Lustseuche im Alterthume, nebst ausführlichen Untersuchungen über den Venus- und Palluscultus, Bordelle, Νοῦσος θήλεια der Skythen, Paederastic und andere geschlechtlichen Ausschweifungen der Alten, als Beiträge zur richtigen Erklärung ihrer Schriften für Aerzte, Philologen und Alterthumsforscher*. 3. Abdruck. Halle: H. W. Schmidt, Halle, 1882.

Soury 1899: Jules Soury, *Le système nerveux central. Structure et fonctions. Histoire critique des théories et des doctrines*. Paris: Georges Carré et C. Naud, 1899.

Sprengel 1846: Kurt Sprengel, *Versuch einer pragmatischen Geschichte der Arzneikunde*, Vierte Auflage mit Berichtigungen und Zusätzen von Julius Rosenbaum, Erster Band: *Aelteste Geschichte der Medicin bis zur empirischen Schule*. Leipzig: Gebauersche Buchhandlung, 1846.

***Virchow's Jahresbericht* 1866–1904**: "Geschichte der Medizin und der Krankheiten", in Rudolf Virchow und August Hirsch (herausgegeben von –), *Jahresbericht über die Leistungen und Fortschritte in der gesammten Medicin* 1–38 (1866–1904).

von Haller 1771–1772: Albertus von Haller, *Bibliotheca botanica. Qua scripta ad rem herbariam facientia a rerum initiis recensentur*, 2 volumes. Tiguri: apud Orell, Gessner, Fuessli, et Socios, 1771–1772.

von Haller 1774–1775: Albrecht von Haller, *Bibliotheca chirurgica qua scripta ad artem chirurgicam facientia a rerum initiis recensentur*. Tomus I: *Tempora ante Annum MDCCX*; Tomus II: *Ab Anno MDCCX ad nostra tempora*. Bernae: apud Em. Haller, et Basileae: apud Joh. Schweighauser, 1774–1775.

von Haller 1774–1777: Albrecht von Haller, *Bibliotheca anatomica qua scripta ad anatomen et physiologiam facentia a rerum initiis recensentur*. Tomus I: *Ad Annum MDCC*; Tomus II: *Ab Anno MDCCI ad MDCCLXXVI*. Tiguri: apud Orell, Gessner, Fuessli, et Socc., 1774–1777.

von Haller 1776–1788: Albrecht von Haller, *Bibliotheca medicinae practicae qua scripta ad partem medicinae practicam facientia a rerum initiis recensentur*. Tomus I: *Ad Annum MDXXXIII*; Tomus II: *Ab Anno 1534. ad. A. 1647*; Tomus III: *Ab Anno 1648. ad A. 1685*; Tomus IV: *Ab Anno 1686 ad A. 1707*. Bernae: apud Em. Haller, et Basileae: apud Joh. Schweighauser, 1776–1788.

von Siebold 1901: Eduard Caspar Jacob von Siebold, *Versuch einer Geschichte der Geburtshilfe*, Zweite Auflage, Erster Band. Tübingen: Franz Pietzcker, 1901.

Wellmann 1891: Max Wellmann, "Die Medicin bis in die zweite Hälfte des zweiten Jahrhunderts", in Franz Susemihl, *Geschichte der griechischen Literatur in der Alexandrinerzeit*, Erster Band. Leipzig: B.G. Teubner, 1891, pp. 777–828.

Diels' Catalogue of Greek Medical Manuscripts in two parts (1905 and 1906) with a Supplement (1908)

Introduction

Diels' catalogue of manuscripts is reproduced here *ad litteram*. Its presentation has been modified, however, for clarity purposes. Whereas items in Diels follow each other so as to form blocks of continuous text, in the present work they are presented in the form of a list, where each line corresponds to one item. The typographic device used in Diels (boldface) to highlight city names, has been maintained. City and library names here are aligned on the left margin while the list of manuscripts related to each such city and library is indented. If the holdings of a library comprise several collections, the same principle of indentation has been used. The several collections are distinguished at the first level of indentation, with the items under each such collection further indented. An example of this layout is as follows:

Rom:

- Palat. 192; s. XV. f. 1.
- Reg. Suec. 182; s. XV. f. 16.
- Urbin.
  - 64*; s. X—XI. f. 116 (» ἐκ τοῦ κατὰ τὸν Ἱππ. ὅρκου, καθ' ὅσον οἷόν τε Χριστιανῷ ὀμόσαι«).
  - 68; s. XIV. f. 4 (*Ilbergs Coll. in dessen Besitz*).
- Vatic.
  - 276; s. XII. f. 1 (*Ilbergs Coll. in dessen Besitz*).
  - 277; s. XIV. f. 25 (*Ilbergs Coll. in dessen Besitz*).
  - 278; a. 1512. f. 27^{v}.
  - 2238; s. XV. f. 180.
  - 2304 (olim 2217); s. XV. f. 1.

Since the original layout of Diels' pages could not be exactly reproduced by way of this variant presentation of data, references to Diels pages have been included. For ease of recognition, these references are placed in the external margin of the pages. They appear between brackets ([ ]) and comprise two elements: an identifier which refers to the first or second issue of Diels' catalogues (I or II, respectively, published in 1905 and 1906) or the supplement (N for *Nachtrag* = *Supplement*; published in 1908), and a number in Arabic numerals (from 3 to 151) referring to the page of Diels' catalogues. The marginal reference [I.3], for example, thus refers to page 3 of part I (about Hippocrates and Galen, published in 1905).

The Manuscripts of Greek Physicians

Part I

Hippocrates and Galen

Hippocrates

Under the title **Zeichenerklärung** (*Table of Symbols*), Diels' catalogue includes some abbreviations and *sigla*, the list of which appears on page 2 of the first issue of the catalogue (1905). Those abbreviations, utilized precisely in the present reproduction of Diels are the following with their respective explicitation:

*	=	die Hds. enthält nur Exzerpte.
[ ]	=	die Hds. ist nur aus Ackermann's *Hist. litteraria Hippocratis* (Kühn Med. Gr. Opp. XXI, 1 ff.) und *Hist. litt. Cl. Galeni* (Kühn M. G. O. I, XVII ff.) oder aus Littré (Œuvr. compl. d'Hippocr. Par. 1839—61. 10 Bde.) bekannt.
J.	=	Galenus, editio Iuntina 1528 (Exemplar der Vatikanischen Handbibliothek).
K.	=	Kühn.
L.	=	Littré.

*	=	the manuscript contains only extracts.
[ ]	=	the manuscript is known only through Ackermann's *Hist. litteraria Hippocratis* (Kühn Med. Gr. Opp. XXI, 1 sq.) and *Hist. litt. Cl. Galeni* (Kühn M. G. O. I, XVII ff.) or Littré (Œuvr. compl. d'Hippocr. Par. 1839—61. 10 vols).
J.	=	Galen, Iuntina 1528 edition (copy of the Vatican Library).
K.	=	Kühn.
L.	=	Littré.

Athen: nr. 1477; s. XV. (προηγεῖται τὸ π. ἀγμῶν).
Jerusalem: Bibl. patriarch. 102; s. XVIII. f. 1 (»Συγγράμματα Ἱππ.«).
Göttingen: Hist. nat.

3 (impress. Hipp. omnia opera Venet. 1526. »Das Handexemplar des Janus Cornarius aus Zwickau ... vgl. Kühlewein im Hermes 27 (1892) p. 302 Anm. 3.«).

4 (Impress. Hipp. libri omnes Basil. 1538. »Handexemplar des Joh. Opsopoeus ... vgl. Kühlewein, Hermes 27 (1892) p. 303«).

Königsberg Pr.: Kgl. u. Univ. Bibl.

1) Dietz-Nachlaß I 1—3 [hs. Verz. von J. Fl. Lobeck]: impress. Hipp. Opera t. I, II, III Kühn mit Fr. R. Dietz' (1804—36) Kollationen zu sämtl. Schriften
2) Dietz-Nachlaß I 4: impress. Ἱπποκράτους π. ἱρ. νούσου βιβλ. rec. Dietz (Lips. 1827), Handexemplar des Editors mit dessen Kollationen mehrerer Hss. Vgl. Galeni de diss. musc. et de consuetud. libri ed. Dietz (Lips. 1832) praef. p. IX.

Konstantinopel: Bibl. d. Serail 11; s. XV.
Leipzig: Lipsiens. 61; s. XIX. (»Lectiones cod. Hauniensis 224 in folio, qui Hipp. opera continet collata cum editione C. G. Kuehnii verglichen von O. D. Bloch Kopenhagen 1825. Vorn ein halbes Blatt in zwei Kolumnen geschrieben: ‚Ex editione Van der Linden. Observ. crit. a Coraës mihi missae.' Am Schlusse zwei Blätter mit einer Abschrift des cod. 109 (Bl. 6), geschrieben von F. Jacobs, München 2. Aug. 1818«).
Leyden: B. P. 670; s. XVI. (»Handschriftl. Bemerkungen des Vulcanius, wie es scheint«).
Mailand: Ambros. (»Handschriftl. Bemerkungen aus 3 Aldinen

1) S. Q. J. VII. 9: fol. 6—30^{v}.
2) S. Q. E. VIII. 13: f. 6—30^{v}.
3) S. Q. E. VIII. 14: f. 1—30^{v}«.).

Padua: Bibl. S. Joann. in Viridario, ad dextr. plut. XVII. (*Verbleib unbekannt.*).
Rhodope: Βιβλ. μον. Μπατσκόβου (»Χειρόγραφον Ἱππ. ἐν παραφράσει«).
Rom: Barberin. 276; s. — (?).
Wien: Vindobon. 69 B 101 (»Handschriftliche Bemerkungen aus einer Basileens. des Hipp., dem Handexemplar des Cornarius. Zu περὶ διαίτης p. 81–109 Bas., zu π. ἱερῆς νούσου p. 122–128«).

[Diels I.4]

Περὶ ἀρχαίης ἰητρικῆς.
De prisca medicina.

L. I 570—636.
Kühlew. I 1–30.

Inc. Ὁκόσοι ἐπεχείρησαν περὶ ἰητρικῆς.
Expl. βέλτιστον δέ ἐστι τὸ προσωτάτω τοῦ ἀνεπιτηδείου ἀπέχον.

Bologna: Bonon. 3632*; s. XV. f. 28.
Cambridge: Cantabrig. Caius Coll. 50; s. XV/XVI. f. 6ᵛ.
Florenz: Laurent. plut. 74, 1; s. XV. p. 12.
Kopenhagen: Hauniens. ant. fund. reg. 224; s. XVI.
Leyden: Voss. fol. 10; s. XVI.
Mailand: Ambros. L 110 Sup.; s. XVI. f. 235ᵛ.
München: Monacens. 71; a. 1531.
Oxford: Baroccian. 204; s. XV. f. 12ᵛ.
Paris: Parisin.
1868*; s. XV. f. 379ᵛ—381. 397 (imperf. L. IV 76).
2140; s. XII—XIII. f. 13.
2141; s. XV. f. 11ᵛ.
2142; s. XIII—XIV. f. 17.
2143; s. XIV. f. 15ᵛ.
2144; s. XIV. f. 17.
2145; s. XV. f. 19ᵛ.
2253; s. XI. f. 117ᵛ.
2255; s. XV. f. 62ᵛ.
2332*; s. XV. f. 204ᵛ.
[2545 (?) = 2145?].
Rom:
Urbin. 68. s. XIV. f. 20 (*Coll. Ilbergs p. 568—580, 5 L. in dessen Besitz*).
Vatic.
277; s. XIV. f. 29ᵛ (*Coll. Ilbergs p. 568—590 L. in dessen Besitz*).
278; a. 1512. f. 30 (Inscr. περὶ ὑπάρξεως ἰητρικῆς· ὅρος ἰητρικός; *Coll. Ilbergs p. 568—578, 11 L. in dessen Besitz*).
Venedig: Marcian. 269; s. XI. f. 16.

Περὶ ἀέρων, ὑδάτων, τόπων.
De aëre, aquis et locis.

L. II 12—93.
Kühlew. I 33—71.

Inc. Ἰητρικὴν ὅστις βούλεται.
Expl. καὶ οὐχ ἁμαρτήσῃ.

Holkham: nr. 282; s. XVI. nr. 9.
Mailand: Ambros. S. Q. T. VIII 9 (Ed. Basil. mit Randbemerkungen zu π. ἀέρων etc.).
Modena: Mutinens. 220 (II H 5); s. XV. f. 63^v.
München: Monacens. 71; a. 1531.
Paris: Parisin.
2146; s. XVI. f. 103^v.
[2254].
2255; s. XV. f. 376 et 393.
Rom:
Barberin. I 5; s. XV. f. 237^v.
Palat. 192; s. XV. f. 26.
Vatic. 276; s. XII. f. 63^v. (*Collat. Ilbergs in dessen Besitz*).
Venedig: Marcian. App. cl. V 14; s. XVI. f. 11 = [Nanian. 248].

Προγνωστικόν. [Diels I.5]
Prognosticon.

L. II 140—190.
Kühlew. I 78—108.

Inc. Τὸν ἰητρὸν δοκέει μοι.
Expl. γνώσῃ τοῖσιν αὐτέοισι σημείοισι.

Bologna: Bonon. 3632; s. XIV. f. 36.
Cambridge:
[Ashmol. 7751; s. —]
[Caius Coll.]
[355; s. XV/XVI. f. 117.]
[954; s. —.]
[1134; s. —.]
[Cantabrig. 2329; s. —.]
[Cath. Metens. 226; s. —.]

[Pembroch. 2055; s. —.]
[St. Petri 1866; s. —.]
Dublin: [Coll. Trinit. 502; s. —]
Escurial: Scorial.
Υ III 17; s. XVI. f. 135 (c. comm. Gal.)
Φ III 7; s. XIV. f. 9 (c. comm. Gal.)
Φ III 12; s. XV. f. 9 (Exc.) et f. 457.
Florenz:
Laurent. plut.
74, 1; s. XV. p. 164 (*Collat. Ilbergs in dessen Besitz*).
74, 11; s. XIII. p. 171 (»Libri III«).
75, 3; s. XII. p. 239b.
[75, 10; s. —]
Riccard. 44 (K II 5); s. XV—XVI. f. 13v.
Gallipoli: Ἐκκλ. ἁγ. Νικολάου 38; s. XIV. f. 81v.
Holkham: nr. 282; s. XVI. no. 3.
Jerusalem: Bibl. Mar-Saba 498; s. XVIII. f. 25 (Ἐξήγησις τῶν προγνωστικῶν Ἱππ.).
Kopenhagen: Hauniens. ant. fund. reg. 224; s. XVI.
Leyden:
Scal. 71; s. XVI. f. 57—91.
Voss. fol. 10; s. XVI.
London:
(Brit. Mus.)
Harleian. (Brit. Mus.) 6295; s. XV (XIV). f. 89.
Regius (Brit. Mus.) 16. C. XVI; s. XVI. f. 48.
[1734, 4; s. —]
Stowe (Brit. Mus.) 1073; s. XVI. f. 62v.
Medical Society H Hi 17 = We 30; s. XV in. f. 12.
Madrid: Matrit. bibl. nac. 4634 (olim N 112); s. XV. f. 36.
Mailand: Ambros.
A 156 Sup.; s. XVI. f. 13.
B 113 Sup.; s. XIV in. f. 171v.
Q 13 Sup.*; s. — f. 4 (Frgm. Inc. ἢ ὁ ἕτερος τοῦ ἑτέρου. Expl. ἐπιγενομένων σημείων).
München: Monac. 71; a. 1531.
Oxford:
Bodleian.
Auct. T II 3*; s. XVIII.
Baroccian.
76*; s. XV—XVI. f. 300—301v (Exc. initii. Expl. πυρετοῦ θάνατον προσημαίνουσι).
204; s. XV. f. 179.

Bodleian. [2753 (sic Kühn prf. p. XLVII); s. —]
Laudian.
[1013; s. —].
[1257; s. —].
[1355; s. —].
Miscell. 132; s. XVI. f. 58b.
Coll. Merton.
[687; s. —].
[688; s. —].
[689; s. —].
[Eccl. Wigorn. 1760; s. —]
Padua: Bibl. S. Joannis in Viridario, ad dextr. plut. XVII. (*Verbleib unbekannt.*)
Paris:
Parisin.
36; s. XIV—XV. f. 17.
396*; s. XIII. f. 460 (prooem.).
1883; s. XIV. f. 66^{v} (»Libri III«).
1884; a. 1503. f. 78^{v}.
2140; s. XII—XIII. f. 184.
2141; s. XV. f. 167.
2142; s. XIII—XIV. f. 292^{v}.
2143; s. XIV. f. 169.
2144; s. XIV. f. 208.
2145; s. XV. f. 268^{v}.
2146; s. XVI. f. 14^{v}.
2168; s. XVI. (comm. Gal.).
2219*; s. XV. f. 105.
2228; s. XII. f. 26.
2229; s. XIII. f. 26.
2253; s. XI. f. 1.
[2254; s. XV.]
2255; s. XV. f. 386.
2256; s. XV. f. 23.
2257; s. XVI. f. 129 (comm. Gal.).
2266; s. XIV (comm. Gal.).
2269; s. XV. f. 68.
2316*; s. XV. f. 154^{v}.
2330; s. XV. f. 69.
2332*; s. XV (XIV).
2545 (? = 2145?; cf. Kühn l. l.)
[2828 (? = 2228?); s. —]

[3170 (?); s. —]
Suppl. 446; s. X. f. 68.

Rom:

Barberin. 136 (= I 11); s. XVI. f. 47.

Ottobon.

157 B; s. XV. f. 23^v.

192*; s. XVI—XVII. f. 16 (Inc. Εἰσὶ δὲ τὰ δώδεκα ζώδια).

Palat.

143; s. XV. f. 137.

192; s. XV. f. 9 (Lib. I et II).

199; s. XIII. f. 18.

Urbin.

64; s. X—XI. f. 96.

68; s. XIV. f. 201^v.

Vatic.

276; s. XII. f. 9^v (*Collat. Ilbergs in dessen Besitz*).

277; s. XIV. f. 227^v (*Coll. Ilbergs in dessen Besitz*).

278; a. 1512. f. 466.

283; s. XIV. f. 4.

294; s. — f. 70^v (»Διαγνωστικά«).

2254; s. X—XI. f. 21 (Init. mutil. *R. Reitzensteins Coll. p. 158, 6—190, 9 L. in Ilbergs Besitz*).

Sens: Miscell. 187*; s. XVII. f. 328.

Turin: Taurin. 156 b II 10*; s. XVI. f. 115^v.

Venedig: Marcian. 269; s. XI. f. 228.

Wien: Vindob. med.

16 (ol. 35); s. XV. f. 185—201 (marg.)

44; s. XV—XVI. f. 232—304^v (Sine auct. nomine. Expl. τεσσαρακοστὴν ἑξηκοστὴν ὅρον ἱστάμενος).

[Diels I.8]

Περὶ διαίτης ὀξέων.
De diaeta (regimine) acutorum.

L. II 224—376. Νόθα II 394—529.
Kühlew. I 109—145. Νόθα 146—179).

Inc. (224) Οἱ ξυγγράψαντες τὰς Κνιδίας καλεομένας γνώμας.
Expl. (376) οὐ δεῖ λούειν.

Νόθα Inc. (394) Καῦσος γίγνεται ὁκόταν.

Expl. (529) ταμιεύου καὶ θεράπευε.

Florenz: Laurent. plut. 74, 1; s. XV. p. 169b.
Holkham: nr. 282; s. XVI. no. 4 (Inscr. ἱππ. πρὸς τὰς κνιδίας γνώμας ἢ περὶ πτισάνης).
Karlsruhe: Caroliruhens. 449; s. XV—XVI. f. 62—73ᵛ (= Kühn Med. Gr. Op. XXII p. 26—36. Initium deest).
Kopenhagen: Hauniens. ant. fund. reg. 224; s. XVI.
Leyden: Voss. fol. 10. s. XVI.
München: Monacens. 71; a. 1531 (Inscr. Περὶ διαίτης ὀξέων, οἱ δὲ περὶ πτισάνης, οἱ δὲ πρὸς τὰς κνιδίας γνώμας).
Oxford: Baroccian. 204; s. XV. f. 185.
Paris: Parisin.
2140; s. XII—XIII. f. 190ᵛ.
2141; s. XV. f. 172.
2142; s. XIII—XIV. f. 302ᵛ.
2143; s. XIV. f. 175ᵛ.
2144; s. XIV. f. 215.
2145; s. XV. f. 277ᵛ.
2146; s. XVI. f. 22.
2148; s. XV. f. 50.
2253; s. XI. f. 37.
2254; s. XV. f. 12.
2332*; s. XIV. f. 231.
[2545 (? = 2145?)].
Rom:
Palat. 192; s. XV. f. 13ᵛ (Πρὸς τὰς Κνιδίας γνώμας ἢ περὶ πτισάνης).
Urbin. 68; s. XIV. f. 209ᵛ.
Vatic.
276; s. XII. f. 14ᵛ.
277; s. XIV. f. 234ᵛ.
278; a. 1512. f. 480ᵛ.
294; s. — f. 88ᵛ.
Venedig: Marcian. 269; s. XI. f. 237.
[**Wien:** Vindob. Lamb. VI 85].

Ἐπιδημιῶν Α' καὶ Γ'. [Diels I.10]
De morbis popularibus I et III.

L. Lib. 1: II 598—716. Lib. 3: III 24—148.
Kühlew. I 180—245.

Lib. 1

Inc. Ἐν Θάσῳ φθινοπώρου περὶ ἰσημερίην.
Expl. ἐκρίθη τελέως ἐνδεκαταίη.

Lib. 3

Inc. Πυθίων ὃς ᾤκει.
Expl. τῇ εἰκοστῇ τετάρτῃ ἀπέθανεν. φρενῖτις.

Athen: nr. 1488; s. XIX. (Lib. I)
[**Dublin:** Bibl. Narcissi cod. Brit. 502].
Florenz: Laurent. plut. 74, 1; s. XV. p. 295b.
Holkham: nr. 282; s. XVI. no. 10.
Kopenhagen: Hauniens. ant. fund. reg. 224; s. XVI.
Leyden: Voss. fol. 10. s. XVI.
Modena: Mutinens. 233 (III H 5); s. XVI. f. 33.
München: Monacens. 71; a. 1531.
Oxford: Baroccian. 204; s. XV. f. 333^{v}.
Padua: Bibl. Joann. Rhodii. (*Verbleib unbekannt*).
Paris: Parisin.
2140; s. XII—XIII. f. 349.
2141; s. XV. f. 293^{v}.
2142; s. XIII—XIV. f. 466.
2143; s. XIV. f. 321.
2144; s. XIV. f. 343^{v}.
2145; s. XV. f. 487.
2146; s. XVI. f. 110.
2165; s. XVI. f. 1. (pars tantum c. comm. Gal.).
2174; s. XVI. f. 1. (L. I. III. c. c. Gal.).
2229*; s. XIII.
2253; s. XI. f. 130^{v} (Lib. I et III init.).
2254; s. XV. f. 256^{v}.
[2332*; s. XV.]
Rom:
Palat. 192; s. XV. f. 114.
Urbin. 68; s. XIV. f. 360^{v}.
Vatic.
276; s. XII. f. 67^{v}.
277; s. XIV. f. 397.
278; a. 1512. f. 824^{v}.
[**Venedig:** Marcian. ? (Liber III). Marcian. ap. Montf. I 472].

Περὶ τῶν ἐν κεφαλῇ τρωμάτων.
De capitis vulneribus.

L. III 182—260.
Kühlew. II 1—29.

Inc. Τῶν ἀνθρώπων αἱ κεφαλαί.
Expl. ὥσπερ καὶ ἐν τῇ πρίσει γέγραπται.

Florenz: Laurent. plut. 74, 7; s. IX f. 74 (Expl. τοῦ βέλεος ἐν τῷ ὀ⟨στέῳ⟩ = L. III 246, 2).
Holkham: nr. 282; s. XVI. no. 8.
München: Monacens. 71; a. 1531.
Paris: Parisin.
2146; s. XVI.
2247; s. XVI. f. 73v.
2248; s. XVI. f. 105v.
[2254 (?)].
2255; s. XV. f. 389v.
Rom:
Palat. 192; s. XV. f. 64.
Vatic. 276; s. XII. f. 57.

Κατ' ἰητρεῖον. [Diels I.11]
De officina medici.

L. III 272—336.
Kühlew. II 30—45.

Inc. Ἢ ὅμοια ἢ ἀνόμοια.
Expl. ὡς μήτε διαναγκάζηται μηδὲ ἐνσείηται.

Cambridge: Cantabrig.
Caius-Coll. 76; s. XV/XVI. f. 213 (?)
Bibl. Univ. L. L. 5, 4; s. — (»très moderne«).
Florenz: Laurent. plut.
74, 1; s. XV. p. 204b.
74, 7; s. IX. f. 9.
Holkham: nr. 282; s. XVI. no. 5.
Kopenhagen: Hauniens. ant. fund. reg. 224; s. XVI.
Modena: Mutinens. 227 (II H 12); s. XVI. f. 39v.
München: Monacens. 71; a. 1531.

Oxford: Baroccian. 204; s. XV. f. 227.
Paris: Parisin.
1849; s. XIV. f. 175v. (c. comm. Gal.)
2140; s. XII—XIII. f. 234.
2141; s. XV. f. 205.
2142; s. XIII—XIV. f. 347v.
2143; s. XIV. f. 219.
2144; s. XIV. f. 250v.
2145; s. XV. f. 336v.
2146; s. XVI. f. 41v.
2247; s. XVI. f. 13.
2248; s. XVI. f. 18.
2254; s. XV. f. 78.
2255; s. XV. f. 366v.
[2287 (?)].
[2545 (?) = 2145?].
Rom:
Palat. 192; s. XV. f. 23v.
Urbin. 68; s. XIV. f. 255.
Vatic.
276; s. XII. f. 26v.
277; s. XIV. f. 279v.
278; a. 1512. f. 584.
Venedig: Marcian. 269; s. XI. f. 293 Bv.

Περὶ ἀγμῶν.
De fracturis.

L. III 412—562.
Kühlew. II 46—110.

Inc. Ἐχρῆν τὸν ἰητρόν.
Expl. τεκμαίρεσθαι ἀπὸ τῶν πρόσθεν γεγραμμένων.

Athen: nr. 1477; s. XVI.
Florenz: Laurent. plut.
74, 1; s. XV. p. 193b.
74, 7; s. IX. f. 13.
Holkham: nr. 282; s. XVI. nr. 6.
Kopenhagen: Hauniens. ant. fund. reg. 224; s. XVI.

Leyden: Voss. fol. 10; s. XVI.
Mailand: Ambros. C 85 Sup.; s. XV—XVI.
Modena: Mutinens. 227 (II H 12); s. XVI. f. 21.
München: Monacens. 71; a. 1531.
Oxford: Baroccian. 204; s. XV. f. 214.
Paris: Parisin.
  1849; s. XIV. f. 147v (c. comm. Gal.).
  2140; s. XII—XIII. f. 220.
  2141; s. XV. f. 195.
  2142; s. XIII—XIV. f. 333.
  2143; s. XIV. f. 205v.
  2144; s. XIV. f. 240.
  2145; s. XV. f. 317v.
  2146; s. XVI. f. 44v.
  2247; s. XVI. f. 16.
  2248; s. XVI. f. 23v.
  2254; s. XV. f. 57.
  [2332*; s. XV. f. 239v].
  [2545 (?) = 2145?].
Rom:
  Palat. 192; s. XV. f. 54v.
  Urbin. 68; s. XIV. f. 240.
  Vatic.
    276; s. XII. f. 27v.
    277; s. XIV. f. 265.
    278; a. 1512. f. 552.
Venedig: Marcian. 269; s. XI. f. 275v.

Περὶ ἄρθρων.
De articulis.

L. IV 78—326.
Kühlew. II 111—244.

Inc. Ὤμου δὲ ἄρθρον.
Expl. κατὰ λόγον τὸν πρότερον.

Cambridge: Cantabrig. Caius Coll. 50; s. XV/XVI. f. 45v.
Florenz: Laurent. plut.
  74, 1; s. XV. p. 36b.

74, 7; s. IX. f. 33^{v}. (Inscr. Περὶ ἄρθρων ἐμβολῆς).
Holkham: nr. 282; s. XVI. no. 7.
Kopenhagen: Hauniens. ant. fund. reg. 224; s. XVI.
Leyden: Voss. fol. 10; s. XVI.
Mailand: Ambros. L 110 Sup.; s. XVI. f. 251^{v}.
Modena: Mutinens. 233 (III H 5); s. XVI. f. 159^{v}.
München: Monacens. 71; a. 1531.
Oxford: Baroccian. 204; s. XV. f. 36.
Paris: Parisin.
[1444 (?)].
1849; s. XIV. f. 111 (c. comm. Gal.)
1868; s. XV. f. 375^{v}—376^{v}. 382. 391 (cf. L. IV 76).
2140; s. XII—XIII. f. 38.
2141; s. XV. f. 35.
2142; s. XIII—XIV. f. 44^{v}.
2143; s. XIV. f. 39^{v}.
2144; s. XIV. f. 44^{v}.
2145; s. XV. f. 58.
2146; s. XVI. f. 61.
2247; s. XVI. f. 35.
2248; s. XVI. f. 51^{v}.
[Diels I.12] [2254 (?)].
2255; s. XV. f. 119^{v}.
[2332*; s. XV. f. 210^{v} (»Ἐν τῷ περὶ ἄρθρων ὤμου«)].
[2545 (?) = 2145?].
Rom:
Palat. 192; s. XV. f. 71.
Urbin. 68; s. XIV. f. 38^{v}.
Vatic.
276; s. XII. f. 37^{v}.
277; s. XIV. f. 61.
278; a. 1512. f. 103.
Venedig: Marcian. 269; s. XI. f. 47.

Μοχλικός.
Vectiarius.

L. IV 340—394.
Kühlew. II 245—274.

Inc. Ὀστέων φύσις· δακτύλων.
Expl. ὁμοιότατα ἐκπίπτουσιν.

Florenz: Laurent. plut. 74, 1; s. XV. p. 185.
Kopenhagen: Hauniens. ant. fund. reg. 224; s. XVI.
Leyden: Voss. fol. 10; s. XVI.
Mailand: Ambros. C 85 Sup.; s. XV—XVI.
München: Monacens. 71; a. 1531.
Oxford: Baroccian. 204; s. XV. f. 203b.
Paris: Parisin.
  2140; s. XII—XIII. f. 209^{v}.
  2141; s. XV. f. 186^{v}.
  2142; s. XIII—XIV. f. 322 *und* 82.
  2143; s. XIV. f. 195^{v}.
  2144; s. XIV. f. 231.
  2145; s. XV. f. 303.
  2247; s. XVI. f. 79.
  2248; s. XVI. f. 117.
  2254; s. XV. f. 41.
  [2332*; s. XV. f. 237].
Rom:
  Urbin. 68; s. XIV. f. 229.
  Vatic.
    277; s. XIV. f. 254.
    278; a. 1512. f. 528^{v}.
Venedig: Marcian. 269; s. XI. f. 261^{v}.

Ἀφορισμοί.
Aphorismi.

L. IV 458—608.

Inc. Ὁ βίος βραχύς.
Expl. ταῦτα χρὴ νομίζειν ἀνίατα.

Antwerpen: Antverp. 426; s. XVI. f. 92^{v}.
Athen:
  nr. 1486; a. 1793 (Ἑρμηνεῖαι εἰς τοὺς ἀφ. καταστρωθεῖσαι εἰς κοινὴν φράσιν παρὰ Μπαλάνου Βασιλοπούλου).
  nr. 1498; s. XVIII. (*Wie in* nr. 1486).

nr. 1500 (Μάρκου τοῦ Κυπρίου Μετάφρασις τῶν Ἱππ. ἀφ. μετά τινος ἐπιστασίας καὶ ἑρμηνείας ἐκ τῆς τοῦ Γαλ. διδασκαλίας συλλεγείσης).

Athos:

Βιβλ. μον. Ἐσφιγμένου

41; s. XV. f. 1 (c. comm. anon.).

2323. 310; s. XVIII.

Βιβλ. μον. Ἰβήρων 4671. 551*; s. XVII. (Ἀφορισμοὶ ἀπὸ τοῦ β' τμήματος τοῦ Ἱππ.).

Βιβλ. μον. Παντελεήμονος

5796. 289; s. XVIII. p. 830. (Ἀφορισμοὶ ἀπὸ τοῦ β' τμήματος τοῦ Ἱππ.).

6342. 835; s. XVII.

Berlin: Phillips.

1532 (ol. Meerman. 225); s. XVI. f. 154 (Anon. comm. in Hipp. Aph.).

1537 (ol. Meerman. 233)*; s. XV. f. 199v.

Bologna: Bonon.

3232; s. XV. f. 28v (Expl. λιμὸς γὰρ ξηραίνει τὰ σώματα).

3636; s. XIV—XV. f. 152 (»cum scholiis; praemittitur f. 151v explicatio locutionis Ἀφορισμὸς Philothei«).

Cambridge:

Cantabrig. Caius Coll.

50; s. XV—XVI. f. 238v (Expl. τὰ δ' ἐναντία δυσχερῶς. τέλος τοῦ α').

355; s. XV—XVI. f. 92 *und* 120 (Inc. ἐν δὲ τοῖσι παροξυσμοῖς. Expl. μᾶλλον βλάψεις sect. 7).

[962].

[Pembroch. 2055].

[St. Petri 1866]

[**Dublin:** Coll. Trinit. 502].

Erlangen: Erlangens. 90; s. XVI. (»Addita est inde ab aph. XXIV. explicatio Philothei.« Inc. Τὰ διακαῆ καὶ ζέουσαν. Expl. τέλος τῶν λειπομένων Θεοφίλου φιλοσ. εἰς τοῦ Ἱππ. ἀφορισμούς).

Escurial: Scorial.

Φ. III. 7; s. XIV. f. 67 (cum comm. Gal.).

Φ. III. 12; s. XV. f. 443v.

Ψ. III. 17; s. XVI. f. 23 (cum comm. anon.) *und* f. 127 (c. comm. Gal.).

y. I. 8; s. XVI. f. 1.

Florenz:

Laurent. plut.

59, 14*; s. XV. f. 100v (frgm.).

[73, 7].

[73. 8].

[73. 22].

74, 1; s. XV. p. 155.

74, 11; s. XIII. f. 131.
74, 13; s. XV. p. 5 (c. comm.).
Riccard.
41 (K II 2); s. XVI. f. 13 (IV 69—83 = L. IV 526—532).
44 (K II 5); s. XV—XVI. f. 1.

Holkham: [Diels I.13]
nr. 282; s. XVI. no. 2 (Expl. καὶ σαρκὶ παρέδωκεν).
nr. 293; s. XV.

Jerusalem: Hierosolym.
bibl. patriarch. 102; s. XVIII. f. 12 (Ἑρμηνεία εἰς τοὺς ἀφ. Ἱππ., καταστρωθεῖσα εἰς κοινὴν φράσιν παρὰ Μπαλάνου Βασιλοπούλου κτλ.).
Bibl. Mar-Saba
481; s. XVIII. f. 265 (Μετάφρασις τῶν ἀφ. τοῦ Ἱππ. εἰς τὴν κοινὴν διάλεκτον).
498; s. XVIII. f. 1.

Karlsruhe: Caroliruh. 449; s. XV—XVI. f. 1 (Sectio III—VII).

Kopenhagen: Hauniens. ant. fund. reg. 224; s. XVI.

Leyden: Scal. 71; s. XVI. f. 1.

London:
Addit. 6898 (Brit. Mus.); s. XIII (XIV). f. 160ᵛ (c. scholiis; Inc. ⟨ἐπε⟩ιδή⟨π⟩ερ ἐνταῦθα σκοπὸν ἔχει ὁ Γαληνός).
Arundel. (Brit. Mus.) 538; s. XV. f. 1.
Harleian. (Brit. Mus.)
5626; s. XV—XVI. f. 86 (Libri II—VI. L. IV 470—576, 1; Expl. τοῖσι σπληνώδεσι δυσεντερίη γενομένη ἀγαθόν).
6295; s. XV (XIV sec. catal.) f. 157 (c. comm. pleniore).
Stowean. (Brit. Mus.) 1073; s. XVI. f. 6 (Expl. χολῇ καὶ αἵματι καὶ φλέγματι καὶ σαρκὶ παρέδωκεν).
Medical Society H Hi 17 = We 30; s. XV. f. 1.

Madrid: Matrit. Bibl. nac. 4634 (ol. N 112); s. XV. f. 2.

Mailand: Ambros.
A 156 Sup.; s. XVI. f. 1 (Expl. πάνυ πολλὴ θανάσιμος).
T 19 Sup.; s. —

Modena: Mutinens. 233 (III H 5); s. XVI. f. 13.

München: Monacens.
71; a. 1531.
287*; s. XIV ex. f. 153 (Ἱππ. πρόγνωσις π. τῶν δ' ὡρῶν = Aph. III 11—14).
525*; ante a. 1336. f. 155ᵛ—163ᵛ (Ex l. III—VI).

Neapel: Neapolit. 91 II C 33; s. XV.

[**Norfolk:** nr. 3189].

Oxford:
Auct. F. Inf. II 3; s. XVIII.

Baroccian. 204; s. XV. f. 169b.
[Laudian.]
[1013].
[1252].
[1355].
[Coll. Merton.]
[687].
[688].
[689].
[722].
Miscell. 132; s. XVI. f. 4b.
Roe. XIV (260); s. XV. f. 87^{v}.
[Coll. Novi]
[1130.]
[1134].
[Eccl. Wigorn. 768].

Padua:
Bibl. Joann. Rhodii. (*Verbleib unbekannt*).
S. Joann. in Viridario (dextr. plut. XVII. *Verbleib unbekannt*).

Palermo: Panormit. Bibl. naz. XIII C 3; s. XVI. f. 49—55 (c. comm.).

Paris:
[Coislin. 1018 (?)].
Parisin.
36; s. XIV—XV. f. 30.
1297; s. XVI. f. 63.
[1848?].
1883; s. XIV. f. 74^{v} (c. comm. Theophil.; init. mutil.).
1884; a. 1503. f. 158 (c. comm. Gal.).
2140; s. XII—XIII. f. 174.
2141; s. XV. f. 159^{v}.
2142; s. XIII—XIV. f. 277.
2143; s. XIV. f. 160^{v}.
2144; s. XIV. f. 188.
2145; s. XV. f. 255.
2146; s. XVI. f. 2.
2147*; s. XVI. (ἐξήγησις Στεφάνου. Inc. ἐπὶ περιπνευμονίῃ φρενῖτις).
[2148; s. XV.].
2149; s. XVI. f. 1 (c. comm. Theophili).
2150; a. 1584 (c. interpretat. Damascii).
[2154; s. XIV.].
2161; s. XV. (c. comm. Gal.).

2168; s. XIV. (c. comm. Gal.).
2178*; s. XIV.
2219; s. XV. (init. mutil. Inc. οἱ ὑγιεινὰ τὰ σώματα).
2222; s. XV. (c. Meletii comm.).
2223; s. XVI. (c. Meletii comm.).
2224*; s. XV.
2228; s. XIV—XI. f. 95 (c. comm. Theophili).
2229*; s. XIV. f. 33.
[2250; s. XVII.].
2255; s. XV. f. 381.
2256; s. XV. f. 9.
2257; s. XVI. f. 1 (c. comm. anon.) *und* f. 120 (Gal. in Aph. comm.; des. in aph. αἱ λεπταὶ καὶ ἀκριβέες).
2258; s. XVI.
2259; s. XVI.
2260*; s. XVI. f. 1 (c. comm. anon.; frgm.).
2266; s. XIV. f. 93 (c. comm. Gal.).
2268; s. XVI. f. 1 (c. Gal. comm.).
2278; s. XVI (c. comm. Gal. in fine mutil.).
2296; s. XVI (c. comm. Theophil.).
2316; s. XV. f. 9 (c. comm. breviss.).
2330; s. XV. f. 1.
[2545 (?) = 2145?].
2596; s. XIV. f. 194 (sect. I.; frgm.).
[2671 (?); s. XV (c. comm. Theophil.).]
[3140 (?)].

Suppl.
64; s. XV—XVII. f. 207 (pars comm. Theophili).
446; s. X. f. 45.
447; s. XIV. f. 1 (c. comm. Gal.)
682; s. X—XIX. f. 85 (c. interpr. Damascii).

Pistoja: Pistoriens. 141 (308); s. XVI. f. 1 (c. comm. Gal.)

Rom:
Angelic. 80 (C 1. 11); s. XV. f. 233.
Barberin.
I 5; s. XV. f. 1 (c. comm. Gal.; Expl. θανάσιμον τὸ τοιοῦτον).
I 11 (= 136); s. XVI. f. 2.
Ottobon.
150; s. XVI. f. 47.
157 A; s. XVI. f. 1.
157 B; s. XV. f. 1.

Palat.

128; s. XV. f. 26ᵛ (aphorismi XIV priores c. Gal. comm.).

143; s. XV. f. 150 (Libri I—III et V in fine mutil.).

192; s. XV. f. 1ᵛ (Aph. ult. Περὶ ἐγκεφάλου ἐσφακελισμένου).

199; s. XIII. f. 47 (c. comm.).

279; s. XIV—XV. f. 1 (sectt. duae primae c. scholiis) *und* f. 31ᵛ (sectiones VI c. comm. Gal.)

297; s. XV—XVI (Liber VII c. scholiis anon.).

[Diels I.14] Reg. Suec. 182; s. XV. f. 58 (sectio prima).

Urbin.

64; s. X—XI. f. 1.

68; s. XIV. f. 189 (sectio I—VI).

Vatic.

276; s. XII. f. 1ᵛ.

277; s. XIV. f. 217.

278; a. 1512 f. 441.

279; s. XII. f. 95 (c. comm. Theophil.; *Verbleib unbekannt*).

280; s. XV. f. 154ᵛ.

294; s. — f. 106ᵛ.

Turin: Taurinens. B V 33 (179b II 33); s. XVI. f. 326. (*Durch Feuer stark beschädigt.*)

Venedig:

[Bibl. S. Anton.].

Marcian. 269; s. XI. f. 215.

Bibl. monast. St. Michael. 104; s. — (»Aphorismata«. *Verbleib unbekannt.*)

Wien: Vindob.

med.

28; s. XV. f. 140—156ᵛ (Expl. ξε'. ἐπὶ λευκῷ φλέγματι ὕδρωψ ἐπιγίνεται).

31; s. XV ex. f. 166ᵛ (I 1. 2 = L. IV 458, 1—12).

48; s. XIV—XV. f. 172—196 (Expl. τὰ καταμήνια ταύτῃ ἐκλέλοιπεν. γυναιξὶν ὁκόσῃισιν ἐντὸς μα... L. IV 544, 15. 16?).

49; s. XVI. f. 2—21 (Expl. εὐνοῦχοι οὔτε ποδαγριῶσιν οὔτε φαλακροὶ γίγνονται L. IV 570, 5.).

histor. 130; s. XV—XVI. f. 182—200 (Expl. ὅταν ὁμοῦ τε πῦον καὶ χολὴν ἀναβήσσῃ).

phil. 179; s. XV. f. 123ᵛ (π. καιρ. πρόγνωσις = Aph. III 11—14 L. IV 490—492).

lat. 4772 (tab. cod. III 382); s. XV. f. 9 (Expl. ξβ'. ἐπὶ σφακελισμοῦ ἀπόστασις ὀστέου).

Ὅρκος. [Diels I.17]
Iusiurandum.

L. IV 628—632.

Inc. Ὄμνυμι Ἀπόλλωνα.
Expl. ἐπιορκοῦντι τἀναντία τουτέων.

Athos: Βιβλ. μον. Ἰβήρ. 4302. 182; s. XVI. f. 8 B.
Bologna: Bonon. 3632*; s. XV. f. 28 (»Ἐκ τοῦ κατὰ τὸν Ἱππ. ὅρκου, καθόσον οἷόν τε Χριστιανῶι ὀμόσαι«).
Cambridge: Cantabrig. Caius Coll. 50; s. XV/XVI. f. 1.
Escurial: Scorial.
  Σ. II. 5; s. XV. f. 28ᵛ.
  y. I. 8; s. XVI. f. 2.
Florenz: Laurent. plut.
  74, 1; s. XV. p. 9b.
  74, 3; s. XII. p. 188b.
  74, 13; s. XV. p. 4.
Kopenhagen: Hauniens. ant. fund. reg. 224; s. XVI. Sequitur ἕτερος ὅρκος Ἱπποκράτους (Inc. Αὐτὸν ἐν ἀχράντοισι. Expl. ὀλβιόδωρον ὑγείην = Hipp. I 74 Kuehlew. *Vgl.* Kuehn, *Additam. ad Fabricii elenchum medicorum vet.* XV. [Lips. 1828] p. 11).
Leyden: Voss. fol. 10; s. XVI.
London:
  Arundel. (Brit. Mus.) 538; s. XV. f. 19.
  Stowean. (Brit. Mus.) 1073; s. XVI. f. 2.
Mailand: Ambros. B 113 Sup.; s. XIV. in. f. 2. ibid.* f. 203ᵛ (Inscr. *wie im* Bonon. 3632. »Textus hac forma 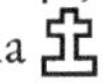 scriptus«). [Diels I.18]
Modena: Mutinens. 61 (III B 9); s. XV. f. 29ᵛ.
München: Monacens. 71; a. 1531. f. 11.
Oxford:
  Baroccian. 204; s. XV. f. 9 (Iuriiurando se applicat »ἕτερος ὅρκος Ἱπποκράτους«. Inc. αὐτὸν ἐν ἀχράντοισιν. Expl. ὀλβιόδωρον ὑγίειαν. »A corrupt form of the metrical »oath« printed in Kühlew. Hipp. opp. I p. 74«. Scott).
  Auct. F. Infra II 3; s. XVIII.
  Miscell. 132; s. XVI. f. 1.
Paris:
  Parisin.
    2047; s. XV. f. 16.
    2140; s. XII—XIII. f. 9ᵛ.

2141; s. XV. f. 8^{v}.
2142; s. XIII—XIV. f. 12^{v}.
2143; s. XIV. f. 11.
2144; s. XIV. f. 13.
2145; s. XV. f. 14.
2146; s. XVI. f. 1.
2148; s. XV. f. 1.
[2254 (?)].
2255; s. XV. f. 55.
[2545 (? = 2145?)].
2596; s. XIV. f. 185^{v}.
Suppl. gr. 608; s. XVI. f. 178^{v}.

Rom:
Palat. 192; s. XV. f. 1.
Reg. Suec. 182; s. XV. f. 16.
Urbin.
64*; s. X—XI. f. 116 (» ἐκ τοῦ κατὰ τὸν Ἱππ. ὅρκου, καθ' ὅσον οἷόν τε Χριστιανῷ ὀμόσαι«).
68; s. XIV. f. 4 (*Ilbergs Coll. in dessen Besitz*).
Vatic.
276; s. XII. f. 1 (*Ilbergs Coll. in dessen Besitz*).
277; s. XIV. f. 25 (*Ilbergs Coll. in dessen Besitz*).
278; a. 1512. f. 27^{v}.
2238; s. XV. f. 180.
2304 (olim 2217); s. XV. f. 1.

Venedig: Marcian. 269; s. XI. f. 12.
Wien: Vindob.
phil. 219; s. XV. f. 140 (*Ilbergs Coll. in dessen Besitz*).
lat. 4772 (tab. cod. III 382); s. XV. f. 105.

Νόμος.
Lex.

L. IV 638—643.

Inc. Ἰητρικὴ τεχνέων μὲν πασέων.
Expl. πρὶν ἢ τελεσθῶσιν ὀργίοισιν ἐπιστήμης.

Bologna: Bonon. 3632*; s. XV. f. 28.
Cambridge: Cantabrig. Caius Coll. 50; s. XV/XVI. f. 1^{v}.

Escurial: Scorial. y. I. 8; s. XVI. f. 1.
Florenz:
Laurent. plut. 74, 1; s. XV. p. 9b.
Marucell. A 109; s. —
Kopenhagen: Hauniens. ant. fund. reg. 224; s. XVI.
Leyden: Voss. fol. 10; s. XVI.
London:
Arundel. (Brit. Mus.) 538; s. XV. f. 53^{v}.
Stowean. (Brit. Mus.) 1073; s. XVI. f. 3^{v}.
Mailand: Ambros.
B 113 Sup.; s. XIV in. f. 1.
L 110 Sup.; s. XVI. f. 233^{v}.
München: Monacens. 71; a. 1531.
Oxford:
Baroccian. 204; s. XV. f. 9.
Auct. F. Infra II 3; s. XVIII.
Miscell. 132; s. XVI. f. 2b.
Paris: Parisin.
1868; s. XV. f. 377.
2140; s. XII—XIII. f. 9^{v}.
2141; s. XV. f. 8^{v}.
2142; s. XIII—XIV. f. 13.
2143; s. XIV. f. 11^{v}.
2144; s. XIV. f. 13.
2145; s. XV. f. 14^{v}.
2146; s. XVI. f. 1^{v}.
2148; s. XV. f. 1.
[2254 (?)].
2255; s. XV. f. 56.
[2545 (? = 2145?)].
Rom:
Urbin. 68; s. XIV. f. 4.
Vatic.
276; s. XII. f. 1^{v} (*Ilbergs Coll. in dessen Besitz*).
277; s. XIV. f. 25^{v} (*Ilbergs Coll. in dessen Besitz*).
278; a. 1512. f. 28.
Venedig: Marcian. 269; s. XI. f. 12.

[Diels I.19]

Ἐπιδημιῶν Β'. Δ'—Ζ'.
De morbis popularibus II. IV—VII.

L.
Lib. 2: V 72—138.
Lib. 4: V 144—196.
Lib. 5: V 204—258.
Lib. 6: V 266—356.
Lib. 7: V 364—468.

Lib. 2
Inc. Ἄνθρακες ἐν Κρανῶνι θερινοί.
Expl. συλλέγεται αὐτῷ ἐπὶ τοὺς τιτθούς.
Lib. 4
Inc. Μετ' ἰσημερίην καὶ μετὰ πληϊάδα.
Expl. πυρετοῖς ἐπιβήσσουσιν.
Lib. 5
Inc. Ἐν Ἤλιδι ἡ τοῦ κηπουροῦ γυνή.
Expl. ἔκφρων νύκτα καὶ ἡμέρην ἔθανεν.
Lib. 6
Inc. Ὁκόσῃσιν ἐξ ἀποφθορῆς.
Expl. ἐτελεύτησεν οὐ βραδέως.
Lib. 7
Inc. Μετὰ κύνα οἱ πυρετοί.
Expl. τὰ κρύφημα οὐκ ὁρῶν ἑστῶτα.

[**Dublin:** Bibl. Narcissi cod. Brit. 502].
Florenz: Laurent. plut. 74, 1; s. XV. p. 295b.
Holkham: nr. 282; s. XVI. no. 10.
Kopenhagen: Hauniens. ant. fund. reg. 224; s. XVI.
Leyden: Voss. fol. 10; s. XVI.
Modena: Mutinens. 233 (III H 5); s. XVI. f. 33.
München: Monacens. 71; a. 1531.
Oxford: Baroccian. 204; s. XV. f. 333v.
Padua: Bibl. Joann. Rhodii. (*Verbleib unbekannt*).
Paris: Parisin.
2140; s. XII—XIII. f. 349.
2141; s. XV. f. 293v.
2142; s. XIII—XIV. f. 466.
2143; s. XIV. f. 321.
2144; s. XIV. f. 343v.

2145; s. XV. f. 487.
2146; s. XVI. f. 110.
2165; s. XVI. f. 1. (pars tant., c. comm. Gal.).
[2229* (?); s. XIII.]
2254; s. XV. f. 256v
[2332*; s. XV].

Rom:
Palat. 192; s. XV. f. 114.
Urbin. 68; s. XIV. f. 360v.
Vatic.
276; s. XII. f. 67v.
277; s. XIV. f. 397.
278; a. 1512. f. 824v.

Venedig: Marcian 269; s. XI. f. 409 (Libri II. IV. V init. desunt).

Περὶ χυμῶν.
De humoribus.

L. V 476—502.

Inc. Τὸ μὲν χρῶμα τῶν χυμῶν.
Expl. ἐπεὶ δὲ τοῦτο ἰητρεύθη, ἐπιπονώτερος.

Cambridge: Cantabrig. Caius-Coll. 50; s. XV/XVI. f. 81v.
Florenz: Laurent. plut. 74, 1; s. XV. p. 58b.
Kopenhagen: Hauniens. ant. fund. reg. 224; s. XVI.
Leyden: Voss. fol. 10; s. XVI.
Mailand: Ambros.
C 85 Sup.; s. XV—XVI.
L 110 Sup.; s. XVI. f. 270. [Diels I.20]
Modena: Mutinens. 220 (II H 5); s. XV. f. 2.
München: Monacens. 71; a. 1531.
Oxford: Baroccian. 204; s. XV. f. 60b.
Paris: Parisin.
2140; s. XII—XIII. f. 62v.
2141; s. XV. f. 57v.
2142; s. XIII—XIV.
2143; s. XIV. f. 62.
2144; s. XIV. f. 71.
2145; s. XV. f. 96v.

2253; s. XI. f. 65.
2255; s. XV. f. 165.
[2254 (?)].
[2332*; s. XV. f. 213].
[2545 (? = 2145?)].

Rom:
Urbin. 68; s. XIV. f. 72.
Vatic.
277; s. XIV. f. 91.
278; a. 1512. f. 164ᵛ.

Tübingen: Tubingens. Bibl. Univ.
23*; s. XVI. (Scholia in Hipp. π. χυμῶν).
37*; a. 1584. no. xx, 13 (*Wie im* Tubing. 23).

Venedig:
[Bibl. S. Anton.]
Marcian. 269; s. XI. f. 74.

[**Wien:** Vindob. med. 28* (?); s. XV. (Π. χ. ἐκ τῶν Ἱππ.)].

Προρρητικὸς Α'.
Praesagiorum liber I.

L. V 510—572.

Inc. Οἱ κωματώδεες ἐν ἀρχῇσι.
Expl. ἀκρίτως καταμωλυνθέντα φλαῦρα.

Florenz: Laurent. plut.
[25, ?].
74, 1; s. XV. p. 276b.

Jerusalem: Bibl. Mar-Saba 498; s. XVIII. f. 37 (Ἱππ. προρρητικῶν ἐξήγησις).

Kopenhagen: Hauniens. ant. fund. reg. 224; s. XVI.

Mailand: Ambros. A 156 Sup.; s. XVI. f. 20.

München: Monacens. 71; a. 1531.

Oxford: Baroccian. 204; s. XV. f. 307.

Paris: Parisin.
[2030; s. XVI.(?)].
2140; s. XII—XIII. f. 324ᵛ.
2141; s. XV. f. 274.
2142; s. XIII—XIV. f. 442.
2143; s. XV. f. 298ᵛ.

2144; s. XIV. f. 323^{v}.
2145; s. XV. f. 453^{v}.
2166; s. XVI. f. 89. (c. comm. Gal.).
[2253 (?)].
2254; s. XV. f. 207^{v}.
[2266 (?)].
[2269 (?)].
[2332*; s. XV. f. 251^{v}].
[2545 (? = 2145?)].

Rom:
Urbin. 68; s. XIV. f. 337^{v}.
Vatic.
277; s. XIV. f. 372^{v}.
278; a. 1512. f. 773^{v}.
283; s. XIV. f. 9.

[**Venedig:** Marcian.].

Κωακαὶ προγνώσεις.
Coa praesagia.

L. V 588—732.

Inc. Οἱ ἐκ ῥίγεος περιψυχόμενοι.
Expl. πυρετὸν ὀξὺν μεθ' ἱδρῶτος.

Florenz: Laurent. plut. 74, 1; s. XV. p. 290b.
Kopenhagen: Hauniens. ant. fund. reg. 224; s. XVI.
Leyden: Voss. fol. 10; s. XVI.
München: Monacens. 71; a. 1531 (fine mutil.)
Oxford: Baroccian. 204; s. XV. f. 326b.
Paris: Parisin.
2140; s. XII—XIII. f. 342^{v}.
2141; s. XV. f. 288^{v}.
2142; s. XIII—XIV.
2143; s. XIV. f. 315.
2144; s. XIV. f. 338.
2145; s. XV. f. 477^{v}.
2254; s. XV. f. 236^{v}.
[2332*; s. XV. f. 263].
[2545 (? = 2145?)].

Rom:

Urbin. 68; s. XIV. f. 354ᵛ.

Vatic.

277; s. XIV. f. 390ᵛ.

278; a. 1512. f. 810ᵛ.

[**Venedig:** Marcian.].

Περὶ τέχνης.
De arte.

L. VI 2—26.

Th. Gomperz, *Die Apologie der Heilkunst.* Wien 1890.

Inc. Εἰσίν τινες οἳ τέχνην.

Expl. ἢ ἐξ ὧν ἂν ἀκούσωσιν.

Bologna: Bonon. 3632*; s. XV. f. 28.

Cambridge: Cantabrig. Caius Coll. 50; s. XV/XVI. f. 2.

Florenz: Laurent. plut. 74, 1; s. XV. p. 10.

Kopenhagen: Hauniens. ant. fund. reg. 224; s. XVI.

Leyden: Voss. fol. 10; s. XVI.

[Diels I.21] **London:** Arundel. (Brit. Mus.) 538; s. XV. f. 55 (Expl. f. 56 δυνάμενος διὰ σοφίην ἢ πεπαίδευται = VI 2, 18 L.).

Mailand: Ambros. L 110 Sup.; s. XVI. f. 234.

München: Monacens. 71; a. 1531.

Oxford: Baroccian. 204; s. XV. f. 9b.

Paris: Parisin.

1868; s. XV. f. 377.

2140; s. XII—XIII. f. 10ᵛ.

2141; s. XV. f. 9.

2142; s. XIII—XIV. f. 13ᵛ.

[2143 (?); s. XIV.]

2144; s. XIV. f. 14.

2145; s. XV. f. 15.

2148; s. XV. f. 1.

2253; s. XI. f. 75.

[2254 (?)].

2255; s. XV. f. 57.

[2332*; s. XIV. f. 204].

[2545 (? = 2145?)].

Rom:
Urbin. 68; s. XIV. f. 17.
Vatic.
277; s. XIV. f. 26 (*Coll. Ilbergs in dessen Besitz*).
278; a. 1512. f. 29 (*Coll. Ilbergs in dessen Besitz*).
Venedig: Marcian. 269; s. XI. f. 12ᵛ.

Περὶ φύσιος ἀνθρώπου.
De natura hominis.

L. VI 32—68.

Inc. Ὅστις μὲν εἴωθεν.
Expl. ἄλλο τι κακουργῆται ὥνθρωπος.

Athos: Βιβλ. μον. Ἐσφιγμένου 2330. 317; s. XVI.
Cambridge: Cantabrig.
Caius Coll.
50; s. XV/XVI. f. 21.
[959].
Bibl. Univ. L l IV 12*; s. XV. f. 40.
Florenz: Laurent. plut. 74, 1; s. XV. p. 22 (*Coll. Ilbergs in dessen Besitz*).
Holkham: nr. 282; s. XVI. no. 11.
Kopenhagen: Hauniens. ant. fund. reg. 224; s. XVI.
Leyden: Voss. fol. 10; s. XVI.
Mailand: Ambros. L 110 Sup.; s. XVI. f. 241ᵛ.
Modena: Mutinens. 233 (III H 5); s. XVI. f. 127.
München: Monacens. 71; a. 1531.
Oxford: Baroccian. 204; s. XV. f. 21b.
Padua: Bibl. S. Joannis in Viridario, ad dextr. plut. XVII. (*Verbleib unbekannt*).
Paris: Parisin.
1868*; s. XIV. f. 368.
2140; s. XII—XIII. f. 22ᵛ.
2141; s. XV. f. 20 (*Coll. Ilbergs in dessen Besitz*).
2142; s. XIII—XIV. f. 28 (*Coll. Ilbergs in dessen Besitz*).
2143; s. XIV (*Coll. Ilbergs in dessen Besitz*).
2144; s. XIV. f. 29 (*Coll. Ilbergs in dessen Besitz*).
2146; s. XVI. f. 179ᵛ (*Coll. Ilbergs in dessen Besitz*).
2147; s. XVI. f. 6 (Expl. Σχεδὸν δὲ καὶ πάντα ...).
2253; s. XI. f. 81 (*Coll. Ilbergs in dessen Besitz*).

2254; s. XV (*Coll. Ilbergs in dessen Besitz*).
2255; s. XV. f. 90.
2316; s. XV. f. 138ᵛ.
2317*; s. XVI. f. 40. 45.
[2545 (? = 2145?)].
[**Reims:** Bibl. S. Remig. 548].
Rom:
Palat. 192; s. XV. f. 91.
Urbin. 68; s. XIV. f. 30 (*Coll. Ilbergs in dessen Besitz*).
Vatic.
276; s. XII. f. 107 (*Coll. Ilbergs in dessen Besitz*).
277; s. XIV. f. 43 (*Coll. Ilbergs in dessen Besitz*).
278; a. 1512. f. 59 (*Coll. Ilbergs in dessen Besitz*).
Venedig:
Marcian. 269; s. XI. f. 28.
App. cl. V 19; s. XV. f. 475.

[Diels I.22]

Περὶ διαίτης ὑγιεινῆς.
De salubri diaeta.

L. VI 72—86.

Inc. Τοὺς ἰδιώτας ὧδε χρή.
Expl. ἐν τῇσι νούσοισιν ὠφελέεσθαι.

Cambridge: Cantabrig. Caius Coll. 50; s. XV/XVI. f. 27b.
Florenz: Laurent. App. 2*; s. XV. f. 106ᵛ (Περὶ διαίτης γυναικῶν. Inc. Τὰς γυναῖκας ὧδε χρὴ διαιτᾶσθαι cf. L. VI 82, 2. Expl. καὶ τὰς σκιατραφίας cf. L. 82, 6).
Holkham: nr. 282; s. XVI. no. 11.
Kopenhagen: Hauniens. ant. fund. reg. 224; s. XVI.
Leyden: Voss. fol. 10; s. XVI.
Mailand: Ambros. L 110 Sup., s. XVI. f. 244ᵛ.
Modena: Mutinens. 213 (III G 9)*; s. XV. f. 235 (Inc. *und* Expl. *wie im* Laurent. App. 2).
München: Monacens. 71*; a. 1531 (Περὶ ἐμέτων. Inc. Ἓξ μῆνας τοὺς χειμερινούς = L. VI 78, 4).
Oxford: Baroccian. 204; s. XV. f. 25b.
Paris:
Parisin.
1868*; s. XV. (Inc. Ὀκόσους δὲ δίψαι = L. VI 84, 15).

[2140; s. XII—XIII. f. —].
[2141; s. XV. f. —].
[2142; s. XIII—XIV. f. —].
[2143; s. XIV. f. —].
[2144; s. XIV. f. —].
[2145; s. XV. f —].
[2146; s. XVI. f. —].
[2147; s. XVI. f. —].
[2253; s. XI. f. —]
[2255; s. XV. f. —].
Suppl. 447*; s. XIV.

Rom:
Reg. Suec. 182*; s. XV. f. 18 (Inscr. *und* Inc. *wie im* Monac. 71).
Urbin. 68*; s. XIV. f. 35.

Venedig: Marcian. 269; s. XI. f. 33v.

Περὶ φυσῶν.
De flatibus.

L. VI 90—114.

Inc. Εἰσί τινες τῶν τεχνέων.
Expl. οὐδαμῶς οὐδὲ πιστότερος.

Escurial: Scorial. Φ. III. 12; s. XV. f. 461.
Florenz: Laurent. plut. 74. 1. s. XV. p. 182 (*Coll. Ilbergs in dessen Besitz*).
Kopenhagen: Hauniens. ant. fund. reg. 224; s. XVI.
Leyden: Voss. fol. 10; s. XVI.
Mailand: Ambros.
B 113 Sup.; s. XIV in. f. 181. (Inscr. ἐκ τοῦ π. φύσεων).
C 85 Sup.; s. XV—XVI. (»De naturis«; *vielmehr Excerpt aus* π. φυσῶν *verm.* Schoene).
Modena: Mutinens. 227 (II H 12); s. XVI. f. 3.
München: Monacens. 71; a. 1531.
Oxford: Baroccian. 204; s. XV. f. 199b.
Paris: Parisin.
2140; s. XII—XIII. f. 206.
2141; s. XV. f. 184.
2142; s. XIII—XIV. f. 319.
2143; s. XIV. f. 192.

2144; s. XIV. f. 228.
2145; s. XV. f. 298.
2253; s. XI. f. 93v (*Coll. Ilbergs in dessen Besitz*).
2254; s. XV. f. 35v.
[2332*; s. XIV. f. 236].
[2545 (? = 2145?)].

Rom:
Urbin.
64*; s. x—XI. f. 100.
68; s. XIV. f. 225 (*Coll. Ilbergs in dessen Besitz*).
Vatic.
[216].
277; s. XIV. f. 250v (*Coll. Ilbergs in dessen Besitz*).
278; a. 1512. f. 520.

Venedig: Marcian. 269; s. XI. f. 257.

Περὶ ὑγρῶν χρήσιος.
De humidorum usu.

L. VI 118—136.

Inc. Ὕδωρ ποτόν, ἁλμυρόν, θάλασσα.
Expl. θέρμη ὠφελέει ἢ βλάπτει.

Paris: Parisin.
2253; s. XI. f. 70v.
[2254 (?); s. XV.].
2255; s. XV. f. 378v.

[Diels I.23]

Περὶ νούσων Α'.
De morbis I.

L. VI 140—204.

Inc. Ὃς ἂν περὶ ἰήσιος.
Expl. ψύχεται πάντα καὶ ἀποθνήσκει.

Cambridge: Cantabrig. Caius Coll. 50; s. XV/XVI. f. 102.
Florenz: Laurent. plut. 74, 1; s. XV. p. 70b.
Kopenhagen: Hauniens. ant. fund. reg. 224; s. XVI.

Mailand: Ambros.
C 85 Sup.; s. XV—XVI.
L 110 Sup.; s. XVI. f. 282ᵛ.
Modena: Mutinens. 220 (II H 5); s. XV. f. 21.
München: Monac. 71; a. 1531.
Oxford: Baroccian. 204; s. XV. f. 74b.
Paris: Parisin.
2140; s. XII—XIII. f. 75ᵛ.
2141; s. XV. f. 70ᵛ.
2142; s. XIII—XIV. f. 107ᵛ.
2143; s. XIV. f. 76ᵛ.
2144; s. XIV. f. 85.
2145; s. XV. f. 116ᵛ.
2148; s. XV. f. 7.
[2254 (?)].
2255; s. XV. f. 191.
[2332*; s. XIV. f. 216].
[2545 (? = 2145?)].
Rom:
Palat. 192; s. XV. f. 18ᵛ.
Reg. Suec. 182*; s. XV. f. 83.
Urbin. 68; s. XIV. f. 86ᵛ.
Vatic.
277; s. XIV. f. 109 (*Coll. Ilbergs in dessen Besitz*).
278; a. 1512. f. 196ᵛ.
Venedig: Marcian. 269; s. XI. f. 91.
Wien: Vindob. med. 4; s. X. f. 88 (*Coll. Ilbergs von VI 140—174, 1 L. in dessen Besitz*).

Περὶ παθῶν.
De affectionibus.

L. VI 208—270.

Inc. Ἄνδρα χρὴ ὅστις ἐστί.
Expl. μᾶλλον βλάπτει ἢ ὠφελέει.

Cambridge: Cantabrig. Caius Coll. 50; s. XV/XVI. f. 159.
Florenz: Laurent. plut. 74, 1; s. XV. p. 106b.
Kopenhagen: Hauniens. ant. fund. reg. 224; s. XVI.
Leyden: Voss. fol. 10; s. XVI.

Mailand: Ambros.
B 126 Sup.; s. XIV. f. 166.
L 110 Sup.; s. XVI. f. 324 (mutil.).
Modena: Mutinens. 220 (II H 5); s. XV. f. 86v.
München: Monacens. 71; a. 1531.
Oxford: Baroccian. 204; s. XV. f. 118.
Paris: Parisin.
2140; s. XII—XIII. f. 117.
2141; s. XV. f. 109.
[2142 (?); s. XIII—XIV.]
2143; s. XIV. f. 111v.
2144; s. XIV. f. 127v.
2145; s. XV. f. 175.
2148; s. XV. f. 26v.
[2254 (?)].
2255; s. XV. f. 265v.
[2332*; s. XIV. f. 222].
Rom: Vatic.
277; s. XIV. f. 155v.
278; a. 1512. f. 298v.
Venedig: Marcian. 269; s. XI. f. 142v.
Wien: Vindob. med. 4; s. X. f. 46 (*Coll. Ilbergs v. VI 208—212, 9 L. in dessen Besitz*).

Περὶ τόπων τῶν κατ' ἄνθρωπον.
De locis in homine.

L. VI 276—348.

Inc. Ἐμοὶ δοκέει ἀρχὴ μὲν οὖν.
Expl. τὰ καταμήνια καλεύμενα.

Holkham: nr. 282; s. XVI. no. 16.
München: Monacens. 71; a. 1531.
Paris: Parisin.
[2142 (?); s. XIII—XIV.]
[2146 (?); s. XVI.]
2253; s. XI. f. 100 (*Coll. Ilbergs v. VI 276—292 L. in dessen Besitz*).
[2254 (?); s. XV.].
[2255 (?); s. XV.]

Rom:

Palat. 192; s. XIV. f. 47 (*Ilbergs Coll. v. VI 276—282, 5 L. in dessen Besitz*).

Vatic. 276; s. XII. f. 134 (*Ilbergs Coll. in dessen Besitz*).

Περὶ ἱερῆς νούσου. *De morbo sacro.* [Diels I.24]

L. VI 352—396.

Inc. Περὶ μὲν τῆς ἱερῆς νούσου.
Expl. ἄλλης βαναυσίης τοιαύτης.

Cambridge: Cantabrig. Caius Coll. 50; s. XV/XVI. f. 94.
Florenz: Laurent. plut. 74, 1; s. XV. p. 66.
Kopenhagen: Hauniens. ant. fund. reg. 224; s. XVI.
Leyden: Voss. fol. 10; s. XVI.
Mailand: Ambros.
C 85 Sup.; s. XV—XVI.
L 110 Sup.; s. XVI. f. 30 (*Dietz' Collation eines der 2 Mediolanenses im Dietz-Nachlaß impress. I 4 der Univ.-Bibl. Königsberg Pr., vgl. oben S. 3*).
Modena: Mutinens. 220 (II H 5); s. XV. f. 14.
München: Monacens. 71; a. 1531.
Oxford: Baroccian. 204; s. XV. f. —
Paris: Parisin.
2140; s. XII—XIII. f. 70v.
2141; s. XV. f. 65v.
2142; s. XIII—XIV. f. 97 (*Ilbergs Coll. in dessen Besitz*).
2143; s. XIV. f. 71v.
2144; s. XIV. f. 80.
2145; s. XV. f. 108v.
[2148; s. XVI. f. 59v.]
2254; s. XV. f. 221v.
2255; s. XV. f. 181.
[2332*; s. XIV. f. 213v].
[2545 (? = 2145?)].
Rom:
Urbin. 68; s. XIV. f. 80v.
Vatic.
277; s. XIV. f. 102 (*Ilbergs Coll. in dessen Besitz*).
278; a. 1512. f. 183.

Venedig: Marcian. 269; s. XI. f. 84ᵛ.
Wien: Vindob. med.
4; s. X. f. 72 (*Ilbergs Coll. in dessen Besitz*).
24; s. XV. f. 1 (*Ilbergs Coll. von VI 368, 10—378, 3 L. in dessen Besitz. Dietz' Coll. im Dietz-Nachlaß impress. I 4 pag. 26 ff. der Univ.-Bibl. Königsberg Pr.*).

Περὶ ἑλκῶν.
De ulceribus.

L. VI 400—432.

Inc. Ἕλκεα ξύμπαντα οὐ χρὴ τέγγειν.
Expl. ἣν δύνηται ἑστάναι.

Cambridge: Cantabrig. Caius Coll.
50; s. XV/XVI. f. 88.
76; s. XV/XVI. f. 206.
[949].
Florenz: Laurent. plut.
74, 1; s. XV. p. 62b.
74, 21*; s. XV. p. 1.
Kopenhagen: Hauniens. ant. fund. reg. 224; s. XVI.
Leyden: Voss. fol. 10; s. XVI.
Mailand: Ambros.
C 85 Sup.; s. XV—XVI.
L 110 Sup.; s. XVI. f. 274.
Modena: Mutinens. 220 (II H 5); s. XV. f. 8.
München: Monacens. 71; a. 1531.
Oxford: Baroccian. 204; s. XV. f. 65.
Paris: Parisin.
2140; s. XII—XIII. f. 66ᵛ.
2141; s. XV. f. 62.
2142; s. XIII—XIV. f. 89ᵛ.
2143; s. XIV. f. 67.
2144; s. XIV. f. 75ᵛ.
2145; s. XV. f. 102ᵛ.
2148; s. XV. f. 57ᵛ.
2149* (?); s. XVI.
[2254 (?)].
2255; s. XV. f. 173ᵛ.

2287; s. XV—XVI. f. 214v.
[2332*; s. XIV. f. 213v].

Rom:
Urbin. 68; s. XIV. f. 76v.
Vatic.
277; s. XIV. f. 97.
278; a. 1512. f. 173.

Venedig: Marcian. 269; s. XI. f. 79v.
Wien: Vindob. med. 47; s. XV. f. 432.

Περὶ αἱμοῤῥοΐδων.
De haemorrhoïdibus.

L. VI 436—444.

Inc. Αἱμοῤῥοΐδων τὸ μὲν νόσημα.
Expl. τὴν ἕδρην ἐξώσας ὡς μάλιστα.

Florenz: Laurent. plut. 74, 1; s. XV. p. 289b.
Kopenhagen: Hauniens. ant. fund. reg. 224; s. XVI.
Leyden: Voss. fol. 10; s. XVI.
Modena: Mutinens. 227 (II H 12); s. XVI. f. 167.
München: Monacens. 71; a. 1531.
Oxford: Baroccian. 204; s. XV. f. 325.
Paris: Parisin.
2140; s. XII—XIII. f. 340v.
2141; s. XV. f. 287v.
2142; s. XIII—XIV. f. 458.
2143; s. XIV. f. 314.
2144; s. XIV. f. 337.
2145; s. XV. f. 476.
[2148; s. XV. f. 57.]
2254; s. XV. f. 234v.
[2332*; s. XIV. f. 262v].

Rom:
Urbin. 68; s. XIV. f. 353v.
Vatic.
277; s. XIV. f. 389v.
278; a. 1512. f. 808.

[Diels I.25] Περὶ συρίγγων.
De fistulis.

L. VI 448—460.

Inc. Σύριγγες γίνονται μέν.
Expl. ὡς θερμότατα διερρήθησαν καταπλάττεσθαι.

Florenz: Laurent. plut. 74, 1; s. XV. p. 287b.
Kopenhagen: Hauniens. ant. fund. reg. 224; s. XVI.
Leyden: Voss. fol. 10; s. XVI.
Modena: Mutinens. 227 (II H 12); s. XVI. f. 164.
München: Monacens. 71; a. 1531.
Oxford: Baroccian. 204; s. XV. f. 322.
Paris: Parisin.
    2140; s. XII—XIII. f. 338v.
    2141; s. XV. f. 285v.
    2142; s. XIII—XIV. f. 456.
    2143; s. XIV. f. 311v.
    2144; s. XIV. f. 335v.
    2145; s. XV. f. 473.
    2148; s. XV. f. 56v.
    2254; s. XV. f. 231v.
    [2332*; s. XV. f. 262v].
Rom:
    Urbin. 68; s. XIV. f. 351v.
    Vatic.
        277; s. XIV. f. 387.
        278; a. 1512. f. 803v.

Περὶ διαίτης Α' Β' Γ'.
De victus ratione I—III.

L. VI 466—636

Lib. 1
    Inc. Εἰ μὲν μοί τις ἐδόκεε.
    Expl. ἀδύνατον ἐκ διαίτης ἀλλοιῶσαι.
Lib. 2
    Inc. Χωρέων δὲ θέσιν.

Expl. ἐς τὴν ἀρχαίην δίαιταν ἡσυχῇ.
Lib. 3
Inc. Περὶ δὲ διαίτης ἀνθρωπίνης.
Expl. πλὴν τῶν περιπάτων.

Cambridge: Cantabrig.
Caius Coll. 50; s. XV/XVI. f. 199ᵛ.
Bibl. Univ. L. l. IV. 12; s. XV. f. 40ᵛ.
Florenz: Laurent. plut. 74, 1; s. XV. p. 131b.
Kopenhagen: Hauniens. ant. fund. reg. 224; s. XVI.
Leyden: Voss. fol. 10; s. XVI.
Mailand: Ambros.
B 108 Sup.; s. XIV. in. f. 19 (Libri I. II).
C 85 Sup.; s. XV—XVI.
Modena: Mutinens. 220 (II H 5); s. XV. f. 129ᵛ.
München: Monacens. 71; a. 1531.
Oxford: Baroccian. 204; s. XV. f. 144b.
Paris: Parisin.
36; s. XIV—XV. f. 55.
2140; s. XII—XIII. f. 146.
2141; s. XV. f. 136 (*Coll. Ilbergs in dessen Besitz*).
2142; s. XIII—XIV. f. 231ᵛ.
2143; s. XIV. f. 136.
2144; s. XIV. f. 158ᵛ.
2145; s. XV. f. 217.
2148; s. XV. f. 39.
[2254 (?)].
2255; s. XV. f. 316.
[2332*; s. XIV. f. 224ᵛ].
[2545 (? = 2145?)].
Rom:
Reg. Suec. 182; s. XV. f. 57ᵛ (fine mutil.).
Urbin. 68; s. XIV. f. 159.
Vatic.
277; s. XIV. f. 187 (*Coll. Ilbergs von VI 466—514, 23 L. in dessen Besitz*).
278*; a. 1512. f. 70ᵛ.
278; a. 1512. f. 370.
Venedig: Marcian. 269; s. XI. f. 179 (*Coll. Kühleweins und Ilbergs im Besitz des letzteren*).
Wien: Vindob. med. 4; s. X. f. 174ᵛ (*Coll. Ilbergs in dessen Besitz*).

[Diels I.26] Περὶ ἐνυπνίων (= περὶ διαίτης Δ').
De insomniis.

L. VI 640—662.

Inc. Περὶ δὲ τῶν τεκμηρίων.
Expl. ἐόντα ξὺν τοῖσι θεοῖσιν.

Bern: Bernens. 579*; s. XIV. f. 98—99.
Cambridge: Cantabrig.
Caius Coll. 50; s. XV/XVI. f. 230v.
Bibl. Univ. L. l. IV. 12; s. XVI. f. 39.
Escurial: Scorial. T. II. 14; s. XVI. f. 235 (Expl. ἐς τὴν ἔσω περιφορὴν ἐμπεπτωκέναι).
Florenz: Laurent. plut. 74, 1; s. XV. p. 150b.
Kopenhagen: Hauniens. ant. fund. reg. 224; s. XVI.
Leyden: Voss. fol. 10; s. XVI.
Mailand: Ambros. C 85 Sup.; s. XV—XVI.
Modena: Mutinens. 220 (II H 5); s. XV. f. 164.
München: Monacens. 71; a. 1531.
Oxford:
Baroccian. 204; s. XV. f. 165.
Miscellan. 130; s. XVII. f. 315.
Paris: Parisin.
2140; s. XII—XIII. f. 169.
2141; s. XV. f. 155.
2142; s. XIII—XIV. f. 268v.
2143; s. XIV. f. 155v.
2144; s. XIV. f. 183v.
2145; s. XV. f. 247v.
[2148; s. XVI. f. 48.]
[2254 (?)].
2255; s. XV. f. 356v.
[2332*; s. XIV. f. 227].
[2545 (? = 2145?)].
Rom:
Barberin. I 127; s. XVI. f. 313.
Urbin. 68; s. XIV. f. 183.
Vallicell. 106 (F 83); s. XV—XVI. f. 188v—190 (Expl. ἡ ταραχή).
Vatic.
277; s. XIV. f. 211v.
278; a. 1512. f. 426.

Venedig:

Marcian. 269; s. XI. f. 208.

App. cl. V 14 (ol. Nanian. 248); s. XVI. f. 1 (*Coll. Ilbergs v. VI 640—662 in dessen Besitz*).

Wien: Vindob.

med. 4; s. X. f. 233 (*Ilbergs Coll. in dessen Besitz*).

phil. 192; s. XV. f. 112 (Inc. Ὁκόσα τῶν ἐνυπνίων. *Coll. Ilbergs v. VI 640—662 in dessen Besitz*).

Περὶ νούσων Β' Γ'.
De morbis II et III.

L. VII 8—114. 118—160.

Lib. 2

Inc. Οὐρέεται πολλόν.

Expl. ἐλέχθη καὶ ὑποκλύζειν.

Lib. 3

Inc. Περὶ μὲν οὖν πυρετῶν.

Expl. διὰ τῆς κοιλίης χολὴν ἄγει.

Cambridge: Cantabrig. Caius Coll. 50; s. XV/XVI. f. 102.

Florenz: Laurent. plut. 74, 1; s. XV. p. 70b.

Kopenhagen: Hauniens. ant. fund. reg. 224; s. XVI.

Mailand: Ambros.

C 85 Sup.; s. XV—XVI.

L 110 Sup.; s. XVI. f. 282^{v}.

Modena: Mutinens. 220 (II H 5); s. XV. f. 21^{v}.

München: Monacens. 71; a. 1531.

Oxford: Baroccian. 204; s. XV. f. 74b.

Paris: Parisin.

2140; s. XII—XIII. f. 75^{v}.

2141; s. XV. f. 70^{v}.

2142; s. XIII—XIV. f. 107^{v}.

2143; s. XIV. f. 76^{v}.

2144; s. XIV. f. 85.

2145; s. xv. f. 116^{v}.

2148; s. XV. f. 7.

[2254 (?)].

2255; s. XV. f. 191.

[2232*; s. XIV. f. 216].
[2545 (? = 2145?)].
Rom:
Palat. 192; s. XV. f. 18ᵛ.
Reg. Suec. 182; s. XV. f. 83.
Urbin. 68; s. XIV. f. 86ᵛ.
Vatic.
277; s. XIV. f. 109.
278; a. 1512. f. 196ᵛ.
Venedig: Marcian. 269; s. XI. f. 102.
Wien: Vindob. med. 4; s. X. f. 88 (*Coll. Ilbergs von VII 118 L. in dessen Besitz*).

[Diels I.27]

Περὶ τῶν ἐντὸς παθῶν.
De internis affectionibus.

L. VII 166—302.

Inc. Ἦν ἡ τοῦ πλεύμονος ἀρτηρίη.
Expl. ἐν πτισάνῃ ἑφθῇ λεπτῇ καὶ μέλιτι.

Cambridge: Cantabrig. Caius Coll. 50; s. XV/XVI. f. 172.
Florenz: Laurent. plut. 74, 1; s. XV. p. 114b.
Kopenhagen: Hauniens. ant. fund. reg. 224; s. XVI.
Modena: Mutinens. 220 (II H 5); s. XV. f. 100ᵛ.
Oxford: Baroccian. 204; s. XV. f. 126.
Paris: Parisin.
2140; s. XII—XIII. f. 126.
2141; s. XV. f. 117ᵛ.
2142; s. XIII—XIV. f. 198ᵛ.
2143; s. XIV. f. 118ᵛ.
2144; s. XIV. f. 138ᵛ.
2145; s. XV. f. 188ᵛ.
2148; s. XV. f. 30ᵛ.
[2254 (?)].
2255; s. XV. f. 281ᵛ.
[2332*; s. XIV. f. 223].
Rom:
Urbin. 68; s. XIV. f. 138.
Vatic.
277; s. XIV. f. 166.

278; a. 1512. f. 320.
Venedig: Marcian. 269; s. XI. f. 154.
Wien: Vindob. med. 4; s. X. f. 1 (Inc. L. VII 168, 4 ⟨περιστρέ⟩φηται).

Περὶ φύσιος γυναικείης.
De natura muliebri.

L. VII 312—430.

Inc. Περὶ δὲ τῆς γυναικείης φύσιος.
Expl. ἐν ὕδατι εὐώδει.

Florenz: Laurent. plut. 74, 1; s. XV. p. 263.
Holkham: nr. 282; s. XVI. no. 22.
Kopenhagen: Hauniens. ant. fund. reg. 224; s. XVI.
Leyden: Voss. fol. 10; s. XVI.
Mailand: Ambros.
B 108 Sup.; s. XIV in. f. 1 (L. VII 318, 11—370, 11. 386, 3—416, 12).
C 85 Sup.; s. XV—XVI.
Modena: Mutinens. 227 (II H 12); s. XVI. f. 139^v.
München: Monacens. 71; a. 1531.
Oxford: Baroccian. 204; s. XV. f. 292.
Paris: Parisin.
2140; s. XII—XIII. f. 308.
2141; s. XV. f. 260^v.
2142; s. XIII—XIV. f. 424.
2143; s. XIV. f. 282.
2144; s. XIV. f. 309^v.
2145; s. XV. f. 431^v.
2146; s. XVI. f. 211.
2254; s. XV. f. 183.
[2332*; s. XIV. f. 250^v].
Rom:
Palat. 192; s. XV. f. 105.
Urbin. 68; s. XIV. f. 323.
Vatic.
276; s. XII. f. 124^v (*Tschiedels Coll. in Ilbergs Besitz*).
277; s. XIV. f. 355^v.
278; a. 1512. f. 736^v.

Venedig: Marcian. 269; s. XI. f. 390.
Wien: Vindobon. med. 4; s. X. f. 383v (Expl. προνη⟨στεύσασαν⟩ = L. VII 412, 16).

Περὶ ἑπταμήνου.
De septimestri partu.

L. VII 436—452.

Inc. Οἱ δὲ ἑπτάμηνοι.
Expl. τὰ γὰρ ἐπὶ σώμασι τάδε γράφω.

Florenz: Laurent. plut. 74, 1; s. XV. p. 260.
Holkham: nr. 282; s. XVI. no. 14 (Inc. Περὶ δὲ ἑπταμήνων ὁ λόγος. Expl. ταῦτα οὖν πρότερον ἐννοούμενος).
Kopenhagen: Hauniens. ant. fund. reg. 224; s. XVI.
Mailand: Ambros. C 85 Sup.; s. XV—XVI.
Modena: Mutinens. 227 (II H 12); s. XVI. f. 134.
München: Monacens. 71; a. 1531.
Oxford: Baroccian. 204; s. XV. f. 288b.
Paris: Parisin.
- 2140; s. XII—XIII. f. 304.
- 2141; s. XV. f. 257v.
- 2142; s. XIII—XIV. f. 420.
- 2143; s. XIV. f. 278v.
- 2144; s. XIV. f. 306.
- 2145; s. XV. f. 426v.
- 2146; s. XVI. f. 206v.
- 2254; s. XV.
- [2546 (? = 2146?)].

Rom:
- Palat. 192; s. XV. f. 102v.
- Urbin. 68; s. XIV. f. 319v.
- Vatic.
  - 276; s. XII. f. 112 (*Tschiedels Coll. in Ilbergs Besitz*).
  - 277; s. XIV. f. 351v.
  - 278; a. 1512. f. 727v (Inc. *und* Expl. *wie im* Holkham. nr. 282).

Venedig: Marcian. 269; s. XI. f. 385.

Περὶ ὀκταμήνου. [Diels I.28]
De octimestri partu.

L. VII 452—460.

Inc. Περὶ δὲ ὀκταμήνου γενέσιος.
Expl. ἤνπερ ἐς τελευταίην περίοδον καταστῇ.

Florenz: Laurent. plut. 74, 1; s. XV. p. 262.
Holkham: nr. 282; s. XVI. no. 15 (Inc. Φημὶ δισσὰς ἐφεξῆς κακοπαθείας γιγνομένας. Expl. ἄρχονται ἐν τούτῳ τῷ χρόνῳ).
Kopenhagen: Hauniens. ant. fund. reg. 224; s. XVI.
Mailand: Ambros. C 85 Sup.; s. XV—XVI.
Modena: Mutinens. 227 (II H 12); s. XVI. f. 137^{v}.
München: Monacens. 71; a. 1531.
Oxford: Baroccian. 204; s. XV. f. 290b.
Paris: Parisin.
2140; s. XII—XIII. f. 306.
2141; s. XV. f. 259.
2142; s. XIII—XIV. f. 422^{v}.
2143; s. XIV. f. 280^{v}.
2144; s. XIV. f. 308.
2145; s. XV. f. 429.
2146; s. XVI. f. 207^{v}.
2254; s. XV. f. 180^{v}.
[2546 (? = 2146?)].
Rom:
Palat. 192; s. XV. f. 103.
Urbin. 68; s. XIV. f. 321^{v}.
Vatic.
276; s. XII. f. 122^{v} (*Tschiedels Coll. in Ilbergs Besitz*).
277; s. XIV. f. 353^{v}.
278; a. 1512. f. 733.
Venedig: Marcian. 269; s. XI. f. 388.

Περὶ γονῆς.
De genitura.

L. VII 470—484.

Inc. Νόμος μὲν πάντα κρατύνει.
Expl. ἐς τὸν λόγον ὃν ἔλεγον.

Bologna: Bonon. 3632; s. XV. f. 46.
Cambridge: Cantabrig. Caius Coll. 50; s. XV/XVI. f. 30v.
Florenz: Laurent. plut. 74, 1; s. XV. p. 27b.
Holkham: nr. 282; s. XVI. no. 13 (Expl. ἐν τῇσι μήτρῃσιν τῆς γυναικός).
Karlsruhe: Caroliruh. 449; s. XV/XVI.
Kopenhagen: Hauniens. ant. fund. reg. 224; s. XVI.
London: Arundel. (Brit. Mus.) 538; s. XV. f. 45.
Mailand: Ambros. L 110 Sup.; s. XVI. f. 245v.
Modena: Mutinens.
218 (II H 3); s. XVI. f. 110v.
233 (III H 5); s. XVI. f. 139v.
München: Monacens. 71; a. 1531.
Oxford: Baroccian. 204; s. XV. f. 27.
[**Padua:** Bibl. Canonicor. Lateranens.].
Paris:
[Coislin. 335].
Parisin.
1868; s. XV. f. 368.
2140; s. XII—XIII. f. 28.
2141; s. XV. f. 25v.
2142; s. XIII—XIV. f. 44v.
2143; s. XIV. f. 31.
2144; s. XIV. f. 34v.
2145; s. XV. f. 43.
2146; s. XVI. f. 198v.
[2147 (?); s. XVI.]
[2254 (?)].
2255; s. XV. f. 101.
2256*; s. XIV (frgm.).
2320; s. XVI. f. 1.
[2332*; s. XIV. f. 208].
Rom:
Palat. 192; s. XV. f. 101.

Reg. Suec. 182; s. XV. f. 20v.
Urbin. 68; s. XIV. f. 35.
Vatic.
276; s. XII. f. 117v.
277; s. XIV. f. 49v.
278; a. 1512 f. 75.
1759; s. XV (XVII?). f. 235v (Frgm. Inc. Νόμος μέν. Expl. ἔξωθεν σαρκώδεις).

Venedig:
Marcian.
269; s. XI. f. 35v.
282; s. XV.
296; s. XV.
App. cl. V 14 (ol. Nanian. 248); s. XV. f. 19.

Wien: Vindob. med. 13; s. XV. f. 1 (Inscr. Περὶ γεννήσεως ἀνθρώπου καὶ περὶ γονῆς. Inc. Νόμος μέν. Expl. f. 4v ταῦτα αἰσχυνόμεθα καὶ κρύπτειν σπουδάζομεν).

Περὶ φύσιος παιδίου. [Diels I.29]
De natura pueri.

L. VII 486—542.

Inc. Ἦν ἡ γονὴ μείνῃ.
Expl. οὗτος ὁ λόγος ὧδε εἰρημένος ἅπας τέλος ἔχει.

Cambridge: Cantabrig. Caius Coll.
50; s. XV/XVI. f. 33v.
76; s. XV/XVI. f. 220 (Inc. ἡ τροφὴ καὶ ἡ αὔξησις τῶν παιδίων = L. VII 514, 6).

Florenz: Laurent. plut.
59, 14; s. XV. f. 227b (Frgm. c. comm. Joannis [Damasceni?]. Ed. Dietz, Scholia in Hipp. et Gal. II 205—235).
74, 1; s. XV. p. 29b.

Holkham: nr. 282; s. XVI. no. 12.

Karlsruhe: Caroliruhens. 449; s. XV/XVI (fine mutil.).

Kopenhagen: Hauniens. ant. fund. reg. 224. s. XVI.

Leyden: Voss. fol. 10; s. XVI.

London: Arundel. (Brit. Mus.) 538; s. XV. f. 21.

Mailand: Ambros. L 110 Sup.; s. XVI. f. 246v.

Modena: Mutinens. 233 (III H 5); s. XVI. f. 144.

München: Monacens. 71; a. 1531.

Oxford: Baroccian. 204; s. XV. f. 29.

Paris: Parisin.
- 1868; s. XIV. f. 369ᵛ.
- 2140; s. XII—XIII. f. 30.
- 2141; s. XV. f. 27ᵛ.
- 2142; s. XIII—XIV. f. 36.
- 2143; s. XIV. f. 32ᵛ.
- 2144; s. XIV. f. 36ᵛ.
- 2145; s. XV. f. 46ᵛ.
- 2146; s. XVI. f. 187.
- 2147; s. XVI. f. 1 (imperf.).
- [2254 (?)].
- 2255; s. XV. f. 104ᵛ.
- [2332*; s. XIV. f. 208].
- [2545 (? = 2145?)].

Rom:
- Palat. 192; s. XV. f. 95.
- Reg. Suec. 182; s. XV. f. 34.
- Urbin. 68; s. XIV. f. 38ᵛ.
- Vatic.
  - 276; s. XII. f. 111ᵛ.
  - 277; s. XIV. f. 52.
  - 278; a. 1512 f. 80ᵛ.

Venedig:
- Marcian. 269; s. XI. f. 38ᵛ.
- App. cl. V 9; s. XV. f. 473.

Περὶ νούσων Δ'.
De morbis liber IV.

L. VII 542—614.

Lib. 4 Inc. Τοῦ ἀνθρώπου ἐς τὴν γένεσιν ἀπὸ πάντων τῶν μελέων.
Expl. ὅτι τὰ σημήϊα αὐτοῦ τάδε.

Cambridge: Cantabrig. Caius Coll. 50; s. XV/XVI. f. 102.
Florenz: Laurent. plut. 74, 1; s. XV. p. 70b.
Kopenhagen: Hauniens. ant. fund. reg. 224; s. XVI.
Mailand: Ambros.
- C 85 Sup.; s. XV—XVI.
- L 110 Sup.; s. XVI. f. 282ᵛ.

Modena: Mutinens. 220 (II H 5); s. XV. f. 71.
München: Monacens. 71; a. 1531.
Oxford: Baroccian. 204; s. XV. f. 74b.
Paris: Parisin.
2140; s. XII—XIII. f. 75v.
2141; s. XV. f. 70v.
2142; s. XIII—XIV. f. 107v.
2143; s. XIV. f. 76v.
2144; s. XIV. f. 85.
2145; s. XV. f. 116v.
2148; s. XV. f. 7.
[2254 (?)].
2255; s. XV. f. 191.
[2332*; s. XIV. f. 216].
[2545 (? = 2145?)].
Rom:
Palat. 192; s. XV. f. 18v.
Reg. Suec. 182*; s. XV. f. 83.
Urbin. 68; s. XIV. f. 86v.
Vatic.
277; s. XIV. f. 109.
278; a. 1512. f. 196v.
Venedig: Marcian. 269; s. XI. f. 129.

Γυναικείων Α' Β'.
De mulierum affectibus.

L. VIII 10—232. 234—406.

Lib. 1
Inc. Τὰ δὲ ἀμφὶ γυναικείων νούσων.
Expl. ἐς ὕδωρ ὑπόγλυκυ.
Lib. 2
Inc. Ῥόος λευκὸς ἐν τῇσι γεραιτέρῃσι.
Expl. ἐν οἴνῳ διακλυζέσθω.

Florenz: Laurent. plut. 74, 1; s. XV. p. 207b.
Holkham: nr. 282; s. XVI. no. 24 *und* 25.
Kopenhagen: Hauniens. ant. fund. reg. 224; s. XVI.
Leyden: Voss. fol. 10; s. XVI.

Mailand: Ambros. C 85 Sup.; s. XV—XVI.
Modena: Mutinens. 227 (II H 12); s. XVI. f. 44.
[Diels I.30] **München:** Monacens. 71; a. 1531.
Oxford: Baroccian. 204; s. XV. f. 229b.
Paris: Parisin.
2140; s. XII—XIII. f. 237v.
2141; s. XV. f. 207v.
2142; s. XIII—XIV. f. 351.
2143; s. XIV. f. 222.
2144; s. XIV. f. 253.
2145; s. XV. f. 341.
2146; s. XVI. f. 241v.
[2242 (?)].
2254; s. XV.
2256; s. XV. f. 83.
[2332*; s. XIV. f. 241].
[2548 (?)].
Rom:
Palat. 192; s. XV. f. 153 (Lib. I fine mutil.).
Urbin. 68; s. XIV. f. 258v.
Vatic.
276; s. XII. f. 141v (*Tschiedels Coll. in Ilbergs Besitz*).
277; s. XIV. f. 282v.
278; a. 1512. f. 591.
Venedig: Marcian. 269; s. XI. f. 298.
Wien: Vindob. med. 4; s. X. f. 241 (Expl. pro διακλυζέσθω sic: διανιζέσθω ὃς ἂν περὶ ἰήσιος ἐθέλῃ ἐρωτᾶν: — γυναικείων β'. *Vgl.* Περὶ νούσων lib. I in.).

Περὶ ἀφόρων.
De sterilibus.

L. VIII 408—462.

Inc. Περὶ μὲν τῶν γινομένων τῇσι γυναιξίν.
Expl. καταλείποντα προβολὴν τῷ σιδήρῳ.

Florenz: Laurent. plut. 74, 1; s. XV. p. 250.
Kopenhagen: Hauniens. ant. fund. reg. 224; s. XVI.
Leyden: Voss. fol. 10; s. XVI.
Mailand: Ambros. C 85 Sup.; s. XV—XVI.

Modena: Mutinens. 227 (II H 12); s. XVI. f. 115ᵛ.
München: Monacens. 71; a. 1531.
Oxford: Baroccian. 204; s. XV. f. 276.
Paris: Parisin.
  2140; s. XII—XIII. f. 291ᵛ.
  2141; s. XV. f. 248.
  2142; s. XIII—XIV. f. 406ᵛ.
  2143; s. XIV. f. 267.
  2144; s. XIV. f. 295.
  2145; s. XV. f. 409.
  [2146; s. XVI. f. 307ᵛ.]
  2254; s. XV. f. 170ᵛ.
  [2545 (? = 2145?)].
Rom:
  Palat. 192; s. XV. f. 31.
  Urbin. 68; s. XIV. f. 308ᵛ.
  Vatic.
    276; s. XII. f. 178ᵛ (*Tschiedels Coll. in Ilbergs Besitz*).
    277; s. XIV. f. 338ᵛ.
    278; a. 1512. f. 699ᵛ.
Venedig: Marcian. 269; s. XI. f. 368ᵛ (*Kühleweins Coll. in Ilbergs Besitz*).

Περὶ παρθενίων.
De virginum morbis.

L. VIII 466—470.

Inc. Ἀρχή μοι τῆς συνθέσιος.
Expl. μᾶλλον ταῦτα πάσχουσιν.

Florenz: Laurent. plut. 74, 1; s. XV. p. 262b.
Holkham: nr. 282; s. XVI. no. 21.
Kopenhagen: Hauniens. ant. fund. reg. 224; s. XVI.
Mailand: Ambros. C 85 Sup.; s. XV—XVI.
Modena: Mutinens. 227 (II H 12); s. XVI. f. 139.
München: Monacens. 71; a. 1531.
Oxford: Baroccian. 204; s. XV. f. 291b.
Padua: Bibl. S. Joannis in Viridario, ad dextr. plut. XVII. (*Verbleib unbekannt.*)
Paris: Parisin.
  2140; s. XII—XIII. f. 307.

2141; s. XV. f. 260.
2142; s. XIII—XIV. f. 423ᵛ.
2143; s. XIV. f. 281ᵛ.
2144; s. XIV. f. 309.
2145; s. XV. f. 430ᵛ.
2146; s. XVI. f. 210ᵛ.
2254; s. XV. f. 182.
[2332*; s. XIV. f. 249ᵛ].
[2545 (? = 2145?)].

Rom:
Palat. 192; s. XV. f. 104ᵛ.
Urbin. 68; s. XIV. f. 322ᵛ.
Vatic.
276; s. XII. f. 124 (*Tschiedels Coll. in Ilbergs Besitz*).
277; s. XIV. f. 355.
278; a. 1512 f. 735.

Venedig: Marcian. 269; s. XI. f. 389.

[Diels I.31]

Περὶ ἐπικυήσιος.
De superfoetatione.

L. VIII 476—508.

Inc. Ὁκόταν ἐπικυΐσκηται γυνή.
Expl. πίνειν καὶ καθαριεῖται.

Florenz: Laurent. plut. 74, 1; s. XV. p. 256b.
Kopenhagen: Hauniens. ant. fund. reg. 224; s. XVI.
Leyden: Voss. fol. 10; s. XVI.
Mailand: Ambros. C 85 Sup.; s. XV—XVI.
Modena: Mutinens. 227 (II H 12); s. XVI. f. 128.
München: Monacens. 71; a. 1531.
Oxford: Baroccian. 204; s. XV. f. 284.
Paris: Parisin.
2140; s. XII—XIII. f. 300.
2141; s. XV. f. 254.
2142; s. XIII—XIV. f. 415ᵛ.
2143; s. XIV. f. 275.
2144; s. XIV. f. 302.
2145; s. XV. f. 420ᵛ.

2146; s. XVI. f. 201v.
2254; s. XV. f. 170v.
[2332*; s. XIV. f. 248v.]
[2545 (? = 2145?)].

Rom:

Palat. 192; s. XV. f. 36.
Urbin. 68; s. XIV. f. 315.
Vatic.
276; s. XII. f. 119 (*Ilbergs Coll. in dessen Besitz*) *und* 184v (*Tschiedels Coll. in Ilbergs Besitz*).
277; s. XIV. f. 347v.
278; a. 1512. f. 717v.

Venedig:

Marcian. 269; s. XI. f. 379v.
App. cl. V 14 (ol. Nanian. 248); s. XVI. f. 22v (Expl. βάπτεειν δὲ τὰς μήλας = L. VIII 496, 9).

Περὶ ἐγκατατομῆς ἐμβρύου (I).
De exsectione foetus.

Περὶ ἐγκατατομῆς παιδίου (II).
De exsectione pueri.

L. VIII 512—518.

I Inc. Περὶ δὲ τῶν μὴ κατὰ τρόπον.
Expl. ἐσθιέτω δὲ σιτία μέτρια.

II Inc. Ἐγκατατομὴν παιδίου ποιήσεις οὕτως.
Expl. = I.

Florenz: Laurent. plut. 74, 1; s. XV. p. 207 *und* 276 (I. II).
Holkham: nr. 282; s. XVI. no. 26 *und* 27 (I. II).
Kopenhagen: Hauniens. ant. fund. reg. 224; s. XVI (I. II).
Leyden: Voss. fol. 10; s. XVI (I. II).
Mailand: Ambros. C 85 Sup.; s. XV—XVI.
Modena: Mutinens. 227 (II H 12); s. XVI. f. 42 *und* 163 (I. II).
München: Monacens. 71; a. 1531 (I. II).
Oxford: Baroccian. 204; s. XV. f. 229 *und* 306b (I. II).

Paris: Parisin.
2140; s. XII—XIII. f. 237 *und* 323^{v} (I. II).
2141; s. XV. f. 207 *und* 273^{v} (I. II).
[2142; s. XIII—XIV. f. 350^{v}] *und* 441 (I. II).
2143; s. XIV. f. 221^{v} *und* 298 (I. II).
2144; s. XIV. f. 252^{v} *und* 323 (I. II).
2145; s. XV. f. 340 *und* 452^{v} (I. II).
2146; s. XVI. f. 318 (II).
2254; s. XV. f. 82^{v} *und* 206^{v} (I. II).
[2257 (?)].
[2332*; s. XIV. f. 241 (I).]
[2545 (? = 2145?)].
Rom:
Palat. 192; s. XV. f. 39^{v} (II ?)
Urbin. 68; s. XIV. f. 257 *und* 337 (I. II).
Vatic.
276; s. XII. f. 187^{v} (II).
277; s. XIV. f. 282 *und* 372 (I. II).
278; a. 1512. f. 589^{v} *und* — (I. II).
Venedig: Marcian. 269; s. XI. f. 297 (I).
Wien: Vindob. med. 14; s. XVI. f. 47 (II).

Περὶ ἀνατομῆς.
De anatome.

L. VIII 538—540.

Inc. Ἀρτηρίη ἐξ ἑκατέρου.
Expl. ἡ φύσις διετάξατο.

Bologna: Bonon. 3632; s. XV. post f. 46.
Holkham: nr. 282; s. XVI. no. 20.
München: Monacens. 71; a. 1531.
Paris: Parisin.
2146; s. XVI. f. 333^{v}.
[2254 (?)].
2255; s. XV. f. 369^{v}.
Rom:
Palat. 192; s. XV. f. 30.
Vatic. 276; s. XII. f. 169^{v} (*Tschiedels Coll. in Ilbergs Besitz*).

Περὶ ὀδοντοφυΐης.
De dentitione.

[Diels I.32]

L. VIII 544—548.

Inc. Τὰ φύσει εὔτροφα.
Expl. δύσπνοιαν ἐπιφέρει.

Holkham: nr. 282; s. XVI. no. 23.
München: Monacens. 71; a. 1531.
Paris: Parisin.
2146; s. XVI. f. 227ᵛ.
[2254 (?)].
2255; s. XV. f. 369ᵛ.
Rom:
Palat. 192; s. XV. *nach* f. 30.
Vatic. 276; s. XII. f. 133 (*Tschiedels Coll. in Ilbergs Besitz*).

Περὶ ἀδένων.
De glandulis.

L. VIII 556—574.

Inc. Περὶ δὲ ἀδένων οὐλομελίης.
Expl. πνεύμονι καὶ ἀποπνίγονται.

Holkham: nr. 282; s. XVI. no. 19.
München: Monacens. 71; a. 1531.
Paris: Parisin.
2146; s. XVI. f. 331.
[2254 (?)].
2255; s. XV. f. 371.
Rom:
Palat. 192; s. XV. f. 45ᵛ.
Vatic. 276; s. XII. f. 195. (*Coll. Tschiedels in Ilbergs Besitz*).

Περὶ σαρκῶν.
De carnibus.

L. VIII 584—614.

Inc. Ἐγὼ τὰ μέχρι τοῦ λόγου τοῦδε.
Expl. ἐγὼ φράσω ἐν ἄλλοισιν.

Holkham: nr. 282; s. XVI. no. 18[b].
München: Monacens. 71; a. 1531.
Paris: Parisin.
2146; s. XVI. f. 326.
[2254 (?)].
2255; s. XV. f. 367v.
Rom:
Palat. 192; s. XV. f. 42v.
Vatic. 276; s. XII. f. 192 (*Coll. Ilbergs in dessen Besitz*).

Περὶ ἑβδομάδων.
De septimanis.

L. VIII 634—673. IX 433—466.

Inc. Mundi forma sic omnis ornata est.
Expl. De febribus quidem omnibus; de ceteris iam dico.

Berlin: Phillipps. 1529 (ol. Meerm. 220)*; s. XVI. f. 194 (Inc. Ἑπτά εἰσιν ὧραι. Expl. κἂν ἀτύχῃ τὰ τοῦ τέλους; cf. L. VIII 633).
Escurial: Scorial. y. III. 16*; s. XV. f. 1 (Inc. εἰσὶ δὲ ἡλικίαι ἑπτά, ὥς φησιν Ἱππ.; cf. L. VIII 636).
Jerusalem: Bibl. d. hl. Grabes 189*; s. XVIII. f. 299 (229? Ἑπτὰ ἡλικίαι τῶν ἀνθρ.).
Paris: Parisin.
396*; s. XIII. f. 707 (Inc. *und* Expl. *wie im* Berol. Phillipps. 1529).
2142*; s. XIII—XIV. f. 547v (Inc. ... οὐκ ἔχει ἑπτὰ μέρεα. Expl. ἀνὴρ πρεσβύτης γέρων; cf. L. IX 433 s.).

Προρρητικὸν Β′.
Praesagiorum liber II.

[Diels I.33]

L. IX 6—74.

Inc. Τῶν ἰητρῶν προρρήσιες.
Expl. καὶ σαρκωδεστάτοις φύεται.

Florenz: Laurent. plut.
  [25 (?)]
  74, 1; s. XV. p. 276b.
Jerusalem: Bibl. Mar-Saba 498; s. XVIII. f. 37 (Ἱππ. προρρητικῶν ἐξήγησις).
Kopenhagen: Hauniens. ant. fund. reg. 224; s. XVI.
Mailand: Ambros. B 108 Sup.; s. XIV in. f. 12 (Inc. = L. IX 12, 16).
München: Monacens. 71; a. 1531.
Oxford: Baroccian. 204; s. XV. f. 307.
Paris: Parisin.
  [2030 (?)].
  2140; s. XII—XIII. f. 324^v.
  2141; s. XV. f. 274.
  2142; s. XIII—XIV. f. 442.
  2143; s. XIV. f. 298^v.
  2144; s. XIV. f. 323^v.
  2145; s. XV. f. 453^v.
  2148*; s. XV. f. 61^v (Inc. ὅσοι μὲν ἢ γέροντες = L. IX 26, 16).
  [2253 (?)].
  2254; s. XV. f. 207^v.
  [2266 (?)].
  [2269 (?)].
  [2332*; s. XIV. f. 251^v.]
  [2545 (? = 2145?)].
Rom:
  Urbin. 68; s. XIV. f. 337^v.
  Vatic.
    277; s. XIV. f. 372^v.
    278; a. 1512 f. 773^v.
    283; s. XIV. f. 9.
[**Venedig:** Marcian. ?].

Περὶ καρδίης.
De corde.

L. IX 80—92.

Inc. Καρδίη σχῆμα μέν.
Expl. περὶ δὲ καρδίης τοσαῦτα εἰρήσθω.

Holkham: nr. 282; s. XVI. no. 18[a].
München: Monacens. 71; a. 1531.
Paris: Parisin.
2146; s. XVI. f. 324[v].
[2254 (?)].
2255; s. XV. f. 370.
Rom:
Palat. 192; s. XV. f. 41[v].
Vatic. 276; s. XII. f. 191 (*Ilbergs Coll. in dessen Besitz*).

Περὶ τροφῆς.
De alimento.

L. IX 98—120.

Inc. Τροφὴ καὶ τροφῆς εἶδος.
Expl. Ὑγρασίη τροφῆς ὄχημα.

Cambridge: Cantabrig. Caius Coll. 50; s. XV/XVI. f. 86.
Florenz: Laurent. plut. 71, 1; s. XV. p. 61 (*Coll. Ilbergs in dessen Besitz*).
Kopenhagen: Hauniens. ant. fund. reg. 224; s. XVI.
Leyden: Voss. fol. 10; s. XVI.
Mailand: Ambros.
C 85 Sup.; s. XV—XVI.
L 110 Sup.; s. XVI. f. 272[v].
Modena: Mutinens. 220 (II H 5); s. XV. f. 6.
München: Monacens. 71; a. 1531.
Oxford: Baroccian. 204; s. XV. f. 63b.
Paris: Parisin.
2140; s. XII—XIII. f. 62[v].
2141; s. XV. f. 60[v].
2142; s. XIII—XIV. f. 86[v].

2143; s. XIV. f. 65^{v}.
2144; s. XIV. f. 74.
2145; s. XV. f. 100^{v}.
2155; s. XIV. f. 301^{v} (Π. τροφῶν).
2253; s. XI. f. 34 (*Coll. Ilbergs in dessen Besitz*).
2255; s. XV. f. 170^{v}.
[2332*; s. XIV. f. 213].
[2545 (? = 2145?)].

Rom:
Urbin. 68; s. XIV. f. 74^{v}.
Vatic.
277; s. XIV. f. 95 (*Coll. Ilbergs in dessen Besitz*).
278; a. 1512 f. 170.

Venedig: Marcian. 269; s. XI. f. 77^{v}.

Περὶ ὄψιος. [Diels I.34]
De visu.

L. IX 152—160.

Inc. Αἱ ὄψιες αἱ διεφθαρμέναι.
Expl. τὴν ὑπάλειψιν ξυμφέρει ποιέεσθαι.

Cambridge: Cantabrig. Caius Coll. 50; s. XV/XVI. f. 234^{v}.
Florenz: Laurent. plut. 74, 1; s. XV. p. 153.
Kopenhagen: Hauniens. ant. fund. reg. 224; s. XVI.
Leyden: Voss. fol. 10; s. XVI.
Modena: Mutinens. 220 (II H 5); s. XV. f. 168^{v}.
Oxford: Baroccian. 204; s. XV. f. 167b.
Paris: Parisin.
2140; s. XII—XIII. f. 171^{v}.
2141; s. XV. f. 157.
2142; s. XIII—XIV. f. 272^{v}.
2143; s. XIV. f. 158.
2144; s. XIV. f. 186^{v}.
2145; s. XV. f. 251^{v}.
[2146 (?)].
[2148; s. XVI. f. 49^{v}.]
[2254 (?)].
2255; s. XV. f. 361^{v}.

[2332*; s. XIV. f. 230.]
[2545 (? = 2145?)].

Rom:

Urbin. 68; s. XIV. f. 186.
Vatic.
277; s. XIV. f. 214.
278; a. 1512. f. 434.

Venedig:

Marcian. 269; s. XI. f. 211v.
App. cl. V 14; s. XV. f. 10 (Expl. ἠλαιωμένον ἐγκατακαίειν = L. IX 154, 11).

Περὶ ὀστέων φύσιος.
De ossium natura.

L. IX 168—196.

Inc. Ὀστέα χειρὸς εἰκοσιεπτά.
Expl. ἐκ τῶν παρεόντων ἑκάστῳ χρωμάτων.

Florenz: Laurent. plut. 74, 1; s. XV. p. 190.
Kopenhagen: Hauniens. ant. fund. reg. 224; s. XVI.
Leyden: Voss. fol. 10; s. XVI.
Mailand: Ambros. C 85 Sup.; s. XV—XVI.
Modena: Mutinens. 227 (II H 12); s. XVI. f. 7v.
München: Monacens. 71; a. 1531.
Oxford: Baroccian. 204; s. XV. f. 210.
Paris: Parisin.

2140; s. XII—XIII. f. 216.
2141; s. XV. f. 191v.
2142; s. XIII—XIV. f. 328v.
2143; s. XIV. f. 201v.
2144; s. XIV. f. 236.
2145; s. XV. f. 312.
[2247; s. XVI. f. 82.]
[2248; s. XV. f. 128.]
2254; s. XV. f. 51.
[2332*; s. XIV. f. 239.]
[2545 (? = 2145?)].

Rom:

Urbin. 68; s. XIV. f. 237v.

Vatic.
[216].
277; s. XIV. f. 260v.
278; a. 1512 f. 542v.
Venedig: Marcian. 269; s. XI. f. 270.

Περὶ ἰητροῦ.
De medico.

L. IX 204—220.

Inc. Ἰητροῦ μέν ἐστι προστασίη.
Expl. ἐν ἑτέροις γεγραμμένον ἐστίν.

Holkham: no. 282; s. XVI. no. 17.
München: Monacens. 71; a. 1531.
Paris: Parisin.
2146; s. XVI. f. 318v.
2255; s. XV. f. 86v.
Rom:
Palat. 192; s. XV. f. 25.
Vatic. 276; s. XII. f. 188 (*Ilbergs Coll. in dessen Besitz*).

Περὶ εὐσχημοσύνης.
De decenti ornatu.

L. IX 226—244.

Inc. Οὐκ ἀλόγως οἱ προβαλλόμενοι.
Expl. ἐς σύνεσιν καθίστανται.

Cambridge: Cantabrig. Caius Coll. 50; s. XV/XVI. f. 18.
Florenz: Laurent. plut. 74, 1; s. XV. p. 20.
Kopenhagen: Hauniens. ant. fund. reg. 224; s. XVI.
Leyden: Voss. fol. 10; s. XVI.
Mailand: Ambros. L. 110 Sup.; s. XVI. f. 240v.
München: Monacens. 71; a. 1531.
Oxford:
Baroccian. 204; s. XV. f. 20.

[Diels I.35] Roe. XIV (260)*; s. XV. f. 73 (Inc. Χρὴ τὸν ἰατρόν = L. IX 236, 3).
Paris: Parisin.
2140; s. XII—XIII. f. 20v.
2141; s. XV. f. 18.
2142; s. XIII—XIV. f. 25v.
2143; s. XIV. f. 23.
2144; s. XIV. f. 27.
2145; s. XV. f. 31.
[2254 (?); s. XV.].
[2255 (?); s. XV.]
[2332*; s. XIV. f. 206.]
[2545 (? = 2145?)].
Rom:
Urbin. 68; s. XIV. f. 28v.
Vatic.
277; s. XIV. f. 40 (*Ilbergs Coll. in dessen Besitz*).
278; a. 1512 f. 54v.
Venedig: Marcian. 269; s. XI. f. 26.

Παραγγελίαι.
Praeceptiones.

L. IX 250—272.

Inc. Χρόνος ἐστὶν ἐν ᾧ καιρός.
Expl. ᾠδή, τόπος ὀνησιφόρος.

Cambridge: Cantabrig. Caius Coll. 50; s. XV/XVI f. 15v.
Florenz: Laurent. plut. 74, 1; s. XV. p. 18b.
Kopenhagen: Hauniens. ant. fund. reg. 224; s. XVI.
Mailand: Ambros. L 110 Sup.; s. XVI. f. 239v.
München: Monacens. 71; a. 1531.
Neapel: Neapolit. 91 II C 33*; s. XV.
Oxford: Baroccian. 204; s. XV. f. 18.
Paris: Parisin.
2140; s. XII—XIII. f. 19.
2141; s. XV. f. 16v.
[2142 (?); s. XIII—XIV.]
2143; s. XIV. f. 21v.
2144; s. XIV. f. 25.

2145; s. XV. f. 28v.
[2254 (?)].
2255; s. XV. f. 83v.
[2332*; s. XIV. f. 205v.]
[2545 (? = 2145?)].

Rom:

Urbin. 68; s. XIV. f. 26v (*H. Schoenes Coll. von 250, 1—256, 7. 268, 1—272, 3 im Besitz der Akademie*).

Vatic.

277; s. XIV. f. 37v.
278; a. 1512. f. 50v.

Venedig: Marcian. 269; s. XI. f. 23v (*Ilbergs Coll. in dessen Besitz*).

Περὶ κρισίων.
De iudicationibus.

L. IX 276—294.

Inc. Περὶ κρισίων ξυντόμων.
Expl. ἄνευ σπασμοῦ ⟨οὐ λύεται, ἢ αἵματος πολλοῦ ἐκ τῶν ῥινῶν,ἢ ὀδύνης ἐς τὰ ἰσχία⟩.

Holkham: nr. 282; s. XVI. no. 18.
München: Monacens. 71; a. 1531.
Paris: Parisin.

[2146 (?); s. XVI.]
[2254 (?)].
2255; s. XV. f. 379v.

Rom:

Palat. 192; s. XV. f. 40.
Vatic. 276; s. XII. f. 189v (*Tschiedels Coll. in Ilbergs Besitz*).

Περὶ κρισίμων.
De diebus iudicatoriis.

L. IX 298—307.

Inc. Μέγα μέρος ἡγέομαι.
Expl. ἡ κατάστασις τῶν πυρετῶν.

Cambridge: Cantabrig. Caius Coll. 50; s. XV/XVI. f. 236.
Florenz: Laurent. plut.
74, 1; s. XV. p. 154.
74, 31; s. XIV. p. 24 (Π. κρισίμων ἡμερῶν).
Kopenhagen: Hauniens. ant. fund. reg. 224; s. XVI.
Leyden: Voss. fol. 10; s. XVI.
Mailand: Ambros. C 85 Sup.; s. XV—XVI.
Modena: Mutinens. 220 (II H 5); s. XV. f. 169v.
München: Monacens. 71; a. 1531.
Oxford: Baroccian. 204; s. XV. f. 168b.
Paris: Parisin.
2140; s. XII—XIII. f. 172v.
2141; s. XV. f. 158.
2142; s. XIII—XIV. f. 274v.
2143; s. XIV. f. 159.
2144; s. XIV. f. 187v.
2145; s. XV. f. 253.
2146; s. XVI. f. 321.
[2148; s. XVI. f. 50.]
[2254 (?)].
2255; s. XV. f. 363.
[2332*; s. XIV. f. 230v.]
[2545 (? = 2145?)].
Rom:
Urbin. 68; s. XIV. f. 187.
Vatic.
277; s. XIV. f. 215v.
278; a. 1512. f. 436v.
Venedig:
Marcian. 269; s. XI. f. 212v.
App. cl. V 14 (ol. Nanian. 248); s. XV. f. 7.

[Diels I.36] Ἐπιστολαί. Δόγμα Ἀθηναίων. Ἐπιβώμιος. Πρεσβευτικὸς Θεσσαλοῦ.
Epistulae. Decretum Atheniensium. Oratio ad aram. Thessali legati oratio.

L. IX 312—428.

Ep. 1 (L. IX 312, 3—15)
Inc. Βασιλεὺς βασιλέων μέγας Ἀρταξέρξης Παίτῳ χαίρειν. Νοῦσος προσεπέλασεν ἡ καλεομένη λοιμική.

Expl. ἀγαθῇ συνειδήσει. Ἔρρωσο.

— 2 (L. IX 312, 16—314, 25)

Inc. Παῖτος βασιλεῖ βασιλέων τῷ μεγάλῳ Ἀρταξέρξῃ χαίρειν. Τὰ φυσικὰ βοηθήματα.

Expl. τῆς θεοπρεποῦς ἐπιστήμης.

— 3 (L. IX 316, 3—9)

Inc. Βασιλεὺς βασιλέων μέγας Ἀρταξέρξης Ὑστάνει Ἑλλησπόντου ὑπάρχῳ χαίρειν. Ἱπποκράτους ἰητροῦ.

Expl. συμβουλίην οὐ ῥηίδιον. Ἔρρωσο.

— 4 (L. IX 316, 10—16)

Inc. Ὑστάης ὑπ. Ἑλλησπ. Ἱπποκράτει Ἀσκληπιαδῶν ὄντι ἀπογόνῳ χαίρειν. Βασιλεὺς μέγας Ἀρταξέρξης (vel Ἣν ἔπεμψεν ὁ βασιλεύς).

Expl. παραγίνου ξυντόμως. Ἔρρωσο (vel ἵνα πέμψω. Ἔρρωσο).

— 5 (L. IX 316, 17—318, 3)

Inc. Ἱπποκράτης ἰητρὸς Ὑστάνει Ἑλλησπ. ὑπάρχῳ χαίρειν. Πρὸς τὴν ἐπιστολήν (vel Πέμπε βασιλεῖ).

Expl. ἐχθροὺς ὑπάρχοντας τῶν Ἑλλήνων. Ἔρρωσο.

— 6 (L. IX 318, 4—6)

Inc. Ἱπποκράτης Δημητρίῳ ὑγιαίνειν. Βασιλεὺς Περσέων.

Expl. πλέον δύναται. Ἔρρωσο.

— 7 (L. 1X 318, 7—13)

Inc. Βασιλεῖ βασιλέων τῷ ἐμῷ μεγάλῳ δεσπότῃ Ἀρταξέρξῃ Ὑστάνης Ἑλλησπ. ὑπ. χαίρειν. Ἣν ἔπεμψας ἐπιστολήν.

Expl. Γυμνάσβην Διευτύχῃ. Ἔρρωσο.

— 8 (L. IX 318, 14—21)

Inc. Βασιλεὺς βασιλέων μέγας Ἀρταξέρξης Κῴοις τάδε λέγει. Δότε ἐμοῖς ἀγγέλοις.

Expl. νῆσος ἢ πόλις Κῶ.

— 9 (L. IX 318, 22—320, 9)

Inc. Ἀπόκρισις Κῴων. Ἔδοξε τῷ δάμῳ.

Expl. ἀμελήσουσιν ἁμέων.

— 10 (L. IX 320, 10—324, 21)

Inc. Ἀβδηριτῶν ἡ βουλὴ καὶ ὁ δῆμος Ἱπποκράτει χαίρειν. Κινδυνεύεται τὰ μέγιστα.

Expl. τὰ πρὸς τὴν ὑγείην. Ἔρρωσο.

— 11 (L. IX 324, 22—330, 2)

Inc. Ἱπποκράτης Ἀβδηριτῶν τῇ βουλῇ καὶ τῷ δήμῳ χαίρειν. Ὁ πολίτης ὑμέων.

Expl. πόλιος ἐόντα κόσμον. Ἔρρωσθε.

— 12 (L. IX 330, 3—332, 18)

Inc. Ἱπποκράτης Φιλοποίμενι χαίρειν. Οἵ τὴν τῆς πόλιος ἐπιστολήν.

Expl. ὡς οἶσθα. Ἔρρωσο.

— 13 (L. IX 332, 19—336, 7)

Inc. Ἱπποκράτης Διονυσίῳ χαίρειν. Ἢ περίμεινόν με.

Expl. ἐπικλώμενον ὑπ' εὐνοίης. Ἔρρωσο.

[Diels I.37] — 14 (L. IX 336, 8—338, 20)
Inc. Ἱπποκράτης Δαμαγήτῳ χαίρειν. Οἶδα παρὰ σοὶ γενόμενος.
Expl. ὃν ἐπιστέλλω σοι χρονίζει. Ἔρρωσο.
— 15 (L. IX 338, 21—342, 12)
Inc. Ἱπποκράτης Φιλοποίμενι χαίρειν. Σύννους καὶ πεφροντικώς.
Expl. καὶ νοσήσοντας ἰώμενος. Ἔρρωσο.
— 16 (L. IX 342, 13—348, 3)
Inc. Ἱπποκράτης Κρατεύᾳ χαίρειν. Ἐπίσταμαί σε ῥιζοτόμον.
Expl. φαρμάκων σοφίη τέλος. Ἔρρωσο.
— 17 (L. IX 348, 4—380, 10)
Inc. Ἱπποκράτης Δαμαγήτῳ χαίρειν. Τοῦτ' ἐκεῖνο, Δαμάγητε.
Expl. γηθοσύνως πάνυ. Ἔρρωσο.
— 18 (L. IX 380, 11—384, 2)
Inc. Δημόκριτος Ἱπποκράτει εὖ πράττειν. Ἐπῆλθες ἡμῖν.
Expl. τὸν περὶ μανίης λόγον. Ἔρρωσο.
— 19 (L. IX 384, 3—386, 8)
Inc. Ὁ περὶ μανίης λόγος. Μαινόμεθα, ὡς ἔφην.
Expl. ἀκούων οὐδὲν ἔπασχεν.
— 20 (L. IX 386, 9—388, 2)
Inc. Ἱπποκράτης Δημοκρίτῳ εὖ πράττειν. Ἰητρικῆς τέχνης, ὦ Δημόκριτε.
Expl. τὸν περὶ τοῦ ἐλλεβορισμοῦ λόγον. Ἔρρωσο.
— 21 (L. IX 388, 3—392, 3)
Inc. Ἱπποκράτης Δημοκρίτῳ περὶ ἐλλεβορισμοῦ. Τοῖς μὴ ῥηϊδίως.
Expl. αἱ μῆτραι καθάρσεως δέωνται.
— 22 (L. IX 392, 4—22)
Inc. Ἱπποκράτους πρὸς τὸν υἱὸν Θεσσαλόν. Ἱστορίης δὲ μελέτω σοι, ὦ παῖ.
Expl. τῆς τοιῆσδε ἐμπειρίης. Ἔρρωσο.
— 23 (L. IX 392, 23—398, 6)
Inc. Δημόκριτος Ἱπποκράτει περὶ φύσιος ἀνθρώπου. Χρὴ πάντας ἀνθρώπους.
Expl. ἔπαυσε λειτουργίης.
— 24 (L. IX 398, 7—400, 14)
Inc. Ἱπποκράτους ὑγιεινὸν πρὸς Δημήτριον βασιλέα. Ἱπποκράτης Κῷος Δημητρίῳ χαίρειν. Ἡμεῖς καὶ πρότερον σπουδάζοντες.
Expl. διατελῇς ἄνουσος ἐών.
— 25 (L. IX 400, 15—402, 12)
Inc. Δόγμα Ἀθηναίων. Ἔδοξε τῇ βουλῇ καὶ τῷ δήμῳ.
Expl. ἐν Πρυτανείῳ διὰ βίου.
— 26 (L. IX 402, 13—404, 14)
Inc. Ἐπιβώμιος. Ὦ πολλοί.
Expl. φιλοτιμίης μηδὲν ἐλλείποντες.

— 27 (L. IX 404, 15—428, 12)
Inc. Πρεσβευτικὸς Θεσσαλοῦ Ἱπποκράτους υἱοῦ. Προσήκειν ἡγέομαι.
Expl. ὧν ἱμείρομεν εὐμοιρήσομεν.

Berlin: Pap.
6934; s. II—III (Ep. 5 et 11 frgm. Ed. K. Kalbfleisch, Berl. Klassikertexte III [1905] p. 5–9).
7094; s. II—III (Ep. 3. 4. 5 et frgm. 11 Ed. K. Kalbfleisch, Berl. Klassikertexte III [1905] p. 5–9).
Bern: Bernens. 579; s. XIV. f. 61 (Epp. 4—6).
Bologna: Bonon. 3563; s. XVI. f. 89ᵛ (Epp. 1—5. [6—9 man. alt. add. in marg.]. 11—18. 20. 22).
Brüssel: Bruxell. 1871—77; s. — f. 68.
Cambridge: Cantabrig. Bibl. Univ. LL 4, 12; s. XV. f. 39b (Ep. 17 frgm. et 18).
Florenz:
Conventi soppressi 153; s. XVI. f. 74 (Epp. 1—5. 11—18. 20. 22).
Laurent. plut. 74, 1; s. XV. p. 343. [Diels I.38]
Heidelberg: Bibl. Univ.
132; s. XV. no. 14.
398; s. X. no. 16.
Kopenhagen: Hauniens. ant. fund. reg. 224; s. XVI. (Expl. μακρῶν μεγάλοι προσεδεήθησαν = L. IX 424, 16).
Leyden: Voss. 4° 38; s. XV. (Ep. 17).
London: Harleian (Brit. Mus.)
5635; s. XV. f. 128ᵛ (Ep. 17); f. 227ᵛ (Ep. 1; des. haec series f. 229 νούσων παύειν, ἐχθροὺς ἐόντας Ἑλλήνων = Expl. Ep. 5).
6301; s. XV vel XVI. f. 3ᵛ (Ep. 3—9).
Madrid: Matrit. bibl. nac. 4557 (N 119); s. XV ex. f. 94—124.
Mailand: Ambros. B 113 Sup.; s. XIV in. f. 184.
Modena: Mutinens.
54 (III B 2); s. XV. f. 121 (Epp. 1—5. 11—17 usque ad ὠχριακῶς πάνυ).
191; s. XV. (Epp. 1—5. 11—18. 20).
München: Monac. 71; a. 1531 (Πρεσβ.).
Neapel:
Neapolit. 187 (II F 30); s. XVI. f. 50 (Πρεσβ.).
Bibl. dei Gerolamini XXII. I; s. XIV. f. 133ᵛ—135ᵛ (Epp. 10—13).
Bibl. S. Giovanno di Carbonara 27; s. XIV.
Oxford:
Auct. T II 10; s. XV. f. 82b.

Baroccian.
51; s. XV. f. 61^{v} (Epp. 3. 5—9).
204; s. XV. f. 46.
Miscell. 210; s. —.

Paris:

Parisin.
1327; a. 1562 f. 208^{v} (Ep. ad Damaget.)
1760; s. XV. f. 146 (Artax. et Hipp. epp.) et f. 205.
[1884; a. 1403 f. 95.]
[1885; s. XVI. f. 35^{v}.]
2140; s. XII—XIII. f. 414.
2141; s. XV. f. 339.
2142; s. XIII—XIV. f. 530.
2143; s. XIV. f. 375.
2144; s. XIV. f. 390.
2145; s. XV. f. 573.
2146; s. XVI. f. 334.
2253; s. XI. f. 74^{v} (Ἐπιβ.).
2254; s. XV. f. 363.
2255; s. XV. f. 26 (Δόγμ.).
[2332*; s. XIV. f. 277.]
2652; s. XV. f. 78^{v}.
2755; s. XV. f. 161.
3047; a. 1420. f. 5.
3050; s. XV. f. 107.
3052; s. XVI. f. 38 (Epp. Artax. et Hipp.).
Suppl. 205; s. XV—XVI. f. 34.
Bibl. de Paris 4; s. XVI. f. 159^{v}.

Rom:

Palat.
132; s. XV. f. 215^{v} (Epp. 14).
192; s. XV. f. 171.
398; s. X. f. 282 (Epp. 1—24?).
Urbin.
64; s. X—XI. f. 104.
68; s. XIV. f. 418^{v}.
Vatic.
276; s. XII. f. 196^{v}.
277; s. XIV. f. 462.
278; a. 1512 f. 965.
1309; s. XVI. f. 302^{v}.

1354; s. XVI. f. 92ᵛ.
1467; s. XV—XVI. f. 140 (Epp. praecip. Hipp. et Democr.).
Sens: nr. 209; s. XVII/XVIII.
Upsala: Upsal. bibl. acad. 8 (Sparfwenf. 49); s. XV. f. 99 (Epp. 8. 9. 1).
Venedig: Marcian.
269; s. XI. f. 446.
609; s. XVI.
Wien: Vindobon.
med. 24; s. XV. f. 2 (Ep. 1 etc.; expl. f. 3ᵛ ὧν ὁ δι᾽ ἀρετῆς ὑποκαθαρθεὶς ὑγιάζεται ἐγὼ δὴ ...).
phil. 82; s. XV—XVI. f. 158ᵛ—177 (Epp. 1—22?).
[**Wolfenbüttel:** Guelf. August. 18, 1 (? Ep. ad Hystan.)].

Περὶ αἰσθήσεων. [Diels I.39]
De sensibus.

Rom: Angelic. 4 (C. 4. 16)*; s. XVI in. f. 174 (Inc. Αἰσθητήρια δέ ἐστιν ἐν τῷ ἀνθρώπῳ. Expl. καὶ ξηρᾶς κράσεώς εἰσιν).

Περὶ ἀλειμμάτων.
De unguentis.

Paris: Parisin. 2148; s. XV. f. 59.

Περὶ ἀλόης.
De aloe.

Athos: Βιβλ. μον. Ἰβήρων 4338. 218; s. XVI. p. 310.

Περὶ ἀνατομικῶν ἐργαλείων.
De anatomicis ferramentis.

Bologna: Bonon. 3632; s. XV. f. 27ᵛ. (Περὶ ἀνατομικῶν ἐργαλίον κατὰ υπ̄π̄ᵏ ποσα ἡσή ἡστὴν ἰατρικὴν ἐπιστίμην. »Zweifelhaft, ob Hippokr. betreffend. Dialekt nicht ionisch.« Schoene.)

Περὶ γενέσεως ἀνθρώπου.
De generatione hominis.

Zürich: Turicens. C 136; s. XVI. f. 177.

Περὶ γυναικῶν.
De mulieribus.

Kopenhagen: Hauniens. ant. fund. reg. 224; s. XVI.
Rom: Barberin. I 127; s. XVI. f. 250ᵛ. (Inscr. Περὶ διαγνώσεως τῶν κυϊσκουσῶν γυναικῶν καὶ περὶ τῶν ἐν γαστρὶ ἐχουσῶν).

Διαθήκη.
Testamentum.

Athos: Βιβλ. μον. Ξηροποταμοῦ 2432. 99; s. XVII. (Διαθήκη τῶν τριῶν ἰατρῶν Γαλ. Ἱππ. καὶ Διοσκορ.)
Berlin: Berolin. qu. 5 (304); s. XV/XVI. f. 53ᵛ (Διαθήκη τῶν τριῶν ἰατρῶν Γαλ. Ἱππ. καὶ Μελετ. περὶ τῆς τοῦ ἀνθρώπου κατασκευῆς καὶ πῶς δεῖ διεξιέναι τὸν καιρόν).
Florenz: Laurent. plut. 74, 10; s. XIV. f. 13ᵛ.
Wien: Vindob. med.
32; s. XVI. f. 11.
53; s. XVI. f. 8ᵛ—10ᵛ.

[Diels I.40] Λεξικὸν τῶν εἰδῶν.
Lexion specierum (?).

Athos: Βιβλ. μον. Ἰβήρων 4271. 151; s. XV. f. 17a.

Ἱπποκράτους, ἄλλοι δὲ Διοκλέους, ἐπιστολὴ πρὸς Πτολεμαῖον βασιλέα Αἰγύπτου.
Hippocratis vel Dioclis epistula ad Ptolemaeum Aegypti regem.

Ed. Fabricius, Bibl. gr. XII [1724]) p. 585—592.
ex Pauli Aeginetae l. I c. 100 fol. 13ᵛ ed. Aldinae, Venetiis 1528.

Inc. Ἐπειδή σοι συμβαίνει.
Expl. εἰς τροπὰς χειμερινὰς ἡμέραι με΄.

Bologna: Bonon. 3633; s. XV. f. 126.
Paris: Parisin.
2229; s. XIII. f. 25.
2301; s. XII—XIII. f. 124.
Rom: Barberin. I 127; s. XVI. f. 310.
Turin: Taurin. C VI 3 (287 c I 42); s. XV. f. 201 (*Durch Feuer stark beschädigt*).
Venedig: Marcian. App. cl. V 16; s. XVI. f. 146.

Ἐπιστολὴ πρὸς Πτολεμαῖον, βασιλέα περὶ κατασκευῆς ἀνθρώπου.
Ad Ptolemaeum regem epistula de hominis fabrica.

Ed. Ermerins, Anecd. med. gr. (Lugd. Bat. 1840).

Inc. Συνέστηκεν ὁ κόσμος ἐκ στοιχείων τεσσάρων.
Expl. ξηραίνεται τὸ ἐγκέφαλον καὶ γίνεται φρενίτης (bei Ermerins τὸν ἐπίλοιπον χρόνον).

Athos:
Βιβλ. μον. Διονυσίου 3701. 167; s. XV.
Ἰβήρων
4212. 92; s. XVI. f. 367 A.
4501. 381; s. XV. f. 341 A.
5034. 914; s. XVII (Expl. εἰς ἡμέρας τξε' καὶ τέταρτον).
Berlin: Phillipps.
1462; s. XV/XVI. f. 407.
1583; s. XV. f. 94^{v}.
Bologna: Bonon. 3632; s. XV post f. 46.
Leiden: Vulc. 56; s. XIV. f. 131—133.
London: Medical Society AA a 1 = Xa 32; s. XVI. p. 1 (Expl. συνάγεται ὁ ἐνιαυτὸς εἰς ἡμέρας τξε'; *Vgl.* Athos Ἰβήρ. 5034. 914.
Mailand: Ambros. A 95 Sup.; s. XV. f. 95.
Modena: Mutinens. 115 (II D 16); s. XV. f. 12.
Moskau: Mosquens. 439; s. XVI. f. 128.
München: Monacens. 72; s. XVI. f. 216 (Expl. εἰς τὴν κύστιν τὸ ὕδωρ).
Oxford: Canonician. 1; s. XVI. f. 66 (Inc. Οὗτος οὖν ὁ κόσμος συνίσταται ἐκ τεσσ. στοιχ.).
Paris:
Parisin.
1630; s. XIV. f. 202^{v}.
2047; s. XV. f. 13^{v}.
2146; s. XVI. f. 228^{v} (»de partibus corporis humani«).

2253; s. XI. f. 100.
2255; s. XV. f. 371ᵛ.
[2301 (?)].
2315; s. XV. f. 282.
2894; s. XIII. f. 334.
Suppl. 165; s. XV. f. 105.

Rom:
Angelic. 4 (C. 4. 16); s. XVI in. f. 172 (Expl. *wie im* Monacens. 72).
Reg. Suec.
181*; a. 1364. f. 281ᵛ (Inc. Ὁ ἄνθρωπος διαιρεῖται) *und* f. 283 (Inc. Ἀπὸ μηνὸς Νοεμβρίου).
182; s. XV. f. 48 (»de partibus corp. hum.; frgm. initio mutilum.« Inc. Λέγεται δὲ καὶ γαστήρ, ὅτε περιαγής ἐστιν) et f. 60 (»de part. corp. hum.« Inc. Συνέστηκεν ὁ ἄνθρωπος).
Vatic.
1066; s. XVI. f. 7ᵛ.
1276; s. XIII. f. 180 (*Vielleicht dieselbe Epist. wie im* Vatic. 1066).

Venedig: Marcian. App. cl. V, 16; s. XVI. f. 82.

Wien: Vindob.
med.
40; s. XV. f. 125 (Expl. ὁ μὲν ἔξωθεν νευρώδης, ὁ δὲ ἔνδοθεν σαρκώδης).
52; s. XV. f. 67 (Inc. ψυχρά · τὸ δὲ ὕδωρ ψυχρὸν καὶ ὑγρόν. Expl. ἐπὶ τὰς ἁπλᾶς καὶ ἡνωμένας τοῦ νοῦ θεωρίας ἀναγομένη).
theol. 293; s. XVI. f. 92.

[Diels I.41] 'Επιστολὴ Ἱππ[οκράτους] πρὸς Πτολεμαῖον βασιλέα.
Epistula ad Ptolemaeum regem de sanitate tuenda.

Ed. Boissonnade, Anecd. Graeca III 422—428.

Inc. 'Επιμελούμενοι τῆς σῆς ὑγιείας.
Expl. καὶ ἡμῶν τὴν ἔκθεσιν ἀληθῆ.

Heidelberg: Bibl. Univ. 155; s. XV. no. 4.

London:
Addit. (Brit. Mus.) 34,060; s. XV. f. 481 (Expl. τοῖς δὲ μείζοσιν ἐνεργεστέρας).
Harleian. (Brit. Mus.)
5626; s. XV—XVI. f. 80 (Expl. ἔπειτα θερμάνας ἄλειφε καὶ δῆσον).
6295; s. XV (XIV sec. catal.). f. 106 (Expl. εἰσὶ μόνον, ἀλλὰ καὶ ἔξω).

Mailand: Ambros. A 110 Sup.; s. XV—XVI. f. 60ᵛ.

Moskau: Mosquens. 439; s. XVI. f. 128.
Oxford:
Baroccian.
10; s. XV. f. 130 (Expl. *wie im* Londin. Addit. 34060).
150; s. XV in. f. 6v.
Clarkian. 16 (18378); s. XIV. f. 88b.
Ger. Langbainii Advers. 2; s. — f. 69b (Expl. mut. πόνοις καὶ καμάτοις καὶ ἀφροδισίοις).
Paris:
[Coislin. 321 (?)].
Parisin.
1630; s. XV. f. 146.
[1884 (?)].
[2229 (?)].
Suppl. 352; s. XIII. f. 145v.
Turin: Taurin. 177 b II 31; s. XVI. f. 33 (*Verbrannt*).
Wien: Vindob.
med. 52; s. XV. f. 49—55 (Ἐγκύκλιος ἐπιστ. Ἱππ. πρὸς Πτολ. βασ., ὅπως ἐπεισέρχεται τῷ τοῦ ἀνθρώπου σώματι νόσος. Expl. μάλιστα θαρρούντων τῷ ἔθει).
phil. 178; s. XV. f. 345 (Expl. εὖ διάξεις, μέγιστε βασιλεῦ Πτολεμαῖε).

Ἐπιστολὴ Ἱπποκράτους πρὸς Πτολεμαῖον βασιλέα.
Hippocratis ad Ptolemaeum regem epistula.

Athos: Βιβλ. μον. Ἰβήρων 4330. 310; s. XVI. f. 44 B.
Berlin: Phillipps. 1566 (ol. Meerm. 269); s. XVI. f. 1.
Chalke: Βιβλ. μον. Θεοτόκου 82; s. — f. 188v.
Gallipoli: Ἐκκλησ. ἁγ. Νικολάου 38; s. XIV. f. 39.
Mailand: Ambros. B 72 Sup.; s. — f. 116.
Paris:
Coislin. 321; s. XVI. f. 115.
Parisin.
2240; s. XVI. f. 156v.
[2699 (?); s. XVI.]
Suppl. 446; s. X. f. 69v.
Rom:
Palat. 155; s. XVI. f. 119v.
Vatic.
293; s. XVI. f. 219.
690; s. XV. f. 257v.

876; s. XV. f. 4.
1065; s. XIII. f. 98.
1095; s. XV. f. 279v.

Νοήματα καὶ σημειώσεις περὶ ζωῆς καὶ θανάτου.
Sententiae de vita et morte.

Athos: Βιβλ. μον. Ἐσφιγμένου 41; s. XV.
London: Medical Society
AA a 1 = Xa 32; s. XVI. p. 34 (Inc. Ὁ ἐμπειρικώτατος ἁπάντων. Expl. εἰς κ' ἡμέρας ἀποθανεῖται).
HH i 21. 22 = We 28. 29; s. XV. f. 361v (Inc. *und* Expl. *wie im* Lond. AA a 1).
Mailand: Ambros. A 95 Sup.; s. XV. f. 4 (Inc. *und* Expl. *wie im* Lond. Medical Society).
Oxford: Roe 14 (260); s. XV. f. 52 (Inc. *und* Expl. *wie im* Lond. Medical Society).
Paris:
Parisin.
2260; s. XVI. f. 1750 (Expl. εἰς πεντήκοντα ἡμέρας ἀποθανεῖται).
2294; s. XV. f. 95v—96v.
2671; s. XV. f. 264—265v (Sine titulo).
Suppl.
637; s. XV. f. 65 (*Abschrift besitzt Mr. E. O. Winstedt, Oxford*).
675; s. XV. f. 83 (*Wie im* cod. monast. Ἐσφιγμένου Athos).
Wien: Vindobon. med. 8; s. XV. f. 282 (Inc. *wie im* Lond. Medical Society. Expl. εἰς ἓξ ἡμέρας ἀποθανεῖται).

[Diels I.42] [Περὶ ζῴων ?].
De animalibus marinis et terrestribus ad morbos curandos idoneis.

Paris: Parisin. 2510; a. 1384. f. 80.

Περὶ ἥπατος.
De iecore.

Florenz: Laurent. App. 2; s. XV. f. 344.

[Θεραπευτικὴ μέθοδος].
[Medendi methodus].

[**Dublin:** Bibl. Narcissi 1709 (Methodus curandi)].
[**Wien:** Vindob. ap. Lambec. VI 145].

Ἰατροσόφιον.
Jatrosophium.

Athos:
Βιβλ. μον. Ἰβήρων
4294. 174; s. XVII. f. 46 B (Ἰατροσόφιον ἐκλελεγμ. ὑπὸ πολλ. ἰατρικῶν βιβλίων Γαλ. Ἱππ. καὶ ἄλλων πολλ. σοφῶν ἰατρῶν).
4463. 343; s. XIX. (Ἱππ. ἰατρικὸν συνταγμάτιον).
4655. 535; s. XVI. (Ἰατροσ. ἐκλελεγμ. ὑπὸ πολλῶν βιβλίων ἰατρικ. Γαλ. Ἱππ. καὶ Μελετίου Inc. Ὅτι ὁ κόσμος).
Παντελεήμονος 5769. 262; s. XVIII. f. 15 A (Ἰατροσ. ἐκλ. ὑπὸ βιβλίων ... Γαλ. Ἱππ. Μελετ. καὶ Παύλ. τ. Αἰγ.).
Florenz: Laurent. App. 2; s. XV. f. 222 (Ἰατρικὸν Ἱππ. καὶ Γαλ. ἰατρεῖαι διάφοροι).
Jerusalem:
Bibl. patriarch. 148; s. XVI. f. 15ᵛ.
Bibl. Mar-Saba. 432; a. 1662. f. 1 (Ἰ. ... Γαλ. Ἱππ. καὶ Μελ. καὶ ἄλλων ...).
London:
Addit. (Brit. Mus.) 28, 830; s. XVIII. f. 15. (Ἰατροσόφ. ... Ἱππ. καὶ Γαλ. Inc. Παρὶ τῆς πεγουνέας [sic]).
Harleian. (Brit. Mus.) 5626; s. XV (XVI). f. 2 (Ἰατροσόφ. ... Ἱππ. καὶ Γαλ. κτλ.).
Palermo: Panormit. bibl. naz. XIII C 3; s. XVI. f. 1—44ᵛ (Ἰατροσόφ. Ἱππ. καὶ Γαλ. καὶ ἑτέρων φιλοσόφων καὶ ἰατρῶν. Inc. Περὶ ἤθους ἰατρῶν. Ποδαπὸν δεῖ εἶναι τὸν ἰητρόν. Expl. ἐν οὔρῳ, ἐν πτύσμασιν, ἐν ἱδρῶτι) *und* f. 121—238 (Inscr. Ἀνθολόγιον ἰατροσοφικὸν Ἱππ. ... καὶ Γαλ. καὶ ἑτέρων ἰατρῶν).
Paris: Parisin.
Coislin. 335; s. XV. f. 75 (Gal. Hipp. et Melet. iatros. cap. 604).
Parisin. 2419; s. XV. f. 153 (Hipp. ... iatros.).
Suppl.
496; s. XVII. f. 7—9 (Ἰατροσόφ. ἐκ τοῦ Ἱππ. βιβλίου. Inc. Ἡ μὲν ἐν ἀρχῇ τοῦ προπάτορος δέσις. Expl. μελανόχολοι καὶ λευκόχροοι).
684; s. XV—XVIII. f. 211 (Iatrosoph. ex Gal. Hipp. et aliis. Inc. Ἐγὼ Γαληνὸς πεπειραμένος).
Rom: Barberin. III 63 (= 245); s. XVI. f. 394 (Ἰατροσόφ. ... Γαλ. Ἱππ. καὶ Μελετ. περὶ γυναικός).

Wien: Vindob. med.
13; s. — f. 59—128 (Ἰατροσόφ. Ἱππ.).
14; s. —
53; s. XVI. f. 59^{v}—128^{v} (Inc. f. 70 περὶ ἀπηγάνου εἰς κρίον ᾱ. Expl. δὸς πιεῖν μετὰ οἴνου καὶ ὠφελεῖται: — τέλος τῶν οκβʹ κεφαλαίων).

Περὶ ἱδρώτων.
De sudoribus.

Rom: Palat. 143; s. XV. f. 162 (De sudoribus febriculosis).
Wien: Vindob. phil. 178; s. XV. f. 43^{r}—43^{v} (Inc. Οἱ δ' ἱδρῶτες ἄριστοι μέν εἰσιν ἐν ἅπασι τοῖσιν ὀξέοισιν. Expl. πίστει καὶ πόθῳ δοξάζωμεν).

[Diels I.43] Ἱππιατρικά.
Hippiatrica.

Vielleicht nicht hergehörig. Vgl. E. Oder Rhein. Mus. 51 [1896] p. 59s.

Leyden: Voss. 4° 50; s. XV. (Ἱππιατρ. τοῦ σοφοῦ ῥήτορος Ἱερακλέου καὶ Ἱππ. κ. τοῦ σοφ. Γαλ.).
Paris: Parisin.
1995; s. XV. f. 190. (Sostrati et Hipp. collectanea hippiatr.).
2091; s. XV. f. 118 (Hippiatr. ex Onosandro et Hippocrate).

Ἱπποκράτους καὶ Γαληνοῦ φιλοσοφία περὶ τῆς τοῦ ἀνθρώπου κατασκσευῆς.
Hippocratis et Galeni philosophia de natura hominis.

Inc. Ὁ ἄνθρωπος θεός ἐστιν ἐπίγειος, ἐπεὶ καὶ πλάσμα ἐστὶ θεικόν.
Expl. καὶ αἱ φλέβες αὐτοῦ λεπταὶ καὶ τὸ σῶμα λευκόν.

Paris: Parisin.
985; s. XVI. f. 302 (Λέξεις Ἱππ. πρὸς Γαλ. τὸν ἑαυτοῦ μαθητὴν περὶ ἀνθρώπου. Περὶ διαπλάσεως ἀνθρώπου [*Abschrift besitzt Dr. Helmreich*]).
2320; s. XVI. f. 7.
Wien: Vindob. med. 13; s. XV. f. 4^{v}—6^{v}.

Περὶ κυνάγχης νόσου.
De angina.

Florenz: Laurent. App. 2; s. XV.

Περὶ τοῦ τραχήλου τῆς κύστεως.
De collo vesicae.

Florenz: Laurent. App. 2; s. XV. f. 355.

Περὶ λίθων δυνάμεως.
De lapidum virtute.

Paris: Parisin. 2316; s. XV. f. 340^{v}.

Ποταπὸν δεῖ εἶναι τὸν μανθάνοντα.
Qualem oporteat esse discipulum.

Escurial: Scorial.
Φ. III. 11; s. XIV. XV. f. 43 (Inc. πρῶτον μὲν τῷ γένει ἐλεύθερον. Expl. εἰ μὴ μόνον ἡμῖν τοῖς ἰατροῖς).
y. I. 8; s. XVI. f. 1.
Mailand: Ambros. B 113 Sup.; s. XIV in. f. 1 (Inc. Δεῖ εἶναι. Expl. ἰητρῷ ἁρμοδιώτερον).

Λόγος τῶν μηνῶν.
De mensibus.

Oxford: Baroccian. 224; s. XV in. f. 3 (Inc. Πρῶτον μὲν περὶ τῆς ἐγκυκλίου σφαίρας. Expl. περὶ μηνῶν καὶ ὀνήσιμος ἄγαν).

[Περὶ σώματος μορίων ?].
De partibus hominis.

Paris: Parisin. 2419; s. XV. f. 153.
Zürich: Turicens. C 136; s. XVI. f. 117 (de partibus hominis).

[Diels I.44]

[Περὶ νόσων καὶ φαρμάκων ?].
De morbis hominum et remediis.

Paris: Parisin. 2178; s. XV. f. 42.

Περὶ οὔρων.
De urinis.

Athos: Βιβλ. μον. Ἰβήρων 4340. 220; s. XVII.
Escurial: Scorial.
T. II. 12; s. XVI. f. 190.
Φ. III. 12; s. XV. f. 8.
Florenz:
Magliabecch. 1; s. XVI. f. 204 (Inc. Οὖρον δὲ ἄριστον. Expl. τὴν ἀνωμαλίην).
Bibl. Nazion. II. III. 428; s. XVI. f. 204 (*Wie im* Magliab. Expl. ὑφιζάνει κάτω, τοσούτῳ βελτίω γίνεται).
Riccard. 41 (K. II. 12); s. XVI. f. ιϵ. (Inc. *und* Expl. *wie im* Magliabecch.).
Leyden: Voss. fol. 10; s. XVI.
Neapel:
Neapolit. III C 2 (260); s. — f. 1 (Inc. Οὖρον ἄριστόν ἐστιν ὅταν λευκή. *Abschrift besitzt Mr. E. O. Winstedt, Oxford*).
Bibl. dei Gerolamini XXII. I; s. XV. f. 166ᵛ—167 (Inc. Ὁκόσοισιν οὖρα παχέα [= Aph. sect. IV no. 69]. Expl. ἀλλ' αὐτῆς καθ' ἑαυτήν).
Oratorian. 152; s. XIV.
Oxford: Baroccian. 88; s. XV—XVI. f. 47b (Σύνοψις ἀκριβὴς περὶ οὔρων Ἱππ. καὶ Γαλ. Inc. 'Εὰν ἔστι κλόκιον ἀνθρώπου. Expl. σύντομον θάνατον).
Paris: Parisin.
2224; s. XV. f. 42 (Ex Gal. Hipp. etc. de urinis).
2269; s. XV. f. 94.
2294; s. XV. f. 68.
2304; s. XV. f. A (Ex Hipp. etc. de urinis).
2308; s. XV. f. 12ᵛ (Inc. *wie im* Neapol. Bibl. dei Gerolamini).
2320; s. XVI. f. 17ᵛ (Περὶ οὔρων χρηστῶν Ἱππ. καὶ Γαλ. τῶν φιλοσόφων).
Rom:
Palat. 143; s. XV. f. 158.
Reg. Suec. 182; s. XV. f. 40.

[Περὶ ποδός (?)].
De pede.

Rom: Palat. 192; s. XV. f. 56v.

Προγνωστικά.
Prognostica.

Athen: nr. 1504; s. XIX. (Προγν. μυστηριώδη).
Athos: Βιβλ. μον. Ἰβήρων 4463. 343; s. XIX.
Florenz: Laurent. plut. 75, 10; s. XV. p. 1 (Hipp. praenotiones quaedam et signa morborum).
Modena: Mutin. 85 (III C 6); s. XV. f. 95v (Πρόγνωσις π. τῶν δ' ὡρῶν. Inc. Ἂν μὲν χειμὼν αὐχμηρός. Expl. καὶ μελαγχολίαι).
München: Monacens. 276; s. XII. (Προγνωστικὸν ἀῤῥώστων συγγραφὲν Ἱππ. καὶ Γαλ. καὶ Πλάτωνος καὶ σοφ. ἰατρῶν).
Oxford: Baroccian. 88; s. XV—XVI. f. 47 (Ἱππ. καὶ Γαλ. καὶ Παύλου Ἰταλ. etc. διάγνωσις περὶ ἰαλίων ἀρρώστων καὶ τελευτῆς ἀνθρώπων. Inc. Τὸ α̅ ἄσπρον. Expl. σημαίνει θάνατον).
Turin: Taurin. C VI 21 (b VI 18); s. XVI. f. 26v (Π. καιρῶν πρόγνωσις).
[**Wien:** Vindob. 179 (*Wie im* Taurin.)].

Περὶ τῶν κατὰ τὴν πτέρνην. [Diels I.46]
De calce.

Rom: Palat. 192; s. XV. f. 57.

Περὶ πυρετῶν.
De febribus.

Holkham: nr. 282; s. XVI. no. 11.
Leyden: Voss. fol. 10; s. XVI. (Inc. Οἱ πλεῖστοι τῶν πυρετῶν).
München: Monac. 71; a. 1531 (Inc. *wie im* Leydens. Voss.)
Paris: Parisin.
[1667 (?)].
1884; s. XIV. f. 92v (Inc. Τοῦτό σοι τὸ τρίτον ἐπίταγμα).
[1885 (?)].

Rom:

Palat. 400; s. XV. f. 7 (Ex Hipp. et Gal. de febribus. Inc. Ἱππ. ὁ διδάσκαλος ἡμῶν).

Regin. 182; s. XV. f. 16ᵛ (Inc. *wie im* Leydens. Voss.) *und* f. 43ᵛ. 45ᵛ (Inc. *wie im* Parisin. 1884).

Περὶ διαφορᾶς πυρετῶν.
De febrium differentiis.

London: Harleian. (Brit. Mus.) 6295; s. XV (XIV sec. catal.) f. 103 (Inc. πυρετοί· οἱ μὲν δακνώδεις εἰσί. Expl. ἐν οἷς αἱ διαφοραὶ τῶν πυρετῶν).

Περὶ σπληνὸς καὶ στομάχου.
De splene et stomacho.

Athos: Βιβλ. μον. Ξηροποτάμου 2432. 99; s. XVII.

Περὶ τῶν δ' στοιχείων καὶ χυμῶν, δι' ὧν συνίσταται ὁ ἄνθρωπος.
De quattuor elementis et humoribus naturae hominis.

München: Monacens. 72; s. XVI. f. 215.

Rom: Angelican. 4 (C. 4. 16); s. XVI in. f. 171 (Inc. Ἰστέον ἐστιν· ὁ ἄνθρωπος ἐπίσταται [sic!]. Expl. ὅσα δὲ γένηται ἐν χειμῶν⟨ι⟩ ἀπαλλάσσονται).

Wien: Vindob. med. 41; s. XIV—XV. f. 81 (Inc. Ἰστέον ὅτι ὁ ἄνθρωπος συνίσταται ἐκ τεσσάρων στοιχείων. Expl. εἰς τὰς τέσσαρας ἑβδομάδας).

Περὶ στοιχείων.
De elementis.

München: Monacens. 494; s. —. f. 14 (Inc. Στοιχεῖα ἀνθρώπου ἴσχοντα ἰσχόμενα ἐνορμῶντα. Expl. γλυκὺ ἁλυκὸν ὀξῶδες καὶ ἄποιον. *Abschrift in Königsberg, Dietz-Nachlaß XVI 31*).

Neapel: Neapol. bibl. dei Gerolamini XXII. I; s. XV. f. 161ᵛ. *Wie im* Monac.

Paris: Parisin. 1883; s. XIV. f. 35ᵛ.

Περὶ σφυγμῶν. [Diels I.47]
De pulsibus.

Oxford: Baroccian. 131; s. XIV in. f. 477b (Διάγνωσις ἀκριβὴς τῶν σφυγμῶν. Expl. ταῦτα γάρ εἰσιν Ἱπποκράτους καὶ Γαλ. τῶν ἐπισήμων ἰατρῶν).
Paris: Parisin. 2316; s. XV. f. 205 (Interrogationes et responsiones de pulsibus).
Rom: Reg. Suec. 182; s. XV. f. 41v (Inc. Ἥκω δή σοι καὶ τὸ περὶ).

Ἱπποκράτους πρὸς Γαληνὸν αὐτοῦ μαθητὴν
περὶ σφυγμῶν καὶ κράσεων ἀνθρωπίνων σωμάτων.
Hippocratis ad Galenum discipulum liber de pulsibus
et de temperamentis corporis humani.

Inc. Τὸ ἀνθρώπινον σῶμα ἐκ τεσσάρων χυμῶν συνίσταται.

Athos:
Βιβλ. μον. Διονυσίου 3758. 224; s. XVI. p. 985.
Βιβλ. μον. Δοχειαρίου 2917. 243; s. XVII. f. 163 A (Περὶ εἰς πίον τόπον τοῦ κορμίου τοῦ ἀνθρώπου εὑρίσκεται καθένα στοιχίον ἀπο τα τεσσαρα. Ἱπποκράτους πρ. Γαλ. τοῦ αὐτοῦ μαθητήν).
Βιβλ. μον. Ἰβήρων 4302. 182; s. XVI. f. 9b (Λέξεις Ὑπποκράτους ἀρχιατροῦ πρ. τὸν αὐτοῦ μαθ. Γαλ.).
Berlin: Phillipps. 1487; s. XV/XVI. f. 339 (Expl. ἡ τροφὴ αὐτοῦ ξηρὰ καὶ γλυκέα).
Escurial: Scorial. Υ. III. 10; s. XV. f. 26v (Expl. *wie im* Berol. Phill.).
Oxford: Canonician. 1; s. XVI. f. 119b (Inscr. Περὶ τοῦ σώματος τοῦ ἀνθρώπου πῶς συνίσταται. Inc. Τὸ σῶμα τοῦ ἀνθρώπου συνίσταται ἐκ τεσσάρων στοιχείων. Expl. εἰς τὴν ἀναλυτικὴν ἐνέργεια τῶν βρωμάτων τῶν ἐν αὐτῷ).
Paris: Parisin.
Suppl.
728 (Minas IZ); s. XIV. f. 28. (*Vgl.* Costomiris Revue des ét. gr. II [1889] p. 353).
754 (Minas); s. — f. 523 (*Vgl.* Costom. *a. a. O.*).
1254; s. XVI. f. 135 (»Ad Gal. de pulsibus«).
Rom:
Palat. 363; s. XV. f. 108.
Vatic. 285; s. XV. f. 287 (Ἱ. πρ. Γαλ. ... π. διπλάσεως ἀνθρώπου).
Turin: Taurinens. C VI 3 (287c I 42); s. XV. f. 199 (»Ad Gal. suum discip. epistolium quoddam de corpore humano, necnon elementorum brevis expositio.« *Durch Feuer stark beschädigt*).

Περὶ τοῦ σώματος καὶ διατυπώσεως ἀνθρώπου.
De corpore et generatione hominis.

London: Medical Society A A a 1 = Xa 32; s. XVI. p. 12. (Inc. Ἀλλὰ μηδεὶς ὑπολαμβανέτω παντελῶς ἄψυχον εἶναι τὴν γονήν. Expl. κομάτια καὶ μέρη, διακόσια εἴκοσι ἐννέα).

Περὶ διαφορᾶς καὶ παντοίων τροφῶν.
De alimentorum differentiis.

Inc. Πέρδικές εἰσι.
Expl. ὑγρότερος καὶ περιττωματικός.

Berlin: Phillipps. 1527 (ol. Meerm. 217); s. XVI. f. 61.

[Diels I.48] Περὶ ὑαλίων.
De vasis vitreis.

Turin: Taurin. 17 B VII 22 (B I 12); s. XVI. XVIII. f. 48^{v} (*Verbrannt*).

Περὶ ὑδάτων.
De aquis.

Rom: Palat. 192; s. XV. f. 18 (De aqua et balneo).

Ὅτι ὑπαρκτικαί εἰσιν αἱ τέχναι.
Esse re vera artes.

Inc. Δοκέει δέ μοι τὸ μὲν σύμπαν.

Cambridge: Cantabrig. Caius Coll. 50; s. XV/XVI. f. 2.
Leyden: Voss. fol. 10; s. XVI.
Rom: Urbin. 68; s. XIV. f. 17.

Περὶ ὑπάρξεως ἰατρικῆς. Ὅρος ἰητρικῆς.
De substantia artis medicae. Definitio artis medicae.

Cambridge: Cantabrig. Caius Coll. 50; s. XV/XVI. f. 2ᵛ.
Leyden: Voss. fol. 10; s. XVI.
München: Monacens. 71; a. 1531.
Rom:
Urbin. 68; s. XIV. f. 17ᵛ.
Vatic. 278; a. 1512 f. 30.

Φάρμακα.
Remedia.

Athos: Βιβλ. μον. Ἰβήρων 4271. 151; s. XV. f. 85 B (Inscr. Ἡ ἱερὰ Ἱπποκράτους. Inc. Κολοκυνθίδι ἐντεριώνην σκίλλης ὀπτῆς ἀγαρικοῦ).
[**Florenz:** Laur. plut. 73, 1].
London: Medical Society H Hi 17 = We 30; s. XI in. no. 21 Dbg.
Paris: Parisin. 2510; a. 1384 f. 133ᵛ (Hipp. et Gal. antidotum).
Rom: Palat.
297; s. XV—XVI. f. 157ᵛ (de remediis ad partum proficientibus. Inscr. Κυητήριον Ἱππ.).
400; s. XV. f. 399 (de prophylacticis adversus arthriticos affectus ex Hipp. Gal. aliisque).

Περὶ φαρμάκων. [Diels I.49]
De remediis.

Göttingen: Gottingens., Bibl. Univ., Philol.
2; s. XVIII. f. 89 (»ex manuscr. Hadriani Junii Hornani«).
21; s. XVII—XVIII. f. 77 (»ex manuscr. Hadr. Iun. Hornani miss. ex Anglia a Rich. Thomone«).
Leyden:
Voss. 8° 7; s. XVII (descr. Is. Vossius ex Hadr. Iun. Hornani msto.).
Vulc. 108 pars 15*; s. XVI.
Mailand: Ambros.
B 113 Sup.*; s. XIV in. f. 181ᵛ (Inc. Τὰ δὲ περὶ φαρμάκων πρήγματα. Expl. τῶν παραπλησίων).
S. Q. E. VIII 14 (»in eine Aldina eingeschr.« Inc. = Ambr. B 113 Sup. Expl. χρείεσθαι γὰρ αὐτὸς κίνδυνος).

Oxford:

[Coll. Merton. 729].

Orvillian. X 1. 4. 29; s. XVIII in.

Rom:

Urbin. 64; s. X—XI. f. 102.

Vatic. 1133; s. — f. 53.

Περὶ φλεβοτομίας.
De venae sectione.

Mailand: Ambros. C 4 Sup.; s. — f. 244v.

Paris: Parisin.

36; s. XIV—XV. f. 95 (Inc. Ἐν πάσῃ ἡμέρᾳ).

2269; s. XV. f. 126.

2320; s. XVI. f. 13v (Περὶ τοῦ ἐκ ποίων τόπων φλεβοτομεῖν).

Turin: Taurin. 17 B VII 22 (B I 12); s. XVI. f. 30v (Π. φλ. ἐκ Γαλ. Ἱππ. Μελ. (*Verbrannt*).

Venedig: Marcian. App. cl. V 13; s. XIV—XVI. f. 118.

Wien: Vindob. med. 16; s. XV—XVI. f. 1.

[Περὶ χειρουργίας (?)].
[*De chirurgia*].

Paris: Parisin. 2247 (Exc. ex libris chirurgicis).

[Περὶ μελαίνης χολῆς (?)].
De specie atrae bilis.

Leyden: Voss. fol. 10; s. XVI.

Πρόγνωσις περὶ τῶν δ' ὡρῶν.
De IV aetatibus praenotio.

Modena: Mutinens. 85 (III C 6); s. XV. f. 95 (Inc. Ἂν μὲν χειμὼν αὐχμηρός. Expl. κόρυζαι χρόνιαι, ἐνίοισι δὲ καὶ μελαγχολίαι).

München: Monacens. 287; s. XV. f. 153.

Excerpta varia. [Diels I.56]

Athos: Βιβλ. Μον. Ἰβήρων 4310. 190; s. XIII. f. 115a.
Berlin: Phillipps. 1538 (ol. Meerm. 233); s. XV ex.
Florenz:
 Laurent. plut.
  [74, 12].
  75, 19; s. XIV. p. 16b. 19. 20.
 Bibl. naz. II, III. 428; s. XVI. f. 204.
Jerusalem: Bibl. patriarch. 463; s. XVIII. no. 8.
Lesbos: Βιβλ. τῆς τοῦ Λειμῶνος μονῆς 175; s. XVII.
Leyden: Scal. 71; s. XVI. f. 92 (Περὶ τῆς ᾗ χρῆται Ἱπποκράτης διαλέκτου. Sunt 17 regulae grammaticae).
Modena: Mutinens. 61 (III B 9); s. XV. f. 31.
Neapel: Bibl. S. Giovanni di Carbonara 15; s. XIV. f. —
Oxford:
 Bibl. Aedis Christi 34; s. XI. f. 131.
 Auct. (Bodl.) T II 3; s. XVIII.
 Baroccian (Bodl.) 131; s. XIV in. f. 477b und 480.
Paris:
 Parisin.
  2149; s. XVI. f. 176b (Frgm. Inc. Φλεγμαίνει γὰρ τὰ ἕλκεα. Expl. τῆς φύσιος τοῦ ἀνθρώπου).
  [2269].
  2847; s. XVI. f. 139.
 Suppl. 1194; s. XV. f. 1.
Rom:
 Barberin. I 127; s. XVI. f. 336 (Inc. Μετὰ τὸ Πυθαγόραν. Expl. τέθνηκάς μοι).
 Palat.
  126; s. XVI. f. 242.
  129; s. XV. f. 49.
  400; s. XV. f. 171 (Inc. Ὅταν ἀκμάζῃ τὸ νόσημα).
 Urbin. 64; s. X—XI. f. 100—103 (I. Ἐκ τοῦ π. φυσῶν. II. Π. χειρουργίας. III. Π. ἀφανῶν νοσημάτων. IV. Τὸ δι' ἐναντίων συγγίνεται ἡ ἰατρική).
Turin: Taurinens.
 17 B VII 22 (B I 12); s. — f. 48v (Verbrannt).
 179b II 33; s. XVI (Durch Feuer stark beschädigt).
Wien: Vindob. med.
 [8].
 [15].
 [41].

52; s. XV. f. 84—92 (Inc. wie im Palat. 400. Expl. ἕνωσον καὶ χρῆσαι).
[53]

[Diels I.57]

Indices et Lexica.

Paris:
Bibl. Facult. Med. 14; s. XVII. (Lexicon Hipp.).
Parisin.
2254; s. XV. f. 1 (Indicis pars posterior P — Ω.).
2255; s. XV. f. 1 (Indicis pars prior A — Π).
Rom: Palat. 428; s. XV—XVII. f. 1 (Index in Gal., Alex. Aphr. et Hipp. aliquot opuscula).

Laterculi antiqui.

Rom: Vatic.
276; s. XII. f. 1 (ed. Ilberg—Kühlew. Hipp. Opp. I p. XV sq.)
277; s. XIV. f. 11.
Venedig: Marcian.
269; s. XI. f. 1^v (*Wie im* Vatic. 277. Ed. Ilb. — Kühlew. ibid. p. XIX sq.)

Galen

Under the title **Zeichenerklärung** (*Table of Symbols*), Diels' catalogue includes some abbreviations and *sigla*, the list of which appears on page 2 of the first issue of the catalogue (1905). Those abbreviations, utilized precisely in the present reproduction of Diels are the following with their respective explicitation:

*	=	die Hds. enthält nur Exzerpte.
[ ]	=	die Hds. ist nur aus Ackermann's *Hist. litteraria Hippocratis* (Kühn Med. Gr. Opp. XXI, 1 ff.) und *Hist. litt. Cl. Galeni* (Kühn M. G. O. I, XVII ff.) oder aus Littré (Œuvr. compl. d'Hippocr. Par. 1839—61. 10 Bde.) bekannt.
J.	=	Galenus, editio Iuntina 1528 (Exemplar der Vatikanischen Handbibliothek).
K.	=	Kühn.
L.	=	Littré.

*	=	the manuscript contains only extracts.
[ ]	=	the manuscript is known only through Ackermann's *Hist. litteraria Hippocratis* (Kühn Med. Gr. Opp. XXI, 1 sq.) and *Hist. litt. Cl. Galeni* (Kühn M. G. O. I, XVII ff.) or Littré (Œuvr. compl. d'Hippocr. Par. 1839—61. 10 vols).
J.	=	Galen, Iuntina 1528 edition (copy of the Vatican Library).
K.	=	Kühn.
L.	=	Littré.

Jena: Aldina c. nott. Cornarii.
Konstantinopel: Bibl. d. Serail 11; s. XV.
Leipzig: Lipsiens.
57; s. XVIII/XIX (»Vier gelbe Pappbände: Jo. Scaligeri emendatt. in Gal. ex exemplo Guelferbyt. I—IV. Am Schluß 2 lose Hefte eingelegt, das eine d. d. 15. Juli 1616: In Gal. libellum qui inscr. π. ὀστῶν«).
58; s. XVI (?). (»Cornarius in Galenum. Coniecturae Cornarii excerptae ex Aldinae editionis exemplo in bibl. Jenensi asservato«. *Vgl. oben* Jena).
London: Burneian. (Brit. Mus.) 523; s. XVIII. f. 9 (»Emendationes in quosdam Galeni locos ed. Basil. 1538 manu Ant. Askew scriptae«).
[Mailand]: [Ambros. ap. Montf. p. 497].
[Moskau]: [Mosquenses complures].
Ravenna: Ravenn. 70; s. XV.
Rom: Bibl. St. Petri H 45; s. XIII (»Palimpsest very damaged contains Galen; part of his works«. Allen).
Wien: Vindobon. med. 16; s. XV—XVI. f. 329 (ἀρχὴ σὺν θεῷ τῶν διαιρέσεων πασῶν τῶν γαληνείων πραγματειῶν ἀρχόμενος ἀπὸ τοῦ περὶ αἱρέσεων, τελευτῶν δὲ εἰς τὴν θεραπευτικήν. Expl. ἢ διὰ τὰ συναμφότερα).
Wolfenbüttel: Guelferbyt. 364 (Gud. 7 et 18); s. XVI. (Aldina a. 1525 cum emendatt. Scaligeri marg. adscriptis).

Γαληνοῦ + παραφράστου τοῦ Μηνοδότου προτρεπτικὸς λόγος ἐπὶ τὰς τέχνας. [Diels I.59]
Galeni paraphrastae Menodoti suasoria ad artes oratio.

K. I 1—39.
Marquardt Gal. scr. min. I 103—129.
G. Kaibel Berol. 1894.

Inc. Εἰ μὲν μηδ' ὅλως λόγου μέτεστι τοῖς ἀλόγοις.
Expl. τοῦτο δ' αὐτὸ δεικτέον ἐφεξῆς.

Cod. Andr. Asulani, Vorlage d. Aldina 1525 (*Verbleib unbekannt*).
Londinensis und cod. Adelphi (*beide in England benutzt von Goulston, Gal. Opusc. varia, Londini 1640, Anhang. Verbleib unbekannt, Name des letzteren unaufgeklärt; vgl. Kaibel, Gal. Protrept. praef. p. V*).

Περὶ ἀρίστης διδασκαλίας.
De optima doctrina.

K. I 40—52.
Marquardt 3 Gal. scr. min. I 82—92.

Inc. Τὴν εἰς ἑκάτερα ἐπιχείρησιν ἀρίστην εἶναι.
Expl. καὶ τοῦτ' ἐπιτρέπων αἱρεῖσθαι τοῖς μαθηταῖς.

Florenz: Laurent. plut. 74, 3; s. XII. p. 132 (*Collat. H. Schoenes in dessen Besitz*).

Dazu:
a) cod. Adelphi (*Name unaufgeklärt*),
b) Londinensis (*benutzt in England von Goulston, Gal. Opusc. varia, Londin. 1640, Anhang. Verbleib unbekannt. Vgl. Kaibel, Gal. Protrept. praef. p. V.*).

Ὅτι ὁ ἄριστος ἰατρὸς καὶ φιλόσοφος.
Quod optimus medicus sit etiam philosophus.

K. I 53—63. H.
Th. Reinhold Athen 1865/66 p. 110 sq.
Iw. Müller Erlang. 1875;
Gal. scr. min. II 1—8.

Inc. Οἷόν τι πεπόνθασιν οἱ πολλοὶ τῶν ἀθλητῶν.
Expl. τὰ λείποντα δ' αὐτοὺς ἐξευρίσκοντας.

Florenz: Laurent. plut. 74, 3; s. XII. p. 129.
Paris: Parisin.
2164; s. XVI. f. 35.
[2169 (?)].
Rom: Urbin. 67; s. XIV et XV. f. 276 (Expl. λαβόντι μὴ οὐχὶ καὶ τὰς ἄλλας).
Venedig: Marcian. App. cl. V 4; s. XV.

Dazu:
a) cod. J. Scaligeri,
b) cod. Londinensis,
c) cod. Adelphi,
d) cod. Regius (seu Bibliothecae Regis Britannici).
(*b c d in England benutzt v. Goulston, Gal. Opusc. varia, Londin. 1640, Anhang. Verbleib unbekannt, Name von c unaufgeklärt; vgl. Kaibel, Gal. Protrept. praef. p. V.*)

Περὶ αἱρέσεων τοῖς εἰσαγομένοις. [Diels I.60]
De sectis ad eos qui introducuntur.

K. I 64—105.
G. Helmreich, Act. Erlang. II 239—310;
Gal. scr. min. III 1—32.

Inc. Τῆς ἰατρικῆς τέχνης σκοπὸς μὲν ἡ ὑγίεια.
Expl. ἱκανὰ ταῦτα, καταπαύσω τῇδε τὸν παρόντα λόγον.

Florenz: Laurent. plut. 74, 5; s. XIV. p. 123.
Modena: Mutinens. 109 (II D 10); s. XIV—XV. f. 63v.
Moskau: Mosquens.
- 51; s. XV.
- 283; s. XV.
- 464; s. XV. f. 2.
- 466; s. XVI. f. 1.

Paris:
- Parisin.
  - 1883; s. XIV. f. 29v.
  - 2283*; s. XVI.
- Suppl.
  - 35; s. XV—XVI. f. 166.
  - 634; s. XIV. f. 2v.

Rom: Palat. 297*; s. XV—XVI. f. 50 (»de Empiricis et Methodicis«).
Venedig:
- Marcian. 282; s. XV.
- App. cl. V 9; s. XV. f. 492 (Expl. μετὰ ἀκριβείας).

Dazu: cod. Adelphi (*Name unaufgeklärt, in England benutzt v. Goulston, Gal. Opusc. varia, Londin. 1640, Anhang. Verbleib unbekannt*).

Πρὸς Θρασύβουλον περὶ τῆς ἀρίστης αἱρέσεως.
De optima secta ad Thrasybulum liber.

K. I 106—223.

Inc. Ἕκαστον τῶν ἰατρικῶν θεωρημάτων.
Expl. ἀνεμποδίστως τὰς ἰδίας χρείας παρέξεται.

Florenz: Laurent. plut. 74, 3; s. XII. p. 38. (*Collation im Bezitz v. Müllers*).

Dazu:

a) cod. Adelphi (*Name unaufgeklärt*),
b) Venetus,
c) Regius (seu Bibliothecae Regis Britannici),
d) Londinensis
(*b bisher nicht identifiziert, über a c d vgl. unter* Ὅτι ὁ ἄριστ. ἰατρ. κ. φιλόσ.)

Πρὸς Πατρόφιλον περὶ συστάσεως ἰατρικῆς.
De constitutione artis medicae ad Patrophilum liber

K. I 224—304.

Inc. Ἐπεί μοι δοκεῖς, ὦ Πατρόφιλε, θεῖόν τι.
Expl. καὶ τοὺς καθ' ἕκαστον αὐτῶν σκοποὺς τῆς ἰάσεως.

Florenz: Laurent. plut. 74, 3; s. XII. p. 64b (*Collation besitzt G. Helmreich*).

[Diels I.61] Τέχνη ἰατρική.
Ars medica.

K. I 305—412.

Inc. Τρεῖς εἰσιν αἱ πᾶσαι διδασκαλίαι τάξεως ἐχόμεναι.
Expl. Γαληνοῦ περὶ τῶν ἰδίων βιβλίων.

Athos: Athous Βιβλ. μον. Ἰβήρων 4284. 164*; s. XIII (»Τάξις τῶν πραγματειῶν τοῦ Γ. κατὰ αὐτὸν ἐν τῷ τέλει τοῦ Μικρὰ τέχνη ἐπιγεγραμμένου βιβλίου«).
Bologna: Bonon. 3636; s. XIV—XV. f. 1.
Dresden: Dresdens. Da 1; s. XV. f. 24ᵛ.
Florenz: Laurent. plut. 74, 19; s. XIV. p. 11.
Kopenhagen: Hauniens. Bibl. Univ. e donatione variorum 4° 42; s. XVI.
Leipzig: Lipsiens. 55; a. 1561.
Leyden: Voss.
[16; s. —].
4° 17; s. XV.
Mailand: Ambros.
C 102 Inf.; s. — f. 128 (Expl. διὰ βάθους δεόμενα).

G 97 Sup.; s. XVI (XV). f. 56 (Inc. Εἴρηται μὲν οὖν. Expl. βιβλία ἐπιγραφὴν ἔχοντα).
Modena: Mutinens. 97 (III C 18); s. XVI.
Moskau: Mosquens. 466; s. XV. f. 251.
[**Oxford:** Bodleian. cat. mss. Angl.]
[1355.]
[1552.]
Padua: Bibl. Joannis Rhodii. (*Verbleib unbekannt*).
Paris:
Parisin.
1644; s. XV. f. 38.
1883; s. XIV. f. 36v.
2163; s. XIV.
2169; s. XVI. f. 82v.
[2175 (?)].
2265; s. XIII. f. 1.
2270; s. XV—XVI. f. 148.
2271; s. XV. f. 1.
2273; s. XV. f. 3.
2277; s. XV—XVI. f. 2.
[2278 (?)].
2285; s. XVI.
[2304 (?)].
2306; s. XV. f. 360.
2307; s. XVI. f. 554.
[2332*; s. XIV. f. 6].
2333; s. XVI.
Suppl.
496; s. XVII.
634; s. XIV. f. 75 (*Collation im Besitz Helmreichs*).
Ravenna: Ravenn. bibl. Classens. 131, 2, H; s. XV.
Rom:
Palat.
128; s. XV. f. 1.
199*; s. XIII. f. 7.
Reg. Suec. 154; s. XV. f. 1.
Vatic.
285; s. XV. f. 12.
1845*; s. XIII (Inc. γνώρισμα τῆς ἐν πνεύμονι = K. I 350, 5. Expl. τῶν ἰδίων συγγραμμάτων, *vgl.* K. I 412).
Venedig:
Marcian. 275; s. XV. f. 1.

App. cl. V 5; s. XV. f. 431ᵛ (Capita quattuor prima; expl. κατὰ τὴν ἀρετὴν τῶν ἐνεργειῶν).

Warschau: Varsoviens. Bibl. Zamoyski 142; s. XIII (?).

Wien: Vindobon. med. 8; s. XV. f. 318ᵛ (Expl. συστῆναι = K. I 312, 17).

[Diels I.63] Περὶ τῶν καθ' Ἱπποκράτην στοιχείων.

De elementis secundum Hippocratem.

K. I 413—508.

G. Helmreich Erlang. 1878.

Inc. (lib. 1) Ἐπειδὴ τὸ στοιχεῖον ἐλάχιστόν ἐστι μόριον.

Expl. (lib. 2) ὑπάρχῃ τῇ φύσει τῷ βιαίως ἑλκομένῳ.

Cambridge: Cantabrig. Caius Coll. 360; s. XVI. f. 1.

Florenz: Laurent. plut.

74, 5; s. XIV. p. 3.

74, 12*; s. XV. p. 30 (Excerpta e libro I.).

75, 14; s. XV. p. 74 (»De quinque sensibus libri II«.).

Leyden: Scal. 18; s. XVI.

Moskau: Mosquens. 466; s. XV. f. 176ᵛ.

Neapel: Neapolit. 229 III D 15; s. XIV. f. 174ᵛ (Προλεγόμενα εἰς τὸ τοῦ Γαλ. περὶ στοιχείων. Inc. Ἐπειδὴ τὰ ἀνθρώπινα σώματα).

Oxford:

Laudian. C 57 (nunc 58, Bodl. 709); s. XV in. f. 133.

[Coll. Merton. 685; s. —.]

Padua: Bibl. Joann. Rhodii. (*Verbleib unbekannt*).

Paris:

Parisin.

[1097 (?)].

1883*; s. XIV. f. 35ᵛ (»de quattuor elementis«).

2267; s. XIV. f. 255.

2283*; s. XVI.

[Diels I.64] 2317*; s. XVI. f. 21ᵛ (»de quattuor elementis«) *und* f. 43ᵛ (»de elementis et humoribus«).

[2332*; s. XV (XIV). f. 6].

Suppl.

634*; s. XIV. f. 19—21ᵛ. 25. 26. 22ʳ (»Scholia in elementa Hipp. aliosque libros continens«. Inscr. *und* Inc. *wie im Neapol. Abschrift in Helmreichs Besitz.*

Vgl. Costomiris Rev. des ét. gr. II [1889] p. 371s. Kalbfleisch, Gal. de victu attenuante p. VII[i]. VIII).
Rom: Vatic. 282; s. XVI. f. 1.
Turin: Taurin. — (»zitiert bei Montfaucon 1837 ‚Gal. de IV elementis'; nicht verifiziert«).
Venedig:
Marcian. 275; s. XV. f. 31.
[Mon. St. Michael.]

Περὶ κράσεων.
De temperamentis.

K. I 509–694.
G. Helmreich Lips. 1904.

Inc. (lib. 1) Ὅτι μὲν οὖν ἐκ θερμοῦ καὶ ψυχροῦ.
Expl. (lib. 3) κἀπὶ τῶν φαρμάκων αὐτῶν εἴρηται πρόσθεν.

Bologna: Bonon. 3636*; s. XIV—XV. f. 126 (σημεῖα κράσεως χυμῶν. Inc. Σκεπτέον ἐστὶ πάντων. Expl. κατὰ φύσιν οὐδένα τούτων ποιήσει).
Cheltenham: Phillipps. 4614; s. XV (XIV?). f. 1 (Inc. = K. I 635, 9).
Florenz: Laurent. plut. 74, 5; s. XIV. p. 17.
Leyden: Scalig. 18; s. XVI.
Mailand: Trivultian. 685; s. XIV. f. 1 (Init. mutil. inc. νοη]θῆναι = K. I 552, 4).
Moskau: Mosquens. 466; s. XV. f. 183[v].
Neapel: Neapolit. Bibl. dei Gerolamini XXII. I*; s. XV. f. 172 sq. (Inc. Τῶν κράσεων δύο εἰσὶ διαφοραί. Expl. τὸ γεῶδες τοῦ σπέρματος).
Oxford: Laudian. C 57 (nunc 58; Bodl. 709); s. XV in. f. 155b.
Padua: Bibl. Joannis Rhodii. (*Verbleib unbekannt*).
Paris:
[Coislin. ap. Montf. II 447].
Parisin.
2267; s. XIV. f. 71[v].
2283*; s. XVI.
2332*; s. XIV. f. 6.
Suppl. 634*; s. XIV. f. 22 (»Scholia in temperamenta continens«).
Rom:
Ottobon. 311; s. XVI. *hinter* f. 28.
Vatic. 282; s. XVI. f. 15.

Venedig:
Marcian. 275; s. xv. f. 56v.
App. cl. V 4; s. XV.

[Diels I.65]

Περὶ φυσικῶν δυνάμεων.
De facultatibus naturalibus.

K. II. 1—214. 14.
G. Helmreich, Gal. scr. min. III 101—257.

Inc. (lib. 1) Ἐπειδὴ τὸ μὲν αἰσθάνεσθαί τε καὶ κινεῖσθαι.
Expl. (lib. 3) ἢ παντάπασι ἐπισπῶνται βραχύν.

Cambridge: Cantabrig. Caius Coll. 360; s. XVI. p. 85.
Cheltenham: Phillipps. 4614; s. XV (XIV?). f. 15v (*Collation W. Scotts im Besitze der Akademie*).
Florenz: Laurent. plut. 74, 5; s. XIV. p. 55.
Leyden: Scalig. 18; s. XVI.
Mailand: Trivultian. 685; s. XIV. f. 29.
Modena: Mutinens. 175 (II F 10); s. XV.
Moskau: Mosquens. 466; s. XV. f. 219v.
Oxford: Laudian. C 57 (nunc 58; Bodl. 709); s. XV in. f. 208.
Padua: Bibl. Joann. Rhodii. (*Verbleib unbekannt*).
Paris:
[Coislin. ap. Montf. II 447].
Parisin. 2267; s. XV.
Rom:
Ottobon. 311*; s. XV—XVI. *hinter* f. 28 (Π. φύσεως δυνάμεων κεφάλαια).
Vatic. 282; s. XV.
Venedig: Marcian. 275; s. XV.
[**Wien:** Vindob. ap. Lambec. I 181].

[Diels I.66]

Περὶ ἀνατομικῶν ἐγχειρήσεων βιβλία ἐννέα.
De anatomicis administrationibus libri IX.

K. II 215—731.

Inc. (lib. 1) Ἀνατομικὰς ἐγχειρήσεις ἔγραψα μὲν καὶ πρόσθεν.
Expl. (lib. 9) τῇ τῆς εἰκόνος ὁμοιότητι προσαχθέντα, τοὔνομα θέσθαι.

Florenz: Laurent. plut. 74, 10*; s. XIV. p. 13 (Inc. Ἑκάστῳ τῶν ζώων).
Kopenhagen: Hauniens. ant. fund. reg. 225; s. XVI. f. 1.
Leipzig: Lipsiens. 52; s. XVI. f. 57.
Leyden:
Voss. fol. 27*; s. XVI. (Anatomica; non integrum opus. Expl. ὅλον ἐγκεφάλου τὸ καλούμενον ὑπό τινων).
Vulc. 57; s. XVI. (Expl. [l. IV] τῷ δ' ὑποτεταμένῳ τῷ μετὰ τὸ μέτωπον δέρματι μυώδη φύσιν ἐγνώκασι μὲν οἱ περὶ τὰς ἀνα ...).
Mailand: Ambros. C 80 Inf.; s. —. f. 1.
Modena: Mutinens. 226 (II H 11)*; s. XVI. f. 271 (»de anatomia internarum et externarum partium«).
Oxford: Baroccian. 204*; s. XV in. f. 2v (Inc. Ἐν πρώτῳ ἑκάστῳ = l. VI c. 1 = K. II 537, 2).
Padua: Bibl. Joannis Rhodii. (*Verbleib unbekannt*).
Paris: Parisin.
[1819 (? = 1849?)].
1849; s. XIV. f. 9.
Venedig:
Marcian. 279; s. XV. f. 1.
App. cl. V 4; s. XV. (Περὶ ἀνατομῆς τῶν ἐντὸς καὶ τῶν ἐκτός).

Περὶ ὀστῶν τοῖς εἰσαγομένοις. [Diels I.67]
De ossibus ad tirones.

K. II 732—778.

Inc. Προοίμιον. τῶν ὀστῶν ἕκαστον οἷόν τέ ἐστιν αὐτό.
Expl. καὶ εἴ τι τοιοῦτο ἕτερον, οὐκ ἀνάγκη νῦν λέγειν.

Berlin: Phillipps. 1567 (ol. Meerm. 270); s. XVI. f. 1.
Escurial: Scorial. T. III. 7; s. XIII. f. 73.
Florenz: Laurent. plut. 74, 7; s. IX. p. 262.
Grottaferrata: Cryptens. Z Γ VI (series IX cod. 46); s. XIV. f. 1.
Mailand: Ambros.
Q 87 Sup.; s. —. f. 222.
S 3 Sup.; s. —.
Paris: Parisin. Suppl.
634; s. XIV. f. 28 (*Collation in Helmreichs Besitz*).
727; s. XIX. f. 71.
765; s. XVII.

Rom: Barberin.
I 80 (= 273); s. XV. f. 1.
I 118; s. XV. f. 262.
Venedig: Venet. bibl. Andreae de Rubeis (gr.?); s. — (»G. de ossibus.« *Verbleib unbekannt*).

Περὶ φλεβῶν καὶ ἀρτηριῶν ἀνατομῆς.
De venarum arteriarumque dissectione.

K. II 779—830.

Inc. Σύνοψιν φλεβῶν καὶ ἀρτηριῶν ἀνατομῆς.
Expl. πρὶν ἄρξασθαι σχίζεσθαι.

Escurial: Scorialens. T. III. 7; s. XIII. f. 21 (Περὶ φλεβῶν. Inc. Περὶ φλεβῶν ἀνατομῆς μέλλοντες ἐξηγήσασθαι. Expl. ἐφεξῆς δὲ περὶ τῶν ἀρτηριῶν ἐροῦμεν) *und* f. 28 (Περὶ ἀρτηριῶν. Inc. Ἀρχὴ μὲν τούτων ἐστὶν ἡ ἀριστερὰ κοιλία τῆς καρδίας. Expl. κατασχίζεται εἰς τὸ πᾶν σῶμα) *ferner* f. 137v *und* 150.
Grottaferrata: Cryptens. Z Γ VI (series IX cod 46); s. XIV. f. 50.
Paris: Parisin. 2164; s. XVI. f. 76v.
Venedig:
Venet. Bibl. Josephi de Aromatariis (*Verbleib unbekannt*).
[Marcian. 279 (?)].

Περὶ νεύρων ἀνατομῆς.
De nervorum dissectione.

K. II 831—856.

Inc. Ὅτι μὲν οὐδὲν τῶν τοῦ ζῴου μορίων.
Expl. εἰς τὸ κόκκυτος ὀστοῦν καλούμενον τελευτώσας.

Escurial: Scorial. T. III. 7; s. XIII. f. 29v (Περὶ νεύρων. Inc. Ὅτι μὲν οὐδὲν τῶν τοῦ ζῴου μορίων. Expl. συμπράξαντος ἡμᾶς ἀριθμῆσαι ταῦτα) und f. 129 (Inscr. Inc. Expl. wie gewöhnlich).
Grottaferrata: Cryptens. Z Γ VI (series IX, 46); s. XIV. f. 58.
Paris: Parisin.
2164; s. XVI. f. 88.
2219; s. XV. f. 140v.

Venedig: Venet. bibl. Joseph. de Aromatariis. (Verbleib unbekannt.)

Περὶ ὀσφρήσεως ὀργάνου. [Diels I.68]
De instrumento odoratus.

K. II 857—886.

Inc. Ὄσφρησιν ὀνομάζουσιν οἱ Ἕλληνες.
Expl. καίτοι τί λέγω κοιλίας.

Florenz: Laurent. plut. 74, 3; s. XII. f. 98.
Paris: Parisin. 2164; s. XVI. f. 28.
Venedig: Marcian. App. cl. V, 4; s. XV.

Περὶ μήτρας ἀνατομῆς.
De uteri dissectione.

K. II 887—908.

Inc. Περὶ μήτρας ὁ λόγος θέσεώς τε καὶ μεγέθους.
Expl. τῷ περὶ τῆς τοῦ ἐμβρύου ἀνατομῆς.

Mailand: Ambros. C 4 Sup.; s. —. f. 222 (»Lacunae crebrae intercapedinibus indicatae sunt«).
Paris: Parisin.
2165; s. XVI. f. 177[v].
2269; s. XV. f. 165[v].
2270; s. XV—XIV. f. 84[v].
2271; s. XV. f. 128.
Rom: Vatic.
285; s. XV. f. 127.
1845; s. XIII. f. 133.
Venedig: Marcian. App. cl.
V, 5; s. XV. f. 410[v].
V, 9; s. XV. f. 145[v].

Περὶ χρείας τῶν ἐν ἀνθρώπου σώματι μορίων λόγοι ΙΖ'.
De usu partium corporis humani libri XVII.

K. III 1—IV 366.
Lib. IV ed. G. Helmreich, Augsburg 1886.

Inc. (lib. 1) Ὥσπερ τῶν ζῴων ἕκαστον ἓν εἶναι λέγεται.
Expl. (lib. 17) τὴν προσηγορίαν αὐτοῦ μετήνεγκα.

Berlin: Phillipps. 1527 (ol. Meerm. 217); s. XVI. f. 1ᵛ—2ʳ.
Cambridge: Cantabrig. Caius Coll.
47; s. XV. f. o. (Libri VI [init. mut.] — XI.).
[946; s. — (imperf.)].
Florenz: Laurent. plut.
74, 4; s. c. XII. p. 1 (*Teilweise Collation in Helmreichs Besitz*).
74, 9; s. XIV. p. 1 (*Collation des 17. B. im Besitz Helmreichs*).
74, 12*; s. XV. p. 26 (Excerpta ex libris XI. XIV. XVII.)
74, 18; s. XIV p. 1 (*Collation des 17. B. im Besitz Helmreichs*).
London:
Addit. (Brit. Mus.) 11, 888; s. XV. f. 25 (In fine epigr. inc. ἥδε βίβλος σύμπασα. expl. πλέξε φύσηϊ Θεός).
Harleian. (Brit. Mus.) 5652; s. XV vel XVI. (*Am Schlusse dasselbe Epigr. wie im* Addit. 11, 888).
Modena: Mutinens. 219 (II H 4); s. XVI. (*Am Schlusse dasselbe Epigr. wie im* Addit. Brit. Mus. 11, 888. *Collationsprobe [17. Buch] besitzt Helmreich*).
Padua: Bibl. Joann. Rhodii. (*Verbleib unbekannt*).
Paris:
Coislin. 333; s. XIV—XV. (L. I—VIII).
Parisin.
985; s. XV. f. 225 (*Collation Helmreichs in dessen Besitz*).
2148; s. XV. f. 123 (*Collation Helmreichs in dessen Besitz*).
2154; s. XIV. f. 1 (Libri III in. mut. — XVII. ἤ τινα τῶν = K. IV 359, 16. *Collation Helmreichs in dessen Besitz*).
2155; s. XIV. f. 1 (»Superest tantum pagina una«).
2253; s. XI. f. 145 (Libri X. XIV. XV. cuius una pagina superest. (*Collation Helmreichs in dessen Besitz*).
2281; s. XVI. f. 1.
2283*; s. XVI.
Rom:
Palat. 251; s. XV. f. 1.
Passioneian. 2; s. — (Libri XVI).

Urbin. 69; s. X—XI. f. 1 (Expl. f. 195ᵛ προβάλλοντες = K. 364, 19. *Collation Helmreichs in dessen Besitz*).
Vatic. 285; s. XV. f. 209 (Lib. I—III cap. 9).

Venedig:
Marcian. 287; s. XV. f. 1—155ᵛ.
App. cl.
V 9; s. XV. f. 514 (Libri III—XVII; expl. ἥλιον ἢ σελήνην ἤ τινα τῶν ...). [Diels I.69]
V 12; s. X—XIII. XV. f. 38 (unum fol. Inc. ἐνέργεια μὲν οὖν μορίου. Expl. κατασκευῆς διαλέγεται »Hat mit Galen nichts zu tun«. Helmreich. *Abschrift in Helmreichs Besitz*).

Dazu: [Mich. Cantacuzeni].

Περὶ μυῶν κινήσεως βιβλ. Β'.
De motu musculorum libri II.

K. IV 367–464.

Inc. (lib. 1) Ὄργανα κινήσεως τῆς καθ' ὁρμὴν οἱ μύες.
Expl. (lib. 2) τὰ κατὰ μέρος ἐξευρίσκειν δυνήσεται.

Escurial: Scorial. T. III. 7; s. XIII. f. 34. 57v.
Florenz: Laurent. plut. 74, 3; s. XII. p. 192 (Pars l. I = K. IV 367—371, 4).
Modena: Mutinens. 237 (III G 18); s. XVI. f. 249.
Paris: Parisin.
1849; s. XIV. f. 95.
2164; s. XVI. f. 91.
2278; s. XVI. f. 1 (Libri II in fine mut.).
Rom: Reg. Suec. 175; s. XIV. f. 242.
Venedig:
Marcian. 279; s. XV. f. 71—84v.
App. cl. V, 5; s. XV. f. 433v (Expl. ταῖς ἡμέραις ὁ ἄνθρωπος = K. IV 443).

Περὶ τῶν τῆς ἀναπνοῆς αἰτίων. [Diels I.70]
De causis respirationis.

K. IV 465—469.

Inc. Τὰ τῆς ἀναπνοῆς αἴτια ὁ προκείμενος.

Expl. ὥσπερ ἡ νίκη τῆς ἡνιοχικῆς.

Modena: Mutinens. 237 (III G 18); s. XVI. f. 247v.
Paris: Parisin. 2165; s. XVI. f. 187.
Rom: Reg. Suec. 175; s. XIV. f. 240v.
Venedig:
Bibl. Josephi de Aromatariis. (*Verbleib unbekannt*).
Marcian. 276; s. XII. f. 268 (Expl. εἶθ' ἑκάτερον αὐτῶν = K. IV 468, 6).
App. cl. V 5; s. XV. f. 433.

Περὶ χρείας ἀναπνοῆς.
De respirationis usu.

K. IV 470—511.

Inc. Τίς ἡ τῆς ἀναπνοῆς χρεία; ὅτι γὰρ οὐχ ἡ τυχοῦσα.
Expl. ἕκαστον τῶν ἐνταυθοῖ γεγραμμένων ἐκλεξαμένοις.

Florenz: Laurent. plut. 74, 5 s. XIV. p. 94b.
Paris: Parisin. Suppl. 35; s. XV—XVI. f. 132v.
Venedig: Marcian. 281; s. XV. f. 77v—81v.

Περὶ σπέρματος βιβλ. Β'.
De semine libri II.

K. IV 512—651.

Inc. (lib. 1) Τίς ἡ χρεία καὶ τίς ἡ δύναμίς ἐστι τοῦ σπέρματος.
Expl. (lib. 2) καθάπερ ἡμεῖς ἀρτίως ἐνεδείξαμεν.

Moskau: Mosquens. 466; s. XVI. f. 143.
Oxford: Miscell. 20; s. XIV. f. 375 (de spermate ex Aristotele et Galeno. Inc. Καὶ τὸ γεννητικόν).
Paris: Parisin. 2279; s. XVI. f. 155v.

Περὶ κυουμένων διαπλάσεως.
De foetuum formatione.

K. IV 652—702.

Inc. Περὶ τῆς τῶν κυουμένων διαπλάσεως ἐπεχείρησαν.
Expl. τῆς ψυχῆς πραγματείᾳ διῆλθον.

Bologna: Bonon. 3637; s. XIV. f. 2 (Περὶ τῆς τοῦ ἀνθρώπου διαπλάσεως).
Florenz: Laurent. plut.
59, 14; s. XV. p. 213.
74, 3; s. XII. p. 80b.
Paris: Parisin. 2164; s. XVI. f. 1.
Venedig:
Bibl. Josephi de Aromatariis (»Gal. de conformatione fetus«. *Verbleib unbekannt*).
Marcian. App. cl. V, 4; s. XV.

Εἰ κατὰ φύσιν ἐν ἀρτηρίαις αἷμα περιέχεται. [Diels I.71]
An in arteriis natura sanguis contineatur.

K. IV 703—736.

Inc. Ἐπειδὴ τιτρωσκομένης ἀρτηρίας ἡστινοσοῦν.
Expl. ἃ δὴ ἰδεῖν ἦν ἀδύνατον.

Florenz: Laurent. plut. 74, 3; s. XII. p. 91.
Venedig: Marcian. App. cl. V, 4; s. XV.

Περὶ ἀρίστης κατασκευῆς τοῦ σώματος ἡμῶν.
De optima corporis nostri constitutione.

K. IV 737—749.
G. Helmreich, Hof 1901.

Inc. Τίς ἡ ἀρίστη κατασκευὴ τοῦ σώματος ἡμῶν; ἆρά γε ἡ εὐκρατοτάτη.
Expl. συμμετρίᾳ δὲ τῶν ὀργανικῶν.

Cheltenham: Phillipps. 4614; s. XV (XIV) nr. 5.
Hamburg: Uffenbach. 105; s. —. no. 2.

Mailand: Trivultian. 685; s. XV (XIV). f. 75—81.
Modena: Mutinens. 109 (II D 10); s. XIV—XV. f. 69.
Moskau: Mosquens.
465; s. XV. f. 1.
466; s. XVI. f. 84.
Paris: Parisin. 2283*; s. XVI.
Venedig: Marcian. 282; s. XV.

Περὶ εὐεξίας.
De bono habitu.

K. IV 750—756.
Helmreich. Hof 1901.

Inc. Τὸ τῆς ἕξεως ὄνομα κατὰ παντὸς ἐπιφέρειν εἰθίσμεθα.
Expl. ἐπειδὰν ἀπορῶσιν εἰς ἀνάψυξιν διαπνοῆς.

Cheltenham: Phillips. 4614; s. XV (XIV). f. 60.
Mailand: Trivultian. 685; s. XV (XIV). f. 81.
Modena: Mutinens. 109 (II D 10); s. XIV—XV. f. 71ᵛ.
Moskau: Mosquens.
465; s. XV. f. 3ᵛ.
466; s. XVI. f. 87.
Paris: Parisin. 2283*; s. XVI.
Venedig: Marcian. 282; s. XV.

[Diels I.72]

Περὶ οὐσίας τῶν φυσικῶν δυνάμεων.
De substantia facultatum naturalium fragmentum.

K. IV 757—766.
Vgl. unter Περὶ τῶν ἑαυτῷ δοκούντων.

Inc. Καί τις ἴσως δόξει διαφωνίας ἀξιόλογον εἶναι.
Expl. ὅθεν οὐδὲ ὁ Πλάτων αὐτῆς ἐμνημόνευσεν.

Florenz: Laurent. plut. 74, 5; s. XIV. p. 91 (*Collation besitzt Helmreich*).
Mailand: Ambros. Q 3 Sup.; s. XV—XVI. f. 185ᵛ. (Inc. ὥσπερ ὅτι ψυχὴν ἔχομεν = K. IV 760, 3. Subscr. *als Titel* Περὶ τῶν ἑαυτῷ δοκούντων. *Collation Kalbfleischs in dessen Besitz*).

Paris: Parisin. Suppl. 35; s. XV—XVI. f. 129.
Venedig: Marcian. 281; s. XV. f. 75v—76v (Inc. *wie im* Ambros. *Eigne Collation besitzt Helmreich, Plasbergs Collation besitzt Kalbfleisch*).

Dazu: cod. Londinensis; cod. Adelphi. (*Vgl. unter* Ὅτι ὁ ἄριστ. ἰατρ. κ. φιλόσ.)

Ὅτι τὰ τῆς ψυχῆς ἤθη ταῖς τοῦ σώματος κράσεσιν ἕπεται.
Quod animi mores corporis temperamenta sequantur.

K. IV 767—822.
Jw. Müller Erlang. 1880. 85. 86.
Gal. scr. min. II 32—79.

Inc. Ταῖς τοῦ σώματος κράσεσιν ἕπεσθαι.
Expl. τοιοῦτοι δ' Ἀθήνησιν ὀλίγοι.

Florenz: Laurent. plut. 56, 15; s. XV. p. 141.
Moskau: Mosquens.
260; a. 1630. f. 202.
292; s. XVII.
München: Monacens. 109; s. XVI. f. 50 (fine mutil.)
Oxford: Baroccian. 131*; s. XIV in. f. 477b (Expl. μὴ ποιήσῃς τόδε).
Paris: Coislin. 336; s. XVI. f. 98v.
Rom:
Reg. Suec. 154; s. XV. f. 41.
Vallicell. 21 (B 93); s. XIV. f. 65v.
Vatic. 154; s. XVI.
Wien: Vindobon. phil. 303; s. XVI. f. 250—279v.
Zeitz: Cizens. 66; s. XVI. f. 100—116.

Dazu:
cod. Londinensis;
cod. Adelphi. (*Vgl. unter* Ὅτι ὁ ἄριστ. ἰατρ. κ. φιλόσ.)

Περὶ διαγνώσεως καὶ θεραπείας τῶν ἐν τῇ ἑκάστου ψυχῇ ἰδίων παθῶν.
De propriorum animi cuiuslibet affectuum dignotione et curatione.

K. V 1—57.
Marquardt, Gal. scr. min. I 1—44).

Inc. Ἐπειδὴ καὶ δι' ὑπομνημάτων ἔχειν.
Expl. τῶν ἁμαρτημάτων ἐφεξῆς εἰρήσεται.

Bern: Bernens. 691*; s. XV—XVI. f. 80—81 (Inc. Οὐ φαίνεσθαι χρὴ τοῖς τοιούτοις. Expl. ἀπὸ στόματος ὕστερον).
Florenz: Laurent. plut. 74, 3; s. XII. p. 159b. (*Coll. H. Schoenes in dessen Besitz*).
Oxford: Bodleian. Is. Casauboni Advers. 4; f. 2.
[Diels I.73] **Upsala:** nr. 25*; s. XVI. f. 39v (Inc. *und* Expl. *wie im* Bernens. 691).
Venedig: Marcian. 281; s. XV.
Wolfenbüttel: Helmstad. 757. 837; s. XVI.

Dazu:
cod. Adelphi;
cod. Londinensis. (*Vgl. unter* Ὅτι ὁ ἄριστ. ἰατρ. κ. φιλόσ.).

Περὶ διαγνώσεως καὶ θεραπείας τῶν ἐν τῇ ἑκάστου ψυχῇ ἁμαρτημάτων.
De cuiuslibet animi peccatorum dignotione atque medela.

K. V 58—103.
Marquardt, Gal. scr. min. I 45—81.

Inc. Ἡ μὲν δὴ τῶν παθῶν ἐν ἑκάστου ψυχῇ.
Expl. πρὸς τὸ παρὸν ἀρκείσθω.

Florenz: Laurent. plut.
74, 3; s. XII. p. 149b. (*Collat. H. Schoenes in dessen Besitz*).
74, 5; s. XIV. p. 92b.
Paris: Parisin. Suppl. 35; s. XV—XVI. f. 130v.
Venedig: Marcian. 281; s. XV. f. 76v—77 (Expl. νῦν εἶναι μόνην).

Περὶ μελαίνης χολῆς.
De atra bile.

K. V 104—148.

Inc. Περὶ μελαίνης χολῆς ἔνιοι μὲν ἐπὶ πλέον.
Expl. τὴν Ἱπποκράτους γνώμην σοφιζομένων.

Escurial: Scorial. III. R. 3*; s. XI. f. 138 (Ἀντίδοτον Γαλ. ... ὠφελοῦν εἰς τὴν μέλαιναν χολὴν καὶ εἰς τὴν ξανθήν. Expl. ἔχεις καὶ θέλης. ἐστὶν γὰρ ὠφελιμώτατον).
Mailand: Ambros. Q 3 Sup.; s. XV—XVI. f. 231.
Modena: Mutinens. 213; s. XV. f. 161v.
Moskau: Mosquens. 467; s. XVI. f. 96.
Paris: Parisin.
2166; s. XV—XVI. f. 73v.
2269; s. XV. f. 201v.
2270; s. XV—XIV. f. 104v.
2271; s. XV. f. 142v.
2283*; s. XVI.
2332*; s. XIV.
Rom:
Urbin. 70*; s. XV. f. 107 (*Unter demselben Titel wie im* Marc. 279).
Vatic.
285; s. XV. f. 139.
1845; s. XIII. f. 152.
Venedig:
Marcian.
276; s. XII. f. 261.
279*; s. XV. f. 269v—271 (Περὶ μελαγχολίας ἐκ τῶν Γαλ. καὶ Ῥούφου καὶ Ποσειδωνίου, in marg. τοῦ Ἀετίου. Inc. Ὥσπερ ἐν τοῖς φαινομένοις μέλεσιν. Expl. στυπτηρίαν ἐπιπάσομεν τῷ ὄξει).
282; s. XV.
284; s. XV.
App. cl.
V, 5; s. XV. f. 322 *und* f. 416.
V, 9; s. XV. f. 155.

Περὶ χρείας σφυγμῶν.
De usu pulsuum.

K. V 149—180.

Inc. Τίς ἡ χρεία τῶν σφυγμῶν; ἆρά γε ἥπερ.
Expl. Ζητεῖται τῶν ἐνεργειῶν, ἐξευρίσκειν.

Cambridge: Cantabrig. Caius Coll. 355; s. XV/XVI. f. 135.
Escurial: Scorial. Φ III 11; s. XIV. XV. f. 16.

[Diels I.74]

Περὶ τῶν Ἱπποκράτους καὶ Πλάτωνος δογμάτων βιβλία Θ'.
De placitis Hippocratis et Platonis libri IX.

K. V 181—805.
Iw. Müller Lips. 1874.

Inc. (lib. 1 [*im Eingange verstümmelt*) ... τὸ πάμπαν · ἀλλὰ κἀκείνου τὸ συνεχὲς τῷ στέρνῳ διεσεσήπει.
Expl. (lib. 9) ἐν τῇ προειρημένῃ πραγματείᾳ διῆλθον.

Berlin: Hamilton. 270 (401); s. XIII (*Collation bei Petersen diss. Gotting. 1888; vgl. E. Wellmann Rhein. Mus. 40, 30 ff., Kalbfleisch diss. Berol. 1892*).
Cambridge: Cantabrig. Caius Coll. 47; s. XV. no. 111.
Florenz: Laurent. plut.
74, 12*; s. XV. p. 1 (Inc. Εἰ γὰρ ἐν τῷ διανοεῖσθαι).
74, 22; s. XIV. p. 15 (Fragmenta libr. II. III. V. VI.).
Moskau: Mosquens. 467; s. XVI. f. 1 (Libri II—IX).
Paris: Parisin.
2277*; s. XV—XVI. f. 111 (Exc. ex libr. II—IX. Inc. *wie im* Laurent. 74, 12. Expl. ὡς χείροσι τοῦ λογιστικοῦ).
[2278 (? L. II—IX)].
2283*; s. XVI.
Venedig:
Marcian. 284; s. XV. (»Libri VII sine primo«).
Bibl. monaster. S. Michaelis Venet. prope Murianum 132; s. — (Libri VII; desunt primus et initium secundi libri. *Verbleib unbekannt*).

Θρασύβουλος [πότερον ἰατρικῆς ἢ γυμναστικῆς ἐστι τὸ ὑγιεινόν].
Thrasybulus sive utrum medicinae sit an gymnastices hygieine.

K. V 806—898).
G. Helmreich Gal. scr. min. III 33—100.

Inc. Οὐκ ἄλλα μέν, ὦ Θρασύβουλε, παραχρῆμα.
Expl. καὶ φιλοσόφων ἀτιμαζομένου;

Florenz: Laurent. plut. 74, 3; s. XII. f. 110v.
Paris: Parisin. 2164; s. XVI. f. 56.
Venedig: Marcian. App. cl. V, 4; s. XV. f. 256.

Περὶ τοῦ διὰ τῆς σμικρᾶς σφαίρας γυμνασίου.
De parvae pilae exercitio.

K. V 899—910.
Helmreich Augsb. 1878.
Marquardt, Gal. scr. min. I 93—102.

Inc. Πηλίκον ἀγαθόν ἐστιν εἰς ὑγίειαν.
Expl. πρὸς ὠφέλειαν ἄριστα παρεσκευασμένα.

Florenz: Laurent. plut. 74, 3; s. XII. f. 134^{v}.
Mailand: Ambros. Q 3 Sup.; s. XV—XVI. f. 200.
Moskau: Mosquens. 467; s. XVI. f. 102^{v}.
Paris:
Parisin. 2164; s. XVI. f. 37^{v}.
Suppl. 35; s. XV—XVI. f. 98^{v}.
Venedig:
Marcian.
276; s. c. XII. f. 269.
282; s. XV. f. 199^{v}—200^{v}.
284; s. XV.
App. cl. V, 4; s. XV. f. 242 (*H. Schoenes Collationen sämtlicher bekannter Hdss. in dessen Besitz*).

Περὶ ἀφροδισίων. [Diels I.75]
De venereis.

K. V 911—914.

Inc. Ἀφροδισίων μὲν κατὰ μὲν Ἐπίκουρον οὐδεμία χρῆσις.
Expl. καὶ τούτους εἶναι σκοποὺς ἐπ' αὐτοῖς.

Paris: Parisin. 2240*; s. XVI. f. 146^{v}.

Ὑγιεινῶν λόγοι ΣΤ'.
De sanitate tuenda libri VI.

K. VI 1—452.

Inc. (lib. 1) Τῆς περὶ τὸ σῶμα τἀνθρώπου τέχνης.
Expl. (lib. 6) ἕτερος ἐπ' αὐτοῖς εἰρήσεται λόγος.

Berlin: Phillipps. 1566 (ol. Meerm. 269)*; s. XVI. (= K. VI 281 sq.).
Leipzig: Lipsiens. 50; s. XVI. f. 132.
London: Harleian. (Brit. Mus.) 5626*; s. XV—XVI. f. 53ᵛ (Ἐκ τῶν ὑγιεινῶν τοῦ Γαλ. προοίμιον, τί ἐστιν ὑγεία καὶ τίνες οἱ ἄριστα κατεσκευασμένοι. Inc. Τῆς περὶ τὸ σῶμα κτλ. Expl. δίαιτα λεπτύνουσα καὶ χρίσματα μετρίως θερμαίνοντα).
Paris: Parisin.
2172; s. XVI. (fine mutil.)
2283*; s. XVI.
Rom: Reg. Suec. 173; s. XV. f. 233.
Venedig: Marcian.
276; s. XII.
282; s. XV. f. 3.

[Diels I.76]

Περὶ τροφῶν δυνάμεως βιβλία Γ'.
De alimentorum facultatibus libri III.

K. VI 453—748.
Helmreich. Ansbach 1905. Lib. I c. 1—13.

Inc. (lib. 1) Περὶ τῶν ἐν ταῖς τροφαῖς δυνάμεων.
Expl. (lib. 3) ἐν οἷς ἐκ πολλοῦ διατρίβουσιν.

Cheltenham: Phillipps. 4614; s. XV (XIV). f. 141.
Mailand: Ambros. B 108 Sup.; s. XIV in. f. 19 (Libri III = K. VI 533, 9—745, 15/16).
Modena: Mutinens. 217 (II H 2); s. XVI. f. 42 (A lib. I 2 = K. VI 483, 13 usque ad cap. περὶ καθαρτηρίων).
München: Monac. 39*; s. XVI. f. 86 (Γαλ. προοίμιον περὶ τροφῶν δυνάμεως κατὰ στοιχεῖον. Inc. Πολλῶν καὶ λογίων, ὦ μέγιστε βασιλεῦ) *und* f. 121 (Inc. Περὶ πυρῶν ἤτοι ἄρτων).
Oxford: Baroccian. 264*; s. XV in. f. 51b (Ἐκ τοῦ γ' λόγου τοῦ περὶ τροφῶν) *und* f. 54b (Exc. e l. III capp. 27—30. 33. 34. 36. 37. 40—44. 52. 62. 68—71).
Paris:
Parisin.
1883; s. XIV. f. 156ᵛ (Libri II).
2164; s. XVI. f. 111.
2167; s. XVI. f. 1 (Libri II, init. et fin. mut.).
2173; s. XVI. f. 6.

Suppl.
634; s. XIV. f. 142 (*Collation besitzt Helmreich*).
764; s. XIV. f. 151.

Rom:
Palat. 199; s. XIII. f. 84 (Libri II. In fine catal. herbar. purgantium).
Urbin. 70; s. XV. f. 1 (Inc. a l. I c. 7; in fine addit. remedium π. καθαρτηρίων. *Collationsprobe = K. VI 523—553 besitzt Helmreich*).
Vatic. lat. 5763; s. V—VI. f. 30v (*Palimpsest; vgl. Sitz. Ber. d. Berl. Ak. 1902 p. 442 f.* Inc. ἔλλοβα = K. VI 557, 11. Expl. οὐ μὴν ἐπί γε = K. VI 559, 4).

Turin: Taurinens. B I 6 (6b IV 6); s. XVI. f. 191 *und* 230v (*Wie im* Monac. 39 f. 86).

Venedig:
Marcian. 279; s. XV. f. 205—243.
App. cl. V, 11; s. XVI. f. 1 (Inc. mut. = K. VI 483, 13).

Wolfenbüttel: Weissenb. 64; s. V—VI. f. 43—57. 67—74. 82—89. 98—105. 114—137. 146—153. 162—169. 186—193. 218—225. 268—270. 273—275. 305—310 (*Palimpsest*).

Περὶ εὐχυμίας καὶ κακοχυμίας τροφῶν. [Diels I.77]
De probis pravisque alimentorum sucis.

K. VI 749—815.

Inc. Οἱ *συνεχῶς ἐτῶν οὐκ ὀλίγων*.
Expl. *αὖθις ἐμπίπτειν, ἀπεργάζονται*.

Florenz: Laurent. plut. 74, 25; s. XIV. p. 153.
London: Stowe (Brit. Mus.) 1073; s. XVI. f. 98v.
Oxford: Miscell. 132; s. XVI. f. 93b.
Paris:
Parisin. 2164; s. XVI. f. 169.
Suppl. 634; s. XIV. f. 117 (*Collation besitzt Helmreich*).
Venedig: Marcian. 285; s. XV. f. 244.

Περὶ πτισάνης.
De ptisana.

K. VI 816—831.

Inc. Ἐπειδὴ πρὸ μικροῦ τινας εὗρον.

Expl. καὶ τοὺς ἀναγκαίους διορισμούς.

Paris: Parisin. 2267; s. XIV. f. 63.
Rom: Reg. Suec. 173; s. XV. f. 355v.

Περὶ τῆς ἐξ ἐνυπνίων διαγνώσεως.
De dignotione ex insomniis.

K. VI 77 832—835.

Inc. Τὸ ἐνύπνιον δὲ ἡμῖν ἐνδείκνυται.
Expl. καί ποιότητας χυμῶν.

Florenz: Riccard. 44 (K II 5); s. XV—XVI. f. 242.
Leyden: Voss. 4° 45; s. XIV.
Mailand: Ambros. A 156 Sup.; s. XVI. f. 263.
Modena: Mutinens. 213 (III G 9); s. XV. f. 154.
Moskau: Mosquens. 395; s. XVI—XVII. f. 2v.
[Diels I.78] **Oxford:** Miscell. 130; s. XVII. p. 327.
Paris: Parisin.
2165; s. XVI. f. 195.
2269; s. XV. f. 174.
2276; s. XVI. f. 179v.
Rom: Vatic.
283; s. XIV. f. 1 *und* 12.
285 s. XV. f. 202v.
1063; s. XIII. f. 107v.
Venedig: Marcian. cl. V, 5; s. XV. f. 332v.
Wien: Vindobon. med. 30*; s. XV.

Περὶ διαφορᾶς νοσημάτων.
De differentiis morborum.

K. VI 836—880.

Inc. Πρῶτον μὲν εἰπεῖν χρή, τί ποτε νόσημα καλοῦμεν.
Expl. ἐν αὐτοῖς ἐπὶ πλεῖστον γυμνάζεσθαι.

Athen: nr. 1491; s. XVIII. no. 1.

Berlin: Phillipps. 1991 (ol. Meerm. 218); s. XVI. f. 2 (Inc. Τὸ δὲ στέγνωσις = K. VI 842, 2).
Escurial: Scorial. Φ. III. 11*; s. XIV. XV. f. 71.
Florenz: Laurent. plut. 74, 16; s. XIV. p. 1.
Leyden:
Scalig. 18 (?); s. XVI.
Voss. 4° 45; s. XIV.
Mailand: Ambros. G 97 Sup.*; s. XVI (XV). f. 1.
Modena: Mutinens. 237 (III G 18); s. XVI. f. 273.
Paris: Parisin.
2157; s. XV. f. 369.
2167; s. XVI. f. 223.
2169; s. XVI. f. 1.
2283*; s. XVI. f. —.
2316; s. XV. f. 215 (De morborum formis).
2332*; s. XIV. f. 6.
Venedig:
Marcian. 275; s. c. XV. f. 176^{v}.
App. cl. V 4; s. XV.

Περὶ τῶν ἐν τοῖς νοσήμασιν αἰτίων.
De morborum causis.

K. VII 1—41.

Inc. Πόσα μέν ἐστι καὶ τίνα τὰ σύμπαντα νοσήματα κατ' εἴδη.
Expl. τῆς τῶν συμπτωμάτων διαφορᾶς ἐφεξῆς διελθεῖν.

Athen: nr. 1491; s. XVIII. no. 2.
Berlin: Phillipps. 1991 (ol. Meerm. 218); s. XVI. f. 13^{v} (Inscr. Συμπτωμάτων (superscriptum: νοσημάτων) διαφορᾶς λόγος β').
Escurial: Scorial. Φ. III. 11*; s. XIV. XV. f. 73 (Π. αἰτίας νοσημάτων).
Florenz: Laurent. plut. 74, 16; s. XIV. p. 8b.
Leyden: Scalig. 18; s. XVI.
Mailand: Ambros. G 97 Sup.*; s. XVI (XV). f. 8.
Modena: Mutinens. 237 (III G 18); s. XVI. post f. 273.
Oxford: Baroccian. 131*; s. XIV. f. 341 (Προθεωρία Γαλ. τῆς περὶ αἰτίας διαφόρων νοσημάτων · ἀρχὴ οὖν καὶ κρηπὶς πάσης τῆς ἰατρικῆς τέχνης. Inc. Ὑπὲρ αἰτίας θεωρία. Expl. ὑποκειμένου χρήσομεν—).

[Diels I.79] **Paris:** Parisin.
2157; s. XV. f. 376.
2167; s. XVI. f. 235^{v}.
2169; s. XVI. f. 11^{v}.
2283*; s. XVI.
2332*; s. XIV. f. 6.
Venedig:
Marcian. 275; s. c. XV. f. 190.
App. cl.
V, 4; s. XV.
V, 12; s. X—XIII. XV. f. 144^{v} (Inscr. Περὶ αἰτίας παθῶν).
Wien: Vindob. 131*; s. —.

Περὶ τῆς τῶν συμπτωμάτων διαφορᾶς.
De symptomatum differentiis.

K. VII 42—84.

Inc. Τίνα μέν ἐστι καὶ πόσα τὰ σύμπαντα.
Expl. τῇ τῶν ἀμφισβητουμένων κρίσει.

Athen: nr. 1491; s. XVIII. no. 3.
Berlin: Phillipps. 1991 (ol. Meerm. 218); s. XVI. f. 27^{v}.
Cambridge: Cantabrig. Caius Coll. 355; s. XV/XVI. f. 1.
Escurial: Scorial.
Σ. II. 5; s. XV. f. 8 (Expl. εἰρήσεται κατὰ τὸν ἑξῆς λόγον).
Φ. III. 11*; s. XIV. XV. f. 73^{v}.
Florenz: Laurent. plut. 74, 16; s. XIV. p. 15b.
Leyden:
Scalig. 18; s. XVI.
[Vossian. ?; s. —].
Mailand: Ambros.
G 97 Sup.*; s. XVI (XV). f. 15.
Q 3 Sup.; s. XV—XVI. f. 1.
Modena: Mutinens. 237 (III G 18); s. XVI. f. 298^{v}.
Moskau: Mosquens. 466; s. XVI. f. 460.
Paris: Parisin.
2157; s. XV. f. 383.
2165; s. XVI. f. 203.
2169; s. XVI. f. 22.

2283*; s. XVI.
2332*; s. XV. f. 6.

Venedig:
Marcian. 275; s. c. XV. f. 202v.
App. cl. V, 4; s. XV.

Περὶ αἰτίων συμπτωμάτων βιβλία Γ'.
De symptomatum causis libri III.

K. VII 85—272.

Inc. (lib. 1) Τὰς αἰτίας τῶν συμπτωμάτων.
Expl. (lib. 3) ἐνταυθοῖ καταπαύσω τὸν λόγον.

Athen: nr. 1491; s. XVIII. no. 4. 5.
Berlin: Phillipps. 1991 (ol. Meerm. 218); s. XVI. f. 41v.
Cambridge: Cantabrig. Caius Coll. 355; s. XV/XVI. f. 17.
Escurial: Scorial.
Σ. II. 5; s. XVI. f. 25.
Φ. III. 11*; s. XIV. XV. f. 76v *und* 78 (Ex libr. II et III).
Florenz: Laurent. plut.
74, 12*; s. XV. p. 30 (E libro II).
74, 16; s. XIV. p. 19b.
Leipzig: Lipsiens. 51; s. —. f. 1 (Libri I et II).
Leyden:
Scalig. 18; s. XVI.
Voss. fol. 11; s. XVI.
Mailand: Ambros.
G 97 Sup.*; s. XVI (XV). f. 22.
Q 3 Sup.; s. XV—XVI. [Diels I.80]
Paris: Parisin.
1949*; s. XV. f. 418v.
2157; s. XV. f. 390v.
2165; s. XVI. f. 213.
2169; s. XVI. f. 32v.
2283*; s. XVI.
2284; s. XVI.
Venedig:
Marcian. 275; s. c. XV. f. 215.

App. cl.
V, 4; s. XV.
V, 5; s. XV. f. 313.

Περὶ διαφορᾶς πυρετῶν βιβλία Β'.
De differentiis febrium libri II.

K. VII 273—405.

Inc. (lib. 1) Αἱ διαφοραὶ τῶν πυρετῶν αἱ μὲν οἰκειόταται.
Expl. (lib. 2) ἤ τι συναμφότερον πάθωσιν.

Bologna: Bonon. 3632*; s. XV. f. 132 (Exc. de febrium differentiis [?]).
Cambridge: Cantabrig. Caius Coll.
76; s. XV/XVI. f. 142 (Frgm. l. I ex. Inc. προεξηρασμένον τὸ τῆς καρδίας σῶμα. Expl. πυρετῶν ἁπάσας ἐροῦμεν διαφοράς) *und* f. 143.
[949; s. —].
Florenz: Laurent. plut. 75, 14; s. XV. p. 20.
Modena: Mutinens. 237 (III G 18); s. XVI. f. 368 (Quaedam de febribus. Inc. ἔοικεν ὁ ἑκτικὸς πυρετός).
Paris:
Coislin. 334; s. XV. f. 10.
Parisin.
985; s. XV. f. 26.
1883; s. XIV. f. 47v.
2155; s. XIV. f. 307 (Init. et fine mut.).
2156; s. XV. f. 1.
[2157 (?)].
2158; s. XV. f. 1.
2167; s. XVI. f. 188 *und* 202 (de febrium causis).
2178*; s. XV. f. 11v (Exc. de febrium differentiis).
2246; s. XVI. f. 71.
2260; s. XVI. f. 138.
2267; s. XIV. f. 1.
2269*; s. XV. f. 163 (de febri semitertiana).
2272; s. XV. f. 1.
2276; s. XVI. f. 147.
2283*; s. XVI.
2332; s. XIV (XV). f. 401 (de febribus liber I).
Suppl. 446; s. X. f. 31v (de febri).

Rom:
Ottobon. 311; s. XV—XVI. f. 28.
Palat.
54; s. XV—XVI. f. 341.
157*; s. XIV. f. 1 (frgm. de febribus).
400*; s. XV. f. 7 (Inc. Ἱπποκράτης ὁ διδάσκαλος ἡμῶν).
Vatic. 285; s. XV. f. 153.
Venedig: Marcian. 282; s. XV. f. 85v.
[**Wien:**]
[Vindob. ap. Nessel III 27 (?) no. 5].
[38 (?)].

Περὶ τῶν ἐν ταῖς νόσοις καιρῶν. *De morborum temporibus.*

[Diels I.81]

K. VII 33 406—439.

Inc. Οἷόν τι τοῖς ζῴοις ἐστὶν ἡ κατὰ τὰς ἡλικίας διαφορά.
Expl. ἄχρι μὲν γὰρ τοῦδε τοὺς ἐν μέρει διῆλθον μόνους.

[**Florenz:** Laurent. plut. 74, (?)].
Modena: Mutinens. 218 (II H 3); s. XVI. f. 102.
Paris:
Parisin.
2271; s. XV. f. 75.
2283*; s. XVI.
Suppl. 35; s. XV—XVI. f. 110v.
Rom:
Palat. 143; s. XV. f. 172.
Vatic.
285; s. XV. f. 81 (Περὶ τῶν ἐν παροξυσμοῖς καιρῶν).
1845; s. XIII. f. 106 (Inscr. *wie im* Vatic. 285).
Venedig:
Marcian. 282; s. XV. f. 3.
App. cl.
V, 5; s. XV. f. 403 (Inscr. *wie im* Vatic. 285).
V, 9; s. XV. f. 131.

Περὶ τῶν ὅλου τοῦ νοσήματος καιρῶν.
De totius morbi temporibus.

K. VII 440—462.

Inc. Ὅλου τοίνυν τοῦ νοσήματος ἐπινοοῦμεν.
Expl. τοὺς ἀναγινώσκοντας αὐτοῦ τὰ βιβλία.

Escurial: Scorialens. Σ. I. 12; s. XVI. f. 68 (fine mutil. expl. εἰς δύο τὰ πάντα παροξυσμούς).
Florenz: Laurent. plut. 74, 5; s. XIV. p. 121.
Paris:
Parisin.
[2170 (?)]
2269; s. XV. f. 183.
2270; s. XV—XIV. f. 71.
[2272 (?)].
Suppl. 35; s. XV—XVI. f. 121.
Rom: Vatic.
285; s. XV. f. 92.
1845; s. XIII. f. 122ᵛ.
Venedig:
Marcian. 281; s. XV. f. 89.
App. cl.
V́, 5; s. XV. f. 407.
V, 9; s. XV. f. 139ᵛ.

[Diels I.82] Περὶ τύπων.
De typis.

K. VII 463—474.

Inc. Πολλῶν πλατυτέρω (sic) ὑπὲρ τῆς περὶ τύπων.
Expl. καὶ ἑξῆς κύκλος ὁμοίως.

Escurial: Scorialens. Φ. III. 11; s. XIV. XV. f. 43ᵛ.
Florenz: Laurent. plut.
59, 14; s. XV. p. 97.
74, 11*; s. XIII. p. 163 (Inc. Πολλῶν δὴ πλατύτερον).
74, 31; s. XIV. p. 208.

[**Paris:** Parisin.]
[2170 (?)].
[2269 (?)].
[2272 (?)].

Πρὸς τοὺς περὶ τύπων γράψαντας, ἢ περὶ περιόδων.

K. VII 475—512.

Inc. Τοῖς μὲν παλαιοῖς ἰατροῖς ἀπόχρη μόνον.
Expl. ὡς φείδεσθαι προσήκει χρόνου.

Mailand: Ambros. Q 3 Sup.; s. XV—XVI. f. 212.
Paris: Parisin. 2170; s. XVI. f. 248.

Περὶ πλήθους.
De plenitudine.

K. VII 513—583.

Inc. Οὔτε πολλάκις ὀνομάζοντες ἕτερον ὄνομα.
Expl. οἱ δ' ἀραιοὶ σπανιώτερον.

Mailand: Ambros. Q 3 Sup.; s. XV—XVI. f. 238.
Modena: Mutinens. 213 (III G 9); s. XV. f. 175.
Paris: Parisin.
2165; s. XVI. f. 164.
2166; s. XV—XVI. f. 51.
Venedig: Marcian. App. cl. V, 5; s. XV. f. 394^{v}.

Περὶ τρόμου καὶ παλμοῦ καὶ σπασμοῦ καὶ ῥίγους.
De tremore, palpitatione, convulsione et rigore.

K. VII 584—642.

Inc. Ἐπειδὴ Πραξαγόρας ὁ Νικάρχου.
Expl. τοῖς τῆς θεραπευτικῆς μεθόδου γράμμασιν.

Florenz: Laurent. plut. 74, 12*; s. XV. p. 28 (brevissimum frgm.).
Paris:
Parisin.
2269; s. XV. f. 219.
2270; s. XV—XIV. f. 124.
2271; s. XV. f. 107ᵛ.
2283*; s. XVI.
Suppl. 35; s. XV—XVI. f. 77.
Rom: Vatic.
285; s. XV. f. 110.
1845; s. XIII. f. 171ᵛ.
Venedig:
Marcian. 282; s. XV.
App. cl.
V, 5; s. XV. f. 421.
V, 9; s. XV. f. 164.

[Diels I.83]

Περὶ τοῦ παρ' Ἱπποκράτει κώματος.
De comate secundum Hippocratem.

K. VII 643—665.

Inc. Τί ποτε σημαίνει τὸ τοῦ κώματος ὄνομα.
Expl. τῷ »ἄρα φρενιτικοί«, τινὲς δ' οὔ.

Florenz: Laurent. plut. 74, 3; s. XII. p. 188b.

Περὶ μαρασμοῦ.
De marcore.

K. VII 666—704.

Inc. Μαρασμός ἐστι φθορὰ ζῶντος σώματος.
Expl. κατὰ τὴν τέχνην γέγραπται.

Paris: Parisin. 2283*; s. XVI.
Venedig: Marcian.
276; s. XII. f. 68.
282; s. XV.

[**Wien:** Vindob. ap. Lambec. I 181].

Περὶ τῶν παρὰ φύσιν ὄγκων.
De tumoribus praeter naturam.

K. VII 47 705—732.

Inc. Ἔν τι τῶν συμβεβηκότων τοῖς σώμασιν ὑπάρχει.
Expl. ἰδέας ἀρρήτου καταλελειμμένης.

Florenz: Laurent. plut. 74, 5; s. XIV. p. 133.
Paris:
Parisin.
2164; s. XVI. f. 185.
2269; s. XV. f. 180.
Suppl.
35; s. XV—XVI. f. 177^{v}.
634; s. XIV. f. 65 (*Collation besitzt Helmreich*).
Rom: Vatic. 283; s. XIV. f. 20.
Venedig: Marcian. 281; s. XV. f. 91.

Περὶ ἀνωμάλου δυσκρασίας.
De inaequali intemperie.

K. VII 733—752.

Inc. Ἀνώμαλος δυσκρασία γίνεται μὲν καὶ καθ' ὅλον.
Expl. τῇ τῆς θεραπευτικῆς μεθόδου.

Cheltenham: Phillipps. 4614; s. XV (XIV). f. 54^{v}.
Florenz: Laurent. plut. 74, 5; s. XIV. p. 129b.
Mailand: Trivultian. 685; s. XV (XIV). f. 77—83.
Modena: Mutinens. 109 (II D 10); s. XIV—XV. f. 73^{v}.
Oxford: Laudian. C 57 (nunc 58; Bodl. 709); s. XV in. f. 202b. [Diels I.84]
Paris: Parisin. 2283*; s. XVI.
Rom: Vatic. 282; s. XVI. f. 46^{v}.
Venedig: Marcian. 282; s. XV. (*Collationen aller Hdss. außer Phillipps. und Parisin. besitzt Helmreich*).

Περὶ δυσπνοίας βιβλία Γ'.
De difficultate respirationis libri III.

K. VII 753—960.

Inc. (lib. 1) Ὅτι μὲν ἡ δύσπνοια βλάβη τις.
Expl. (lib. 3) ἑτέρων κατεπειγόντων οὐκ ἐπ' ἐκεῖνα μεταβήσομαι.

Cheltenham: Phillipps. 4614; s. XV (XIV). f. 62.
Modena: Mutinens. 237 (III G 18); s. XVI. f. 181.
Oxford:
Baroccian. 220; s. XIII. f. 1 (Libri II et III).
Canonician. 44; s. XV. ex. f. 251 (Libri III; l. II des. δύσπνοια = K. VII 887, 6. l. III Inc. καὶ τὰ λοιπά = K. VII 890, 10).
Paris: Parisin.
2165; s. XVI. f. 118.
2166; s. XV—XVI. f. 35 (Liber I fine mutil.).
Rom: Reg. Suec. 175; s. XIV. f. 179ᵛ.
Venedig:
Marcian. App. cl. V, 5; s. XV. f. 222.
Venet. Bibl. Josephi de Aromatariis. (*Verbleib unbekannt*).

[Diels I.85] Περὶ τῶν πεπονθότων τόπων βιβλία ΣΤ'.
De locis affectis libri VI.

K. VIII 1—452.

Inc. (lib. 1) Τόπους ὀνομάζουσι τὰ μόρια τοῦ σώματος.
Expl. (lib. 6) τῆς προκειμένης πραγματείας, καταπαύσω τὸν λόγον ἐνταῦθα.

Florenz: Laurent. plut.
74, 16; s. XIV. p. 62 (Διαγνώσεις τόπων πεπονθότων; libri VI).
74, 30; s. XIV. p. 1.
Leipzig: Lipsiens. 50; s. XVI. f. 1.
Leyden: Voss. fol. 53; s. XV. (Περὶ διαγνώσεως τ. πεπ. τόπ.).
London: Harleian. (Brit. Mus.) 5651; s. XV—XVI. (c. scholiis).
Mailand: Ambros.
Q 3 Sup.; s. XV—XVI. f. 45.
Q 52 Sup.; s. — (= K. VIII 97—376. Expl. πρὸς αὐτὰ τὸ αἷμα καὶ τὴν ὀρεκτικὴν τῶν).

Modena: Mutinens. 213 (III G 9); s. XV. f. 3 (Expl. φαίνεσθαι τῶν καταμηνίων ἐπεχομένων).
Oxford:
Canonician. 44; s. XV ex. f. 1 (Libri VI; l. III des. τινες = K. VIII 214, 4. l. IV inc. λογικὰς διαγνώσεις = K. VIII 271, 1).
Laudian. C 57 (nunc 58; Bodl. 709); s. XV in. f. 2.
Padua: Bibl. Joannis Rhodii. (*Verbleib unbekannt*).
Paris: Parisin.
2157; s. XV. f. 256.
2161; s. XV. f. 163.
2332*; s. XV (XIV). f. 6.
Rom: Palat. 54; s. XV—XVI. f. 24.
Venedig:
Marcian. 280; s. XV. f. 24—102.
App. cl. V, 5; s. XV. f. 336^{v}.
Wien: Vindob. med.
18; s. XVI. f. 1—256.
22; s. XV. f. 1—195.

Dazu: [Mich. Cantacuzeni].

Περὶ σφυγμῶν τοῖς εἰσαγομένοις. [Diels I.86]
De pulsibus ad tirones.

K. VIII 453—492.

Inc. Ὅσα τοῖς εἰσαγομένοις, φίλτατε Τεῦθρα, χρήσιμον.
Expl. καὶ τάσιν τινὰ τῆς ἀρτηρίας βραχεῖαν.

Berlin: Phillipps. 1524 (ol. Meerm. 214); s. XVI. f. 41 (Expl. σκεψώμεθα = K. VIII 484, 9).
Bologna: Bonon. 3632*; s. XV. f. 63^{v}.
Florenz: Laurent. plut. 74, 5; s. XIV. p. 311 (Expl. καὶ μαίλακος).
Moskau: Mosquens. 466; s. XVI. f. 1.
Paris:
Parisin.
2207*; a. 1299. f. 217.
2260; s. XVI. f. 120^{v}.
2276; s. XVI. f. 199.
2830; a. 1515. f. 175.
Suppl. 446; s. X. f. 95.

Rom:
Palat. 400; s. XV. f. 48.
Reg. Suec. 181*; a. 1364. f. 225 (Inc. Ἐν τοῖς σφυγμοῖς μόνον τοῦ καρποῦ).
Venedig: Marcian. 281; s. XV. f. 72—75ᵛ.
Wien: Vindob. med. 52; s. XV. f. 23—35ᵛ (Expl. ὥστε καὶ μικρὸν εἶναι αὐτὸν καὶ ἀμυδρόν).
Wolfenbüttel: Guelferb. 368 (Gud. 11); s. XVI.

[Diels I.87]

Περὶ διαφορᾶς σφυγμῶν λόγοι Δ'.
De pulsuum differentiis libri IV.

K. VIII 493—765.

Inc. (lib. 1) Εὐξαίμην μὲν ἂν καὶ μαθεῖν καὶ διδάξαι.
Expl. (lib. 4) ἡ περὶ συλλογισμοῦ προτέρων ἀναλυτικῶν.

Florenz: Laurent. plut.
74, 18; s. XIV. p. 189.
74, 28; s. XIV. p. 1.
74, 31*; s. XIV. f. 206ᵛ.
Leyden:
[Voss. 2168; s. —].
Vulc. 43; s. XV.
London: Harleian. (Brit. Mus.) 5625; s. XV (XVI). f. 1.
Mailand: Ambros. O 50 Sup.; s. — (Libri IV; fine mutil. Expl. σαφηνίζεσθαι καὶ μὴ κεναῖς ὑπονοι ...)
Modena: Mutinens. 226 (II H 11); s. XVI. f. 1.
Moskau: Mosquens. 464; s. XV. f. 8.
Oxford: Laudian. C 55 (nunc 57; Bodl. 707); s. XV in. f. 1.
Paris: Parisin.
[2157 (?)].
2161; s. XV. f. 283.
2167; s. XVI. f. 287.
[2276 (?)].
Rom: Vatic.
281; s. XIV. f. 30ᵛ.
1064; s. —. f. 25ᵛ.
Venedig: Marcian. 287; s. XV. f. 157—196.
Wolfenbüttel: Guelferb. 368 (Gud. 11); s. XVI (λόγος δεύτερος π. διαφορ. σφυγμ. Inc. Οὐ τὴν αὐτὴν χρή. Expl. mutil. κινδυνεύω δ' εἰπεῖν ὅτι τὸ τῶν πολλῶν).

Περὶ διαγνώσεως σφυγμῶν λόγοι Δ'.
De dignoscendis pulsibus libri IV.

K. VIII 766—961.

Inc. (lib. 1) Τῆς περὶ τοὺς σφυγμοὺς θεωρίας εἰς τέτταρα.
Expl. (lib. 4) τεττάρων ἑκατέρᾳ βιβλίων ἐσομένη.

Florenz: Laurent. plut.
74, 18; s. XIV. p. 149.
74, 28; s. XIV. f. 114b.
Leyden: Vulc. 43; s. XV.
London: Harleian. (Brit. Mus.) 5625; s. XV (XVI). f. 91.
Modena: Mutinens. 226 (II H 11); s. XVI. f. 86.
Moskau: Mosquens. 464; s. XV. f. 42.
Oxford: [Diels I.88]
Baroccian. 131*; s. XIV. f. 477ᵛ (Διάγνωσις ἀκριβὴς τῶν σφυγμῶν. Expl. Ἱπποκράτους καὶ Γαληνοῦ τῶν ἐπιστήμων [sic] ἰατρῶν).
Laudian. C 55 (nunc 57; Bodl. 707); s. XV in. f. 75b.
Paris: Parisin.
2153; s. XV. f. 81.
[2157 (?).]
[2158 (?)].
2161; s. XV. f. 353ᵛ.
2167; s. XVI. f. 303.
[2276 (?)].
Rom: Vatic.
281; s. XIV. f. 42.
1064; s. —. f. 114.
Venedig: Marcian. 287; s. XV. f. 196ᵛ—224ᵛ.

Περὶ τῶν ἐν τοῖς σφυγμοῖς αἰτίων λόγοι Δ'.
De causis pulsuum libri IV.

K. IX 1—204.

Inc. (lib. 1) Τῶν τοὺς σφυγμοὺς τρεπόντων αἰτίων.
Expl. (lib. 4) τοῖς μεμνημένοις τῶν ἔμπροσθεν εἰρημένων.

Florenz: Laurent. plut.
74, 18; s. XIV. p. 275.

74, 28; s. XIV. p. 199b.
Leyden: Vulc. 43; s. XV.
London: Harleian. (Brit. Mus.) 5625; s. XV (XVI). f. 157 (Inscr. περὶ αἰτίων τῶν σφυγμῶν).
Modena: Mutinens. 226 (II H 11); s. XVI. f. 144.
Moskau: Mosquens. 464; s. XV. f. 67.
Oxford: Laudian. C 55 (nunc 57; Bodl. 707); s. XV in. f. 128.
Paris: Parisin.
[2137 (?)].
2161; s. XV. f. 406.
2167; s. XVI. f. 343.
[2276 (?)].
Rom: Vatic.
281; s. XV. f. 73v.
1064; s. —. f. 141 (Libri III ?).
Venedig: Marcian. 287; s. XV. f. 225—253.

Περὶ προγνώσεως σφυγμῶν λόγοι Δ'.
De praesagitione ex pulsibus libri IV.

K. IX 205—430.

Inc. (lib. 1) Ὅτι μὲν οὐ τῶν μελλόντων ἡ πρόγνωσίς ἐστι μόνον.
Expl. (lib. 4) αὐτάρκως ἐν τοῖς τῶν κρίσεων ὑπομνήμασιν.

Florenz: Laurent. plut.
74, 18; s. XIV. p. 298b.
74, 28; s. XIV. p. 294b.
Leyden: Vulc. 43; s. XV.
London: Harleian. (Brit. Mus.) 5625; s. XV (XVI). f. 226.
Modena: Mutinens. 226 (II H 11); s. XVI. f. 204.
Moskau: Mosquens. 464; s. XV. f. 93.
[Diels I.89] **Oxford:** Laudian. C 55 (nunc 57; Bodl. 707); s. XV in. f. 183 (L. IV lacunos. des. περὶ κρίσεων = K. IX 429, 4).
Paris: Parisin.
[2157 (?)].
2161; s. XV. f. 460v.
2167; s. XVI. f. 387.
[2276 (?)].

Rom: Vatic.
281; s. XV. f. 106.
1064; s. —. f. 201.
Venedig: Marcian. 287; s. XV. f. 254—287.
Wien: Vindob. med. 28 (Θεοφίλου ἐκ τοῦ προγνωστικοῦ Γαλ. π. σφυγμῶν).

Σύνοψις περὶ σφυγμῶν ἰδίας πραγματείας.
Synopsis librorum suorum sedecim de pulsibus.

K. IX 431—549.

Inc. Οἱ πολλοὶ τῶν ἀνθρώπων ὀρέγονται μὲν ἐπιστήμης.
Expl. εἰς σύνοψιν ἀγαγεῖν προτεθήκαμεν.

Cheltenham: Phillipps. 24, 386; s. XV. f. 1 (*W. Scotts Collation u. Abschrift im Besitze der Berl. Akademie*).
Florenz: Laurent. plut. 59, 14; s. XV. f. 178.
Kopenhagen: Hauniens. Bibl. Univ. e donatione variorum Fol. 14; s. XV—XVI. f. 1.
Mailand: Ambros.
C 120 Sup.; s. XVI in. f. 69 *und* 109 (*zweimal in ders. Hds. Bretzls Collation im Besitze der Berl. Akademie*).
D 293 Inf.; s. XV ex. (Expl. κατὰ λόγον ὁ σφυγμὸς φαίνεται. *Bretzls Collation im Besitze der Berl. Akademie*).
D 518 Inf.; s. XVI in. (*Bretzls Collation im Besitze der Berl. Akademie*).
Padua: Bibl. Joann. Rhodii. (*Verbleib unbekannt*).
Paris:
Parisin.
2155; s. XIV. f. 315v (Liber de pulsibus, fine mutil.).
2229; s. XIII. f. 43v (Tract. de pulsibus).
2315; s. XV. f. 393v (Liber de pulsibus).
2332*; s. XV (XIV). f. — (Exc. e l. περὶ σφυγμῶν).
3035; s. XIV. f. 209 (Liber de pulsibus).
Suppl.
446; s. X. f. 33v (de pulsu).
629; s. XIX. f. 59 (Tract. de pulsibus).

Περὶ κρίσεων βιβλία Γ'.
De crisibus libri III.

K. IX 550—768.

Inc. (lib. 1) Εἴτε τὴν ἀθρόαν ἐν νόσῳ μεταβολήν.
Expl. (lib. 3) καὶ οὐδὲν ἔτι τετάρτου λόγου προσδεῖ.

Athos: Βιβλ. μον. Ἰβήρων 4309. 189; s. XIII. f. 174 B.
Leyden: Voss. 4° 45; s. XIV.
London:
Harleian. (Brit. Mus.) 6305; s. XVI (?). f. 6.
[Bibl. eccl. Westmonast. 1100].
Modena: Mutinens. 218 (II H 3); s. XVI. f. 2.
Oxford: Laudian. C 57 (nunc 58; Bodl. 709); s. XV in. f. 262b.
Paris: Parisin.
2246; s. XVI. f. 111.
2272; s. XV. f. 41.
2283*; s. XVI.
2332*; s. XV.
Rom:
Palat.
157; s. XIV. f. 110.
279*; s. XIV—XV. f. 307.
295*; s. XV—XVI. f. 177. (Exc. e ll. II et III).
Vatic. 282; s. XVI. f. 87.
Venedig:
Marcian. 282; s. XV. f. 6v—33.
App. cl.
V, 4; s. XV.
V, 8; s. XIV. f. 10.
[**Wien:** Vindob. ap. Lambec. I 181].

[Diels I.90] Περὶ κρισίμων ἡμερῶν βιβλία Γ'.
De diebus decretoriis libri III.

K. IX 769—941.

Inc. (lib. 1) Τῶν νοσημάτων αἱ λύσεις, ὅσαι μὴ κατὰ βραχύ.
Expl. (lib. 3) καὶ τῶν πραγμάτων αὐτῶν αἱ διαγνώσεις.

Athos: Βιβλ. μον. Ἰβήρων 4309. 189; s. XIII. f. 247 B.
Florenz: Laurent. plut. 74, 12*; s. XV. p. 29 (Exc. e l. II).
London:
Harleian. (Brit. Mus.) 6305; s. XVI (?). f. 83.
Reg. (Brit. Mus.) 16 C XI; s. XVI. f. 1.
Mailand: Ambros. Q 94 Sup.; s. —. f. 29v. [Diels I.91]
Oxford:
Laudian. C 57 (nunc 58; Bodl. 709); s. XV in. f. 319.
[Coll. Merton. 685; s. —].
Paris: Parisin.
2246; s. XVI. f. 172.
2272; s. XV. f. 101v.
2283*; s. XVI.
2332*; s. XV (XIV).
Rom:
Palat. 157; s. XIV. f. 219.
Vatic.
282; s. XVI. f. 121.
300; s. XII—XIII. f. 287v—288v (Inc. Τὰ νοσήματα ἅτινα. Expl. καὶ τοῦ γνῶναι τὰ σημεῖα).
Venedig:
Marcian. 282; s. XV. f. 33—53v.
App. cl.
V, 4; s. XV.
V, 8; s. XIV. f. 62.
XI, 5; s. XIV. f. 92.

Θεραπευτικῆς μεθόδου βιβλία ΙΔ'.
Methodi medendi libri XIV.

K. X 1—1021.

Inc. (lib. 1) Ἐπειδὴ καὶ σύ με πολλάκις, ὦ Ἱέρων.
Expl. (lib. 14) τελευτάτω καὶ οὗτος ὁ λόγος.

Athen: nr. 1494*; s. XVIII. no. 1 (Εἰσαγωγὴ ἐκ τῆς μεγάλης θεραπευτικῆς).
Athos: Athous Βιβλ. μον. Ἰβήρων 4284. 164; s. XIII.
Cambridge: Cantabrig. Caius Coll.
47; s. XV. f. 1 (Lib. I—VI in fine mutil.).
360; s. XVI. p. 161 (Lib. VI—XIV).

Florenz: Laurent. plut.
74, 6; s. XIV. p. 1.
74, 7*; s. IX. p. 81 (Lib. VI c. 5—6).
74, 12*; s. XV. p. 20 (Ex libb. I. II. VII. IX. XII. XIII.).
Leyden:
[Diels I.92] Miscell. 11; s. XIII. f. 29—44 (Init. et fine mutil.; fort. Therapeut. ad Glauconem).
[Vossian. ? (in. et fin. mut.)].
London: Addit. (Brit. Mus.) 6898; s. XIII/XIV. f. 1.
Mailand: Ambros. G 97 Sup.*; s. XVI (XV). f. 57 (Τῆς μεγάλης θεραπευτικῆς λόγος α'. Inc. Τολμηρότατε Θεσσαλέ. Expl. ἐν μὲν δὴ τοῖς τοιούτοις ἅπασι προ ... Esse excerptum hoc opus conicit Schoene).
Messina: Messanens. 111; s. XII (Lib. I).
Moskau: Mosquens.
464; s. XV. f. 127.
466; s. XV. f. 265.
Oxford: Laudian. C 54 (nunc 56; Bodl. 706); s. XV in.
Paris:
Parisin.
2157; s. XV. f. 425 (Libri III primi fine mutil.).
2160; a. 1473. f. 1.
2162; s. XV—XVI. f. 1.
2169; s. XVI. f. 83 (Libri IV).
2171; s. XVI. f. 1.
2232; s. XV. f. 88 (Liber III fine mut.).
[2262 (?)].
2274; s. XV.
2280; s. XVI. f. 1.
2283*; s. XVI (Exc. e θεραπευτικὴ μεγάλη).
Suppl. 634; s. XIV. f. 257 (Lib. I—VI. XIII—XIV).
Rom:
Reg. Suec. 174; s. XIV. f. 1.
Vatic. 1028*; s. —. f. I (»Lib. X c. 10 vel exc. ex hoc capite«).
Venedig:
Marcian.
276; s. XII. f. 74.
284; s. XV.
App. cl. V 4; s. XV.
Monast. S. Michaelis prope Murianum 93; s. XIV. (*Verbleib unbekannt*).
Wien: Vindob. med. 28*; s. XV. f. 17v (Ἀπὸ θεραπευτικῆς ἐκ τοῦ περὶ τραυμάτων. Inc. πῶς τὸ πύον γίνεται λευκόν — τὰ δὲ συμπτώματα ἐν ταῖς ἐνεργείαις · σχολ. τὸ περὶ διαφορᾶς πυρετῶν).

Wolfenbüttel: Guelferbyt. 369 (Gud. 69); s. XVII.

Τῶν πρὸς Γλαύκωνα θεραπευτικῶν βιβλία Β'. [Diels I.93]
Ad Glauconem de medendi methodo libri II.

K. XI 1—146.

Inc. (lib. 1) Ὅτι μὲν οὐ τὴν κοινὴν μόνον.
Expl. (lib. 2) ἡμῖν ὑπομνημάτων ἕκαστον.

Athos: Athous Βιβλ. μον. Ἰβήρων 4271. 151; s. XV. f. 128a.
Cheltenham: Phillipps. 4614; s. XV (XIV). f. 107.
Escurial: Scorial. Φ. III. 11*; s. XIV. XV. f. 80 (Ex l. I).
Florenz: Laurent. plut.
75, 9; s. XV. p. 171.
75, 16; s. XV. p. 148b.
Leipzig: Lipsiens. 53; s. XVI—XVII. p. 1.
Leyden:
B. P. 2 A; s. XVI (c. Steph. interpr. lib. I).
Miscell. 11; s. XIII. f. 29—44 (*Vielleicht zur* Θεραπ. μέθοδ. *gehörig*).
Voss. F° 53; s. XV.
London: Arundelian. (Brit. Mus.); s. XV in. f. 114.
Mailand: Trivultian. 685; s. XV (XIV). f. 86—119.
Modena: Mutinens. 109 (II D 10); s. XIV—XV (Libri II. Expl. φαρμάκων ἐπιτιθέναι τι τῶν πρὸς τὰ ...).
Moskau: Mosquens.
464; s. XV. f. 301v.
466; s. XVI. f. 25.
München: Monacens. 236; s. XV. f. 1.
Padua: Bibl. Joann. Rhodii. (*Verbleib unbekannt*).
Paris:
Parisin.
[2156 (?)].
2157; s. XV. f. 217.
2166; s. XV—XVI. f. 1 (Libri II fine mut.).
2260; s. XVI. f. 386.
2265; s. XIII. f. 76v.
2269; s. XV. f. 1.
[2270 (?)].
2304; s. XV. f. 155v.

2308; s. XV. f. 160ᵛ.

Suppl.

446; s. X. f. 1.

634; s. XIV. f. 39.

764; s. XIV. f. 121.

Rom:

Palat. 54; s. XV—XVI. f. 1.

Vatic.

2182; s. XV. f. 48 (Lib. I in fine mutil.; des. τῆς ἡμέρας ἡ μὲν = K. XI 66).

2254; s. X—XI. f. 1.

Venedig:

Marcian. 280; s. XV. f. 1—22ᵛ.

App. cl. V, 4; s. XV.

Wien: Vindobon. med.

13; s. XV. f. 6ᵛ—23ᵛ (Expl. εἰς μακρὸν κελεύειν καὶ τῶν σπλάγχνων προνοεῖσθαι κατανοοῦντά τε ...).

18*; s. XV. f. 2 (Inc. οὐ δεῖται τὸ πλῆθος. Expl. εἰ δ' ἐξ ἀγενοῦς σίτου λαμβάνεις τὸ ἄλευρον).

Wolfenbüttel: Guelferbyt. 369. 370 (Gud. 69); s. XVII.

[Diels I.94] Περὶ φλεβοτομίας πρὸς Ἐρασίστρατον.
De venae sectione adversus Erasistratum.

K. XI 147—186.

Inc. Ἄξιον εἶναί μοι δοκεῖ ζητήσεως.
Expl. τῆς ἐκ τοῦ κενοῦν ὠφελείας ἔχει.

Mailand: Ambros. B 108 Sup.; s. XIV in. f. 140.
Rom: Urbin. 70; s. XV. f. 80.

Περὶ φλεβοτομίας πρὸς Ἐρασιστρατείους τοὺς ἐν Ῥώμῃ.
De venae sectione adversus Erasistrateos Romae degentes.

K. XI 187—249.

Inc. Ὅτε τὸ πρῶτον ἧκον εἰς Ῥώμην.
Expl. ἢ καθαίρειν ἔτι ὑγιαίνοντας προσήκει.

Mailand: Ambros. B 108 Sup.; s. XIV in. f. 128 (= K. XI 222—249).
Rom: Urbin. 70; s. XV. f. 64.
Venedig: Marcian. 279; s. XV. f. 253—258ᵛ.

Περὶ φλεβοτομίας θεραπευτικὸν βιβλίον.
De curandi ratione per venae sectionem.

K. XI 250—316.

Inc. Τοῖς περὶ φλεβοτομίας σκοπουμένοις.
Expl. περὶ τὸ κέντρον τοῦ μυὸς παντός.

Athos: Athous Βιβλ. μον. Ἰβήρων 4309. 189; s. XIII. f. 371 A.
Bologna: Bonon. 3636*; s. XIV—XV. f. 129ᵛ (cap. IV—XXI. Inc. Ὅτι τοῖς τὰ συνήθη πράττουσι. Expl. ἀλλὰ τηρεῖν καὶ αὖθις ἐπαφαιρεῖν) *und* f. 133 (cap. XXII).
Florenz: Laurent. plut. 74, 22; s. XIV. p. 2b. [Diels I.95]
Mailand: Ambros. B 108 Sup.; s. XIV in. f. 158ᵛ.
Rom: Urbin. 70; s. XV. f. 90.
Venedig: Marcian. 279; s. XV. f. 259—267ᵛ.

Περὶ βδελλῶν, ἀντισπάσεως, σικύας καὶ ἐγχαράξεως καὶ κατασχασμοῦ.
De hirudinibus, revulsione, cucurbitula, incisione et scarificatione.

K. XI 317—322.

Inc. Θηρῶντές τινες τὰς βδέλλας κατακλείουσι.
Expl. καὶ συνάγχας καὶ σφηνώσεις.

Paris: Parisin. 2269; s. XV. f. 178.
Rom: Vatic. 283; s. XIV. f. 2.
Venedig: Marcian. App. cl. II, 171*; s. XV.

Περὶ τῆς τῶν καθαιρόντων φαρμάκων δυνάμεως.
De purgantium medicamentorum facultate.

K. XI 323—342.

Inc. Κατὰ τὴν αὐτὴν αἰτίαν ἐοίκασι.
Expl. ἡ τῶν καθαιρόντων φαρμάκων δύναμις.

Florenz: Laurent. plut.
74, 3; s. XII. p. 60b.
74, 22; s. XIV. p. 1.
Mailand: Ambros. Q 3 Sup.; s. XV—XVI. f. 225.
Modena: Mutinens. 213 (III G 9); s. XV. f. 143 (Expl. καὶ τοὺς καθ' ἕκαστον αὐτῶν τρόπους τῆς ἰάσευς).
Paris:
Parisin. 2165; s. XVI. f. 188.
Suppl. 35; s. XV—XVI. f. 93.
Venedig: Marcian. App. cl.
V, 4; s. XV.
V, 5; s. XV. f. 328.

Τίνας δεῖ ἐκκαθαίρειν καὶ ποίοις καθαρτηρίοις καὶ πότε.
Quos, quibus catharticis medicamentis et quando purgare oporteat.

K. XI 343—356.

Inc. Τοὺς ὑγιεινὰ τὰ σώματα ἔχοντας.
Expl. πάλιν ἑτέρας κενώσεως γίνηται.

Florenz: Laurent. plut. 75, 7; s. XIV. p. 217.
Leyden: Voss. 4° 45; s. XIV.
Modena: Mutinens. 213 (III G 9); s. XV. f. 157.
München: Monacens. 469; s. XV. p. 132—137.
Paris: Parisin.
2165; s. XVI. f. 197.
2166; s. XV—XVI. f. 70.
Rom: Palat. 199*; s. XIII. f. 471.
Venedig: Marcian. App. cl. V, 5; s. XV. f. 334v.

[Diels I.96] Τῷ ἐπιλήπτῳ παιδὶ ὑποθήκη.
Puero epileptico consilium.

K. XI. 357—378.

Inc. Ἐγὼ μὲν ᾤμην, ὦ Καικιλιανέ.
Expl. οὐκ ἀβλαβὲς δὲ τῶν νεύρων.

Mailand: Ambros. C 4 Sup.; s. —. f. 233.

Moskau: Mosquens. 466; s. XVI. f. 78.

Paris:

Parisin.

2269; s. XV. f. 193.

2270; s. XV—XVI. f. 94^{v}.

2271; s. XV. f. 135.

Suppl. 35; s. XV—XVI. f. 109.

Rom: Vatic.

285; s. XV. f. 133.

1845; s. XIII. f. 142^{v}.

Venedig:

Marcian.

282; s. XV. f. 1.

App. cl.

V, 5; s. XV. f. 413^{v}.

V, 9; s. XV. f. 150^{v}.

Περὶ κράσεως καὶ δυνάμεως τῶν ἁπλῶν φαρμάκων βιβλία ΙΑ'.
De simplicium medicamentorum temperamentis et facultatibus libri XI.

K. XI 379—XII 377.

Inc. (lib. 1) Τὰς τῶν ἁπλῶν φαρμάκων δυνάμεις ἀκριβῶς.

Expl. (lib. 11) σηπεδονωδῶν ἑλκῶν ἐχρησάμεθα.

Berlin: Berol. qu. 21 (319); s. XVI. f. 1.

Bologna: Bonon. 2678 (ol. 228); s. XV. f. 67 (Libri VI—XI).

Cambridge: Cantabrig. Bibl. Univ. F. F. 3. 30*; s. XVI. no. 2 (Ἀπὸ τῶν τοῦ Γαλ. ἁπλῶν ἐκλογή τινων κεφαλαίων κτέ.).

Cheltenham: Phillipps.

6665 = 6765*; s. XII. no. 2 (*Wie im* Cantabrig. Inc. Ἀβρότονον· θερμόν ἐστι καὶ ξηρόν. Expl. πεπονθόσι τὴν κύστιν καὶ τοῖς λιθιῶσιν).

6774 (ol. Meerm. 298)*; s. XII. (*Wie im* Cantabr.).

Escurial: Scorial.

C. II. 11; s. XV. f. 37.

C. III. 17; s. XVI. f. 36 (Libri I—V. c. lacunis).

Φ. III. 11*; s. XIV. XV. f. 60—66 (Ex libris I—IV).

Florenz: Laurent. plut. 74, 17; s. XII. p. 133 (Libri X. XI 1—11).

Genf: Genev. bibl. urb. 42; s. XVI. f. 1.

Leipzig: Lipsiens. 51; s. —. f. 41.
Leyden: B. P. 16; s. XV.
Mailand: Ambros.
A 81 Inf.; s. —. f. 1 (A lib. V 2 usque ad l. IX in. πόλιν ἐκείνην τῆς μυρί...).
E 105 Sup.; s. — (A lib. I—V ἐναντίως ἔχειν σπέρματα τὴν δ' αὐ...).
Modena: Mutinens.
78 (II C 11); s. XV.
107 (II D 8); s. XV.
216 (II H 1)*; s. XVI. f. 25 (Frgm. l. VI οὕτως οὖν τὸ ἀφέψημα .... ἀδήκτως ξηραίνει).
München: Monacens. 469; s. XIII. p. 56—131 (Libri VIII et IX).
Neapel: Neapolit. 304 III D 20*; s. XIV. (Frgm. Xenocratis ex libro XI).
Padua: Bibl. Joann. Rhodii. (*Verbleib unbekannt*).
Paris:
[Coislin. ap. Montf. II 448].
Parisin.
2148; s. XV. f. 67 (Libri II fine mutil.)
2156; s. XV. f. 176ᵛ.
2157; s. XV. f. 1.
2158; s. XV. f. 167.
2159; a. 1492.
[2160 (?)].
2170; s. XVI. f. 1.
2279; s. XVI. f. 1 (Libri V).
[2280 (?)].
Rom:
Palat.
31; s. XIV. f. 1 (Lib. III init. mut. — VI. IX—XI. Lib. XI lacunos.).
199*; s. XIII. f. 3 (de lacte ex libro IV).
Urbin. 67; s. XIII. f. 188 (Libri VI—XI) *und* f. 282 [s. XIV. XV.] (Libri I—V).
Vatic. 1066; s. XVI. f. 168 (διαγνώσεις ex libro I) *und* f. 169 (Liber II).
Turin: Taurin. 17 B VII 22 (B I 12); s. XVIII. f. 171 (Initium tantum. *Verbrannt*).
Venedig:
Marcian. 286; s. XV.
App. cl.
V 6; s. XIII. XV. p. 199.
V 9; s. XV. f. 366 (Libri I—V).
Wien: Vindob. med.
1; s. V—VI. f. 1 (*Vgl.* M. Wellmann, Hermes 38, 292—304).
25*; s. XV—XVI. f. 11 (ex libris VI—VIII).
35; s. XV ex. f. 1—236ᵛ (Libri VI—XI 2).
48; s. XIV—XV. f. 46—164 (Libri VI—VIII).

Περὶ συνθέσεως φαρμάκων τῶν κατὰ τόπους βιβλία Ι΄. [Diels I.97]

De compositione medicamentorum secundum locos libri X.

K. XII 378—XIII 361.

Inc. (lib. 1) Ὅτι μὲν οὐ μόνον τὸ θεραπευόμενον πάθος.
Expl. (lib. 10) συλλογὰς καὶ ἀπαλλάττει τῶν πόνων.

Berlin: Phillipps. 1566 (ol. Meerm. 269)*; s. XVI. f. 14 (Lib. X cap. 2).
Florenz: Laurent. plut.
 75, 8; s. XV. p. 9.
 75, 17; s. XIV. p. 4.
[**Oxford:** Eccles. Wigorn. 745]. [Diels I.98]
Padua: Bibl. Joann. Rhodii. (*Verbleib unbekannt.*)
Paris: Parisin.
 Coislin. 387*; s. XI/XII. f. 241^{v} (Εἰς τὸ τοῦ Φίλωνος βοήθημα = K. XIII 267).
 Parisin.
  [2123 (?)].
  2155; s. XIV. f. 2 (Libri I—IX).
  2164; s. XVI. f. 269 (Lib. I. II).
  [2167 (?); s. XVI].
  2173; s. XVI. f. 71.
Rom:
 Palat. 54; s. XV—XVI. f. 103^{v}.
 Reg. Suec. 172; s. XIV. f. 105.
 Urbin. 67; s. XIII. f. 53.
Rosanbo: Bibl. de M. le marquis de Ros. 286; s. XVI. f. 90 (τῶν εἰς ι΄ τὸ δέκατον. Περὶ νεφριτικῶν. Inc. Ὅτι μὲν νεφριτικάς. Expl. ἀναλάμβανε ...).
Venedig:
 Marcian.
  280; s. XV.
  288; s. X.
 App. cl. V, 7; s. XIV. f. 1 (Libri III init. mutil. — X).
[**Wien:** Vindob. ap. Lamb. II c. 6 (L. VI—VIII)].

Περὶ συνθέσεως φαρμάκων τῶν κατὰ γένη βιβλία Ζ'.
De compositione medicamentorum per genera libri VII.

K. XIII 362—1058.

Inc. (lib. 1) Ἔθος ἐστὶ τοῖς νεωτέροις ὀνομάζειν.
Expl. (lib. 7) τάς τε ἁπλὰς τούτων φύσεις.

Berlin: Phillipps. 1529 (ol. Meerm. 220); s. XVI. f. 1 (Inc. μὴ δ' ὅλως δάκνοντα = K. XIII 499, 10 [lib. II 5]. Expl. = lib. VII 16, K. XIII 1047).
Florenz: Laurent. plut. 74, 25; s. XV. p. 1.
Kopenhagen: Hauniens. ant. fund. reg. 225; s. XVI. f. 176 (Inc. *wie im* Berol. Phillipps. Expl. = K. XIII 1058).
Padua: Bibl. Joann. Rhodii. (*Verbleib unbekannt*).
Paris: Parisin.
2156; s. XV. f. 358 (Libri III).
2158; s. XV. f. 312 (Libri III).
Rom: Reg. Suec. 172; s. XIV. f. 1v.
Venedig: Marcian. 285; s. XV. f. 128—211v (Expl. μάλιστα χειμῶνος ἔν γε ταῖς ὁ = K. XIII 1052, 18).

[Diels I.99] Περὶ ἀντιδότων βιβλία Β'.
De antidotis libri II.

K. XIV 1—209.

Inc. (lib. 1) Τὰς ἰωμένας τὰ πάθη.
Expl. (lib. 2) καρύου μέγεθος σὺν ὕδατι ἐπ' ἐνιαυτόν.

Athos: Athous Βιβλ. μον. Ἰβήρων 4339. 219; s. XVIII.
Florenz: Laurent. plut. 74, 5; s. XIV. p. 163.
Kopenhagen: Hauniens. ant. fund. reg. 225; s. XVI. f. 114.
Paris:
Parisin. 2664; s. XVI. f. 218.
Suppl.
35; s. XVI. f. 219.
1193*; s. XVI. f. 17.
Rom: Reg. Suec. 173; s. XV. f. 73.
Venedig: Marcian. 281; s. XV. f. 106.
Wien: Vindob. med. 48*; s. XIV—XV. f. 164v—171v (Ex l. I).

Πρὸς Πίσωνα περὶ τῆς θηριακῆς.
De theriaca ad Pisonem liber.

K. XIV 210—294.

Inc. Καὶ τοῦτόν σοι τὸν περὶ τῆς θηριακῆς.
Expl. τῶν παρὰ θεῶν γενέσθαι σοι εὔχομαι.

Florenz: Laurent. plut. 74, 5; s. XIV. p. 160.
Kopenhagen: Hauniens. ant. fund. reg. 225; s. XVI. f. 170 (Expl. mutil. καὶ οὕτω λοιπὸν ἀκριβῶς).
[**Leyden:** Vossian. 58].
Paris:
Parisin.
2164; s. XVI. f. 191.
2195; s. XIII. f. 467v.
Suppl. 35; s. XV—XVI. f. 185v.
Venedig: Marcian. 281; s. XV. f. 93v.

Περὶ θηριακῆς πρὸς Παμφιλιανόν.
De theriaca ad Pamphilianum.

K. XIV 295—310.

Inc. Πολλάκις ἐπιζητοῦντί σοι, κράτιστε Παμφιλιανέ.
Expl. τηνικαῦτα γάρ εἰσι μάλιστα ἀκμαῖαι.

Mailand: Ambros. B 108 Sup.; s. XIV in. f. 185 (Expl. K. XIV 306, 11).
Paris:
Parisin. 2164; s. XVI. f. 215.
Suppl. 35; s. XV—XVI. f. 215v.
Rom: Urbin. 70; s. XV. f. 104.
Venedig: Marcian.
279; s. XV. f. 267v—269v.
281; s. XV. f. 104v.

Περὶ εὐπορίστων βιβλία Γ'.
De remediis parabilibus libri III.

K. XIV 311—581.

Inc. (lib. 1) Τὴν ἰατρικὴν τέχνην οὐ πόλεσιν.
Expl. (lib. 3) πυριαζέσθω οὕτως.

Athen: nr. 1493*; s. XII ex. no. 1 (Ex libris I et II).
Athos: Athous. Βιβλ. μον. Ἰβήρων 4271. 151; s. XV. f. 19 (Libri II Inscr. Γαλ. θεραπευτικὴ διαφόρων νόσων διὰ τῶν εὐπορίστων φαρμάκων. Inc. Περὶ τῆς ἐξεκκαύσεως κεφαλαλγίας. Expl. γάλα ἵστησιν).
[Diels I.100] **London:** Medical Society H Hi 17 = We 30; s. XV in. no. 40 Dbg. (Liber I. Expl. θαυμάσεις δὲ πάνυ δεξάμενος · τῶν εὐπορίστων ἰαμάτων δὴ πέρας).
Mailand: Ambros.
B 126 Sup.; s. XIV ex. f. 130 (»Liber II = K. XIV 391 et 383, 4—6«).
C 102 Inf.*; s. —. f. 6 (Περὶ ῥεουσῶν τριχῶν = K. XIV 393; liber II 2).
Q 94 Sup.; s. —. f. 8v (Liber II. Inc. Ἐπιζητήσαντός μου. Expl. καὶ καταχρασθὲν ἐπιτιθέμενον).
Moskau: Mosquens. 468; s. XVII. f. 1.
Paris: Parisin. Suppl.
636; s. XVI. f. 3.
684; s. XV—XVIII. f. 5v.
Rom: Urbin. 67; s. XIII. f. 268 (Liber I).

Περὶ τῶν παρὰ τὴν λέξιν σοφισμάτων.
De captionibus penes dictionem.

K. XIV 582—598.
C. Gabler, Rostock 1903.

Inc. Ἀριστοτέλης ὁ φιλόσοφος διδάσκων.
Expl. καὶ δι' αὐτὴν ἐγίγνετο διττὸς ὁ λόγος.

Mailand: Ambros. Q 3 Sup.; s. XV—XVI. f. 207v.

Περὶ τοῦ προγιγνώσκειν πρὸς Ἐπιγένην.
De praegnotione ad Epigenem liber.

K. XIV 599—673.

Inc. Ὅσον μὲν ἐπὶ τοῖς πολλοῖς τῶν ἰατρῶν.
Expl. οὐκ ἔχοντα δύσκολον τὴν πρόγνωσιν.

Florenz: Laurent. plut. 74, 5; s. XIV. p. 104.
Mailand: Ambros. Q 3 Sup.; s. XV—XVI. f. 265.
Paris: Parisin. 2332*; s. XV (XIV).
Rom: Vatic. 1845: s. XVI. f. 197ᵛ.
Venedig: Marcian. 281; s. XV. f. 81ᵛ.

Εἰσαγωγὴ ἢ ἰατρός.
Introductio sive medicus.

K. XIV 674—797.

Inc. Ἕλληνες τῶν τεχνῶν τὰς εὑρέσεις.
Expl. ῥευματίζεσθαι τὰ ἕλκη σπουδάζομεν.

Athen: nr. 1502; s. XVIII. no. 1.
Athos: Athous Βιβλ. μον. Ἰβήρων 4300. 180; s. XVII. f. 172.
Berlin: Phillipps. 1526 (ol. Meerm. 216); s. XVI. (Non sine lacunis).
Dresden: Dresdens. Da 1; s. XV. f. 1.
Escurial: Scorial.
Σ. II. 11; s. XV. f. 1.
Σ. III. 17*; s. XVI. f. 25 *und* f. 94—101 »quae ponenda sunt ante f. 25«.
Φ. III. 11*; s. XIV. XV. f. 47 (περὶ τοῦ πόσοι εἰσὶν οἱ συστησάμενοι τὴν ἐμπειρικήν = K. XIV 683).
Florenz: Laurent. plut. 74, 14; s. XV. p. 26b.
Leipzig: Lipsiens. 52; s. XVI. f. 1.
Modena: Mutinens.
213 (III G 9); s. XV. f. 198ᵛ (Ab initio usque ad cap. περὶ ἐμβροχῶν).
217 (II H 2); s. XIV. f. 34 (Usque ad ὡς δὲ ἐκ τῶν δευτέρων, καὶ = K. XIV 696, 6).
München: Monacens. 109; s. XVI. f. 22 (Cap. V et X desunt). [Diels I.101]
Oxford: Orvillian. X 1. 1. 3; s. XV ex. f. 214 (Capitum divisio ab usitata discrepat).
Paris:
Coislin. 228; s. XI—XIV. f. 96 (pars tantum oper.).

Parisin.
1438; s. XVI. f. 275.
[2113 (?)].
2153; s. XV. f. 1.
2156; s. XV. f. 33.
2158; s. XV. f. 32.
2160; a. 1473. f. 220.
2167; s. XVI. f. 249.
[2169 (?)].
2171; s. XVI. f. 209.
2175; s. XVI. f. 1.
2246; s. XVI. f. 231.
2270; s. XV—XVI. f. 1.
2271; s. XV. f. 41, *und* 95v (de oculorum affectibus = Εἰσ. cap. XVI. XVII).
2280; s. XVI. f. 389.
2282; s. XVI. f. 1.
[2304 (?)].
2306; s. XV. f. 345.
2307; s. XVI. f. 531v.
Suppl. 35; s. XV—XVI. f. 23v.
Ravenna: Bibl. Classens. 131. 2. H; s. XV.
Rom:
Barberin. I 127*; s. XVI. f. 261v (Inc. Ὅτι παρὰ τῷ Γαλ. πρῶτος Ἀπόλλων ἐφεῦρεν ἰατρικήν. Expl. τῶν εἰσφερομένων κοινοτήτων θεωρία).
Urbin. 67; s. XIV. XV. f. 1.
Vatic.
285; s. XV. f. 49.
1845; s. XIII. f. 44v.
Venedig: Marcian. App. cl.
V, 9; s. XV. f. 206v (Expl. τὰ ἕλκη σπουδάζομεν).
V, 10; s. XVI. f. 2.

Γαληνοῦ εἰς τὸ Ἱπποκράτους περὶ φύσιος ἀνθρώπου βιβλίον ὑπόμνημα Α' Β'.
Galeni in Hippocratis de natura hominis lib[rum] commentarii II.

K. XV 1—173.

Inc. Περὶ τῶν καθ' Ἱπποκράτην στοιχείων.
Expl. ὃ Πολύβου φασὶν εἶναι σύγγραμμα.

Florenz: Laurent. plut.
59, 14; s. XV. p. 101.
74, 12*; s. XV. p. 28b.
Modena: Mutinens. 240 (III F 17); s. XV—XVI. f. 8 (Expl. τὰ περὶ τὴν γῆν · οὐ μὴν κεκραμένον γε = K. XV 50, 3).
Rom: Reg. Suec. 173; s. XV. f. 185.
Venedig: Marcian. 282; s. XV (*Ilbergs Collation in dessen Besitz*).

Εἰς τὸ περὶ διαίτης ὑγιεινῆς τῶν ἰδιωτῶν Ἱπποκράτους ἢ Πολύβου ὑπόμνημα.
In Hippocratis vel Polybi opus de salubri victus ratione privatorum commentarius.

K. XV 174—223.

Inc. Ἓν τοῦτό ἐστι βιβλίον ἰδίαν ἐπαγγελίαν ἔχον.
Expl. ἀεὶ φαίνεται τοῦτο γιγνόμενον οὔθ' ὡς ἐπὶ τὸ πολύ.

Florenz: Laurent. plut. 59, 14; s. XV. p. 151.
Paris:
Parisin. 2276; s. XVI. f. 1.
Suppl. 447; s. XIV. f. 229.
Rom: Reg. Suec. 173; s. XV. f. 222.
Venedig: Marcian.
277; s. XV (sine titulo).
278; s. XI. f. 146 (*Ilbergs Collation von Hipp. VI 72—86 L. in dessen Besitz*).
282; s. XV.
285; s. XV (*Ilbergs Collation von Hipp. VI 72—86 L. in dessen Besitz*).
Wien: Vindob. med. 34; s. —. f. 229.

Εἰς τὸ Ἱπποκράτους περὶ τροφῆς ὑπομνήματα Δ'. [Diels I.102]
In Hippocratis librum de alimento commentarii IV.

K. XV 224—417.

Inc. (lib. 1) Τροφὴ καὶ τροφῆς εἶδος μία καὶ πολλαί.
Expl. (lib. 4) τὸ τρέψον ἐκ τῆς κοιλίας, μὴ παραπέμποντος ὑγροῦ τινος **

[cod. Matthiae Corvini].

Ἱπποκράτους περὶ διαίτης ὀξέων νοσημάτων βιβλίον καὶ Γαληνοῦ ὑπόμνημα Α' Β' Γ' Δ'.
In Hippocratis librum de acutorum victu commentarii IV.

K. XV 418—919.

Inc. (lib. 1) Οἱ ξυγγράψαντες τὰς Κνιδίας καλεομένας γνώμας.
Expl. (lib. 4) παρέγκειται δέ τινα καὶ ἀσαφῆ, περὶ ὧν ἐφεξῆς ποιήσομαι τὸν λόγον.

Athos: Athous Βιβλ. μον. Ἰβήρων
  4304. 184; s. XIV/XV. f 130 A.
  4309. 189; s. XIII. f. 42 A.
Escurial: Scorial. Σ. II. 5; s. XV. f. 73 *und* 178—183.
Florenz: Laurent. plut. 75, 5; s. XIV. p. 159.
Mailand: Trivultian. 685; s. XV (XIV). f. 120. 122ᵛ—193.
Moskau: Mosquens. 465; s. XV. f. 33 (Libri I et III).
München: Monacens. 469; s. XV. f. 1—50 (*Collation besitzt Helmreich*).
Paris: Parisin.
  2165; s. XVI. f. 258.
  2276; s. XVI. f. 1.
  2332*; s. XV (XIV).
Rom: Reg. Suec. 173; s. XV. f. 73ᵛ.
Venedig:
  Marcian. 281; s. XV. f. 2—46ᵛ.
  App. cl.
    V, 4; s. XV.
    V, 5; s. XV. f. 89.
    V, 9; s. XV. f. 508 (τμῆμα α'.).
[**Wien:** Vindob. ap. Nessel P. III.]

Dazu:
  [cathedr. Metens. 226].
  Rasarius, Venedig 1562 p. 211ᵛ (»fehlt bei Kühn.« Schoene).

[Diels I.103] Τῶν εἰς τὸ περὶ χυμῶν Ἱπποκράτους ὑπομνημάτων τὸ Α' Β' Γ'.
In Hippocratis de humoribus librum commentarii III.

K. XVI 1—488.

Inc. (lib. 1) Διεφώνησαν πρὸς ἀλλήλους οἱ παλαιοὶ ἐξηγηταί.
Expl. (lib. 3) μετὰ δόξης καλῶς δυνάμεθα καταγινώσκειν.

Escurial: Scorial. Σ. II. 11; s. XV. f. 32.
Leipzig: Lipsiens. 56; s. XIX.
Mailand: Ambros. C 118 Sup.; s. — (non sine lacunis, ut videtur).
Moskau: Mosquens. 466; s. XVI. f. 61—63 (Auctoris nomen deest et discrepat initium; Inc. Χυμοὶ καθ' Ἱππ. εἰσὶ ...; in fine mutil.).
Paris:
Coislin. 163; a. 1560.
Bibl. Facult. Medic. 14; s. XVII. f. 73 (»e cod. Coisl. 163 descr.«).
Parisin. 2177*; s. XVI. f. 1.
Suppl. 2; s. XVI.
[B. R. Paris. 120 ap. Montf. II 902].
Rom: Urbin. 67; s. XIV. XV. f. 33.

Dazu: [C. de Montchal].

Εἰς τὸ Ἱπποκράτους προρρητικῶν βιβλίον πρῶτον ὑπόμνημα Α' Β' Γ'.
In Hippocratis praedictionum librum primum commentarii III.

K. XVI 489—840.

Inc. (lib. 1) Οὐ μὴν οὐδὲ τὴν Ἡροφίλου νομοθεσίαν.
Expl. (lib. 3) τὴν μετάστασιν τῶν λυπούντων γεγονέναι.

Mailand:
Ambros. Q 3 Sup.; s. XV—XVI. f. 129.
Trivultian. 685; s. XV (XIV). f. 193—230 (Libri I et II; lib. II inc. ἂν ᾖ κατὰ μὲν τὴν χρόαν, ὕπωχρον μετρίως = K. XVI 588, 14; expl. ἢ σπόνδυλος ἐγκάθηται, τουτέοισιν = K. 678).
Modena: Mutinens. 237 (III G 18); s. XVI. f. 3.
Paris: Parisin.
2166; s. XV—XVI. f. 89.
2168; s. XV—XVI. f. 172.
2228; s. XIV—XV. f. 66.
Rom: Reg. Suec. 175; s. XIV. f. 89.
Venedig:
Marcian. 281; s. XV. f. 47—71ᵛ.
App. cl. V, 5; s. XV. f. 182ᵛ (Commentarius duplex).

[Diels I.104] Ἱπποκράτους ἐπιδημιῶν α' καὶ Γαληνοῦ εἰς αὐτὸ ὑπόμνημα Α' Β' Γ'.
In Hippocratis epidemiarum librum primum commentarii III.

K. XVII A 1—302.

Ἱππ. ἐπιδ. β' καὶ Γ. εἰς αὐτὸ ὑπ. Α' Β' Γ' Δ' Ε'.
In librum secundum commentarii V.

K. XVII A 303—479.

Ἱππ. ἐπιδ. γ' καὶ Γ. εἰς αὐτὸ ὑπ. Α' Β' Γ'.
In librum tertium commentarii III.

K. XVII A 480—792.

Ἱππ. ἐπιδ. ς' καὶ Γ. εἰς αὐτὸ ὑπ. Α' Β' Γ' Δ' Ε' ΣΤ'.
In librum sextum commentarii VI.

K. XVII A 793—XVII B 344.

In lib. I:
Inc. (lib. 1) Οὐκ ἐν τούτῳ μὲν βιβλίῳ Ἱπποκράτης.
Expl. (lib. 3) ἡ γυνὴ διὰ τὴν ἰσχὺν τῆς φύσεως σωθῆναι.
In lib. II:
Inc. (lib. 1) Ἄνθρακες ἐν Κρανῶνι.
Expl. (lib. 5) αἷμα συλλέγεται αὐτῷ ἐπὶ τοὺς τιτθούς.
In lib. III:
Inc. (lib. 1) Πυθίων ὃς ᾤκει παρὰ Γῆς ἱερόν.
Expl. (lib. 3) εἰδέναι οὓς καὶ ὅτε καὶ ὡς δεῖ διαιτᾶν.
In lib. VI:
Inc. (lib. 1) Ἐλυμήναντο πολλοὶ τῶν ἐξηγητῶν.
Expl. (lib. 6) ποδάγρας τε καὶ ἀρθρίτιδας.

Florenz: Laurent. plut. 74, 25; s. XIV. p. 127. (in librum III.).
Modena: Mutinens. 211 (III G 7); s. XV (in Hipp. de morb. popul. lib. I et III).
München: Monacens. 231; s. XVI. (in libr. I et III).
Padua: Bibl. Joannis Rhodii. (In lib. II epid. *Verbleib unbekannt*).
Paris: Parisin.
2165; s. XVI. f. 1 (in libros III).
2174; s. XVI. f. 1 (in libr. II) *und* f. 106 (in libr. III.).

Rom: Urbin. 64; s. X—XI. f. 48v (Σχόλιον τῆς ἕκτης ἐπιδημίας ἀπὸ φωνῆς Γαλ. VII partes. Inc. Ἄρτι ταῖς μεθόδοις τὰ ὀξέα τῶν νοσημάτων).

Venedig:

Marcian.

283; s. XV. f. 1 (in libr. VI.).

285; s. XV. (in libr. III.).

App. cl.

V, 5; s. XV. f. 249 (in libr. II) *und* f. 311 (in libr. III. libri II.).

V, 15; s. XVI. (in libr. I. liber I; Expl. τῶν ἔνδον τοῦ περιτοναίου μορίων).

Ἱπποκράτους ἀφορισμοὶ καὶ Γαληνοῦ εἰς αὐτοὺς ὑπομνήματα Ζ'.
Hippocratis aphorismi et Galeni in eos commentarii VII.

K. XVII B 345—XVIII A 195.

Inc. (lib. 1) Ὁ βίος βραχύς, ἡ δὲ τέχνη μακρή.
Expl. (lib. 7) θανάσιμον εἶναι τὸ τοιοῦτον νόσημα.

Athos: Athous Βιβλ. μον. Ἐσφιγμένου 41; s. XV (in libros II—VII).

Escurial: Scorial.

Υ. III. 17; s. XVI. f. 127.

Φ. III. 7; s. XIV. f. 67.

Florenz:

Laurent. plut. 74, 8; s. XV. p. 1.

Riccard. 44 (K. II. 5); s. XV—XVI. f. 27.

Jerusalem: [Diels I.105]

Bibl. patriarch. 102; s. XVIII. f. 12 (Ἑρμηνεία εἰς τοὺς ἀφ. Ἱππ., καταστρωθεῖσα εἰς κοινὴν φράσιν παρὰ Μπαλάνου Βασιλοπούλου ... κατὰ τὸν Γαληνόν).

Bibl. Mar-Saba 481; s. XVIII. f. 265 (Μετάφρασις τῶν ἀφ. τοῦ Ἱππ. εἰς τὴν κοινὴν διάλεκτον ... ἐκ τῆς τοῦ Γαλ. διδασκαλίας).

London: Harleian. (Brit. Mus.) 5611; s. XV. f. 1.

Mailand: Ambros. A 156 Sup.; s. XVI. f. 24.

Paris:

Parisin.

1884; a. 1503. f. 158.

2161; s. XV. f. 1.

2168; s. XVI. f. 1.

2219; s. XV. f. 74 (Libri II—VI, init. mutil.).

2257; s. XVI. f. 120.

2266; s. XIII. f. 93.

2268; s. XIV.
2278; s. XVI. f. 1 (initio et fine mutil.).
2332*; s. XV (XIV). f. — (ex libr. I—VI).
Suppl. 447; s. XIV. f. 1.
Pistoja: Pistoriens. 141 (308); s. XVI. f. 1.
Rom:
Palat.
128; s. XV. f. 26v (in aph. XIV primos).
278; s. XIV—XV. f. 31v (in sectiones VI).
385; s. XV—XVI. f. 1 (init. et fine mutil.).
Urbin. 65; s. XIV. f. 1.
Vatic.
279; s. —. f. 31 (*Verbleib unbekannt*).
280; s. XV. f. 1.
283; s. XIV. f. 22.
Venedig:
Marcian.
277; a. 1416.
278; s. XI. f. 1.
285; s. XV.
App. cl.
V, 5; s. XV. f. 2.
V, 9; s. XV. f. 1 (Expl. ἵδρως πολύς = K. XVIII A 176).
V, 10; s. XVI. f. 29.
Wien: Vindob. 34; s. —. f. 1.

Dazu: [Paul. Lips.].

[Diels I.106]

Πρὸς λύκον.
Adversus Lycum.

K. XVIII A 196—245.

Inc. Ἀνεμέσητον μὲν δήπου Λύκῳ.
Expl. ἄνευ τοῦ μεμαθηκέναι πρότερον αὐτά.

Florenz: Laurent. plut. 74, 3; s. XII. p. 2 (*Collation besitzt Helmreich*).
Paris: Parisin. 2164; s. XVI. f. 44v (*Collation besitzt Helmreich*).
Venedig: Marcian. App. cl. V, 4; s. XV.

Πρὸς τὰ ἀντειρημένα τοῖς Ἱπποκράτους ἀφορισμοῖς ὑπὸ Ἰουλιανοῦ βιβλίον.
Adversus ea quae Juliano in Hippocratis aphorismos enuntiata sunt libellus.

K. XVIII A 246—299.

Inc. Ἄμεινον μὲν ἦν, ὥσπερ οἱ νομοθέται τοὺς ψευδῶς.
Expl. ποτὲ δ' ἀναιρῶν αὐτῶν τὰ δόγματα.

Florenz: Laurent. plut. 74, 3; s. XII. p. 12 (*Collation besitzt Helmreich*).
Venedig: Marcian. App. cl. V, 4; s. XV. (»Unvollständig«. Helmreich. *Collation in dessen Besitz*).

Ἱπποκράτους τὸ περὶ ἄρθρων βιβλίον καὶ Γαληνοῦ εἰς αὐτὸ ὑπομνήματα Δ'.
In Hippocratis de articulis librum commentarii IV.

K. XVIII A 300—767.

Inc. (lib. 1) Ὅτι μὲν τὸ βιβλίον ἕπεται τῷ περὶ ἀγμῶν.
Expl. (lib. 4) διὰ τῆς κοινῆς προσηγορίας ἐδήλωσε τῆς σχοινία.

Florenz: Laurent. 74, 7; s. IX. p. 312 (*Collation H. Graevens in H. Schoenes Besitz*).
Paris: Parisin.
1849; s. XIV. f. 111.
2247; s. XVI.
2248; s. XVI.
Venedig: Marcian. 279; s. XV. f. 84v—130v (*Probecollation [p. 300—313 K.] H. Graevens in H. Schoenes Besitz*).

Περὶ τῶν ἐπιδέσμων. [Diels I.107]
De fasciis.

K. XVIII A 768—827.

Inc. Οὐκ ἀσκόπως μοι δοκεῖ ὁ παλαιὸς Ἱπποκράτης.
Expl. διεκβάλλομεν τὰς ἑτέρας ἐπὶ τὴν ζώνην.

Florenz: Laurent. 74, 7; s. IX. f. 286.
Paris: Parisin.
[2245 (?)].

[2247 (?); s. XVI.].
2248 (?); s. XVI.
2383; s. XVI. f. 7.

Ἱπποκράτους προγνωστικὸν καὶ Γαληνοῦ εἰς αὐτὸ ὑπόμνημα Α' Β' Γ'.
In Hippocratis prognosticum commentarii III.

K. XVIII B 1—317.

Inc. (lib. 1) Τὸν ἰητρὸν δοκέει μοι ἄριστον εἶναι πρόνοιαν ἐπιτηδεύειν.
Expl. (lib. 3) τεσσαρακοστὴν ἢ ἑξηκοστὴν ὅρον θέμενος.

Escurial: Scorial.
Υ. III. 17; s. XVI. f. 135.
Φ. III. 7; s. XIV. f. 9.
Florenz:
Laurent. plut.
74, 8; s. XV. p. 173.
74, 31*; s. XIV. p. 199b (Ex libris I. II. III).
75, 5; s. XIV. p. 249.
Riccard.
17 (K. I. 24); s. XVI. f. 111.
44 (K. II. 5); s. XV—XVI. f. 192.
Mailand: Ambros. A 156 Sup.; s. XVI. f. 190.
Modena: Mutinens. 237 (III G 18); s. XVI. f. 93.
Paris: Parisin.
2168; s. XVI. f. 172.
2257; s. XVI. f. 129.
2266; s. XIII. f. 1.
Pistoja: Pistoriens. 141 (308); s. XVI. f. 146.
Rom:
Palat.
157; s. XIV. f. 2.
173; s. XV. f. 1.
Reg. Suec. 175; s. XIV. f. 1.
Vatic.
1063; s. XIII. f. 1.
1858; s. —. f. 234 (Inc. Ὅτι μὲν ἀντί. Expl. εὐθέως ὁμολογουμένου ὡς τα ..).
Venedig:
Marcian. 282; s. XV. f. 53^v—85^v.

App. cl. V, 5; s. XV. f. 145^{v}.
Wien: Vindob. 44; s. XV. XVI. f. 232.

Εἰς τὸ Ἱπποκράτους περὶ ἀγμῶν ὑπόμνημα Α' Β' Γ'. [Diels I.108]
In Hippocratis librum de fracturis commentarii III.

K. XVIII B 318—628.

Inc. (lib. 1) Πρὸ τῆς τῶν κατὰ μέρος ἐξηγήσεως.
Expl. (lib. 3) τὸ ἐκπεπτωκὸς ἄρθρον εἰς τὴν πρόσω χώραν.

Moskau: Mosquens. 466; s. XVI. f. 90 (discrepat init.).
Paris: Parisin. 1849; s. XIV. f. 147^{v}.
Venedig: Marcian. 279; s. XV. f. 130^{v}—163^{v}.

Τὸ Ἱπποκράτους κατ' ἰητρεῖον βιβλίον καὶ Γαληνοῦ εἰς αὐτὸ ὑπόμνημα Α' Β' Γ'.
In Hippocratis librum de officina medici commentarii III.

K. XVIII B 629—925.

Inc. (lib. 1) Ἰατρικὸν ἐπέγραψεν αὐτὸ κατ' ἰητρεῖον.
Expl. (lib. 3) ἵνα μήτε βιαίως μήτε χαλαρῶς ἐπιδεδεμένα ᾖ.

Paris: Parisin. 1849; s. XIV. f. 175^{v}.
Venedig: Marcian. 279; s. XV. f. 163^{v}—202.

Περὶ μυῶν ἀνατομῆς
De musculorum dissectione.

K. XVIII B 926—1026.
Dietz, Lips. 1832.

Inc. Μυῶν ἀνατομὴν ἀμέμπτως μὲν οὐδεὶς ἔγραψεν.
Expl. δοκεῖν εἶναι καθ' ἕκαστον δάκτυλον.

Escurial: Scorial. T. III. 7; s. XIII. f. 1 (Περὶ μυῶν. Inc. Τοῦ λιχανοῦ δακτύλου μετακάρπιον. Expl. περὶ μὲν οὖν τῆς τῶν μυῶν ἀνατομῆς ἱκανὰ τὰ εἰρημένα. *Vgl.* Costomiris Rev. d. étud. gr. II [1889] p. 374) *und* f. 90 (Π. μυῶν ἀνατ. τ. εἰσαγομ.).

[Diels I.109] **Grottaferrata:** Cryptens. Z Γ VI (series IX cod 46); s. XIV. f. 18.
Leipzig: Lipsiens. 54; s. XIX.
Mailand: Ambros. Q 87 Sup.*; s. XIV. XV. f. 222.
Paris: Parisin.
2219; s. XV. f. 124ᵛ.
2283*; s. XVI.
Venedig: Venet. Bibl. Josephi de Aromatariis. (*Verbleib unbekannt*).

Πῶς δεῖ ἐξελέγχειν τοὺς προσποιουμένους νοσεῖν.
Quomodo morbum simulantes sint deprehendendi.

K. XIX 1—7.

Inc. Διὰ πολλὰς αἰτίας ἄνθρωποι πλάττονται νοσεῖν.
Expl. τὰ δὲ σκοτόδινον.

Leyden: Voss. 4° 45; s. XIV.
Modena: Mutinens. 213 (III G 9); s. XV. f. 155.
Paris: Parisin.
2165; s. XVI. f. 195ᵛ.
2269; s. XV. f. 175ᵛ.
Rom: Vatic.
283; s. XIV. f. 1ᵛ.
1063; s. XIII. f. 114ᵛ.
Venedig: Marcian. App. cl. V, 5; s. XV. f. 333ᵛ (*Collation besitzt Helmreich*).

Περὶ τῶν ἰδίων βιβλίων.
De libris propriis.

K. XIX 8—48.
Iw. Müller, Gal. scr. min. II 91—124.

Inc. Ἔργῳ φανερὰ γέγονεν ἡ συμβουλή.
Expl. κριτικὸς καὶ γραμματικὸς ἕν.

Mailand: Ambros. Q 3 Sup.; s. XV—XVI. f. 187.

Περὶ τῆς τάξεως τῶν ἰδίων βιβλίων πρὸς Εὐγενιανόν.
De ordine librorum suorum ad Eugenianum.

K. XIX 49—61.
Iw. Müller, Erlang. 1874.
Gal. scr. min. II 80—90.

Inc. Καλῶς μοι δοκεῖς, ὦ Εὐγενιανέ, γενέσθαι τι.
Expl. ἁπασῶν ἄμεινον ἀναγινώσκειν.

Mailand: Ambros. Q 3 Sup.; s. XV—XVI. f. 197.

Τῶν Ἱπποκράτους γλωσσῶν ἐξήγησις.
Linguarum s[ive] dictionum exoletarum Hippocratis explicatio.

K. XIX 62—157.

Inc. Τὰς παρ' Ἱπποκράτει γλώσσας, ὦ Τεῦθρα.
Lexic. inc. Ἀγκυλιδωτόν.
Expl. ὠχέτευται : ἐκρύσεις καὶ διεξόδους κέκτηται.

[**Amsterdam:** Amstelodam. ?].
Berlin: Phillipps. 1525 (ol. Meerm. 215); s. XVI. (Expl. mutil. ψαφερον ψαδυρὸν ψέφαρα).
Brüssel: Bruxellens. 11345—48; s. XVI. f. 25.
Florenz: Laurent. plut.
74, 1; s. XV. f. 1v.
74, 3; s. XII. p. 22 (*Collation besitzt Helmreich*). [Diels I.110]
Kopenhagen: Hauniens. Bibl. Reg. ant. fund. 224; s. XVI.
Leyden: Voss. Miscell. 1 pars 13; s. XV.
[**Moskau:** Mosquens. ?].
München: Monacens. 71; a. 1531. f. 1.
Oxford:
Baroccian. 204; s. XV. f. 1 (»Consentit plerumque, sed paulo contractius cum Galeni lexico«).
Dorvillian. X 1. 1. 3; s. XV ex. f. 144.
Paris: Parisin.
2140; s. XII—XIII. f. 1.
2141; s. XV. f. 1.
2142; s. XIII—XIV. f. 1 (*Collation Ilbergs von p. 62—78. 156—157 K. in dessen Besitz*).

2143; s. XIV. f. 1v.
2144; s. XIV. f. 1.
2145; s. XV. f. 1.
2255; s. XV. f. 27.
2287; s. XV—XVI. f. 191.

Rom:
Urbin. 68; s. XIV. f. 3.
Vatic. 277; s. XIV. f. 12 (*Collation besitzt J. v. Müller*).

Venedig: Marcian. 269; s. XI.

Dazu: [Cangii].

Εἰ ζῷον τὸ κατὰ γαστρός.
An animal sit quod est in utero.

K. XIX 158—181.

Inc. Ὅπερ φυσικῶς καὶ πᾶσι φιλοσόφοις.
Expl. ὡς ὁ Μακεδὼν Ἀλέξανδρος καὶ ὡς Ἡρακλῆς.

Florenz: Laurent. plut. 74, 3; s. XII. p. 105b.
Paris: Parisin.
2164; s. XVI. f. 14v.
3035; s. XIV. f. 197 (*Kalbfleischs Probecollation p. 158—166, 8 in dessen Besitz*).
Venedig: Marcian. App. cl. V, 4; s. XV.

Περὶ τῆς κατὰ τὸν Ἱπποκράτην διαίτης ἐπὶ τῶν ὀξέων νοσημάτων.
De victus ratione in morbis acutis ex Hippocratis sententia.

K. XIX 182—221.

Inc. Ὁ παροξυσμὸς οὐ μὲν τὴν βίαν.
Expl. πάλιν ἀναγραφῆς ἀξιώσομεν.

Florenz: Laurent. plut. 74, 3; s. XII. p. 141b (Inc. mutil. ἠρεμίαν δὲ καὶ παρηγορίαν. Expl. ἀξιώσομεν).
Rom: Palat. 143; s. XV. f. 164 (Inc. Μελίκρητον δὲ πινόμενον. »Spectare videntur ad Gal. libr. de victus ratione in morb. acut., ex Hipp. sententia.«).

Περὶ φιλοσόφου ἱστορίας.
De historia philosopha.

K. XIX 222—345.
Diels, Doxographi Graeci p. 595—648.

Inc. Ποία πρὸ τοῦ Σωκράτους ἦν ἡ φιλοσοφία κτλ. Τῶν ἐξ ἀρχῆς φιλοσοφησάντων.
Expl. πεπυκνῶσθαι καὶ διὰ τοῦτο πολυχρόνια.

Cheltenham: Phillipps. 23007; s. XV.
Florenz: Laurent. plut.
58, 2; s. XV. p. 78.
74, 3; s. XII. p. 171b.
Oxford: Baroccian. 131; s. XIV. f. 343.

Ὅροι ἰατρικοί. [Diels I.111]
Definitiones medicae.

K. XIX 346—462.

Inc. Τὴν περὶ τῶν ὅρων πραγματείαν πολυωφελεστάτην.
Expl. ἢ αὐλῶν ἢ συμβόλων ἀκούσαντες.

Athos: Athous Βιβλ. μον. Κουτλουμουσίου 3321. 248; s. XVII. (Ὅροι τῶν νοσημάτων).
Berlin: Phillipps. 1526 (ol. Meerm. 216); s. XVI. (Sine titulo).
Bologna: Bonon. 3632; s. XV. f. 129—131.
Cambridge: Cantabrig. Caius Coll.
355; s. XV/XVI. f. 151 (Γαλ. περὶ ὅρων ἰατρικῶν. Inc. Ὅρα σοφὴν σύνταξιν ἐ⟨ν⟩τέρων ὅλων. Expl. τοῖς σώμασιν ἐκ τῶν λαμβανομένων τροφῶν).
[948; s. —].
Florenz: Laurent. plut.
73, 9; s. XVI. f. 5ᵛ
74, 14; s. XV. p. 1.
Kopenhagen: Hauniens. Bibl. Reg. ant. fund. 1648; s. XV.
Leipzig: Lipsiens. 52; s. XVI. f. 40.
London:
Addit. (Brit. Mus.) 11, 888; s. XV. f. 1.
Regius 12 F III; s. XVII. f. 1.
Mailand: Ambros.
B 90 Sup.; s. XVI.

T 19 Sup.; s. —.
Modena: Mutinens. 210 (III G 6); s. XVI. f. 387.
Moskau: Mosquens. 464; s. XV. f. 328v.
München: Monacens.
109; s. XVI. f. 1.
469; s. XV. p. 51—55 (Ἐρωτήματα ἰατρικῆς τέχνης = K. XIX 350—377).
Oxford: Dorvillian. X 1. 1. 3; s. XV ex. f. 191.
Paris:
Parisin.
[2151 (?)].
2167; s. XVI. f. 269v.
2175; s. XVI. f. 50.
[2252 (?)].
2282; s. XVI. f. 53v.
Suppl.
35; s. XV—XVI. f. 1 (*Kalbfleischs Probecollation in dessen Besitz, Schoenes Probecollation der Vorrede im Besitze der Akademie*).
446; s. X. f. 70 (Inc. mutil. — σαντο τὰ κατὰ τὴν ἰατρικὴν = K. p. 348, 1. *Schoenes Collation im Besitze der Akademie, Kalbfleischs Probecollation in dessen Besitz*).
Rom:
Ottobon. 311; s. XV—XVI. f. 112.
Palat. 297; s. XV—XVI. f. 19v.
Vatic.
1614; s. XVI. f. 122.
4423; s. —. f. 1.
Turin: Taurin. 8 B V 31 (B VI 29); s. XVI. f. 3—5 (Inc. Ἐξόμφαλός ἐστι. Expl. ἧλός ἐστι κτλ. *Verbrannt*).
Wien: Vindob. med. 16; s. XV—XVI. f. 287.

Ὅτι αἱ ποιότητες ἀσώματοι.
Quod qualitates incorporeae sint.

K. XIX 107 463—484.

Inc. Οὐδὲν τῶν ἐμῶν ἀγνοεῖν βουλόμενος.
Expl. ἡ κοινωνία πρὸς ἑτέρους, ἀλλ' ἡ λύσις.

Florenz: Laurent. plut. 74, 3; s. XII. p. 136b (*Plasbergs Collation in Kalbfleischs Besitz*).
Mailand: Ambros. Q 3 Sup.; s. XV—XVI. f. 202 (*Kalbfleischs Collation in dessen Besitz*).

Paris:

Parisin. 2164; s. XVI. f. 40 (*Kalbfleischs Probecollation p. 463—469, 6 in dessen Besitz*).

Suppl. 35; s. XV—XVI. f. 102 (*Kalbfleischs Collation in dessen Besitz*).

Venedig: Marcian. App. cl. V, 4; s. XV (*Plasbergs Collation in Kalbfleischs Besitz*).

Περὶ χυμῶν.
De humoribus.

K. XIX 485—496.

Inc. Ὅπερ ἐν κόσμῳ στοιχεῖον, τοῦτο ἐν ζῴοις χυμός.
Expl. τὴν ἐντελῆ διάκρισιν τῆς ἀσθενείας ἀνέθεντο.

Escurial: Scorial. Σ. III. 17; s. XVI. f. 32.
Paris: Parisin.
2156; s. XV. f. 64v.
2158; s. XV. f. 64v.
2760; s. XVI. f. 21.

Περὶ προγνώσεως. [Diels I.112]
De praenotione.

K. XIX 497—511 = Περὶ συστάσεως ἰατρικῆς K. I p. 289—304; *vgl.* Kalbfleisch, Berl. philol. Wochenschrift 1896 p. 59 f.

Inc. Περὶ προγνώσεως τοίνυν ἐφεξῆς λέγωμεν.
Expl. καὶ τοὺς καθ' ἕκαστον αὐτῶν τρόπους τῆς ἰάσεως.

Florenz: Riccard. 44 (K II 5); s. XV—XVI. f. 243v.
Leyden: Voss. 4° 45; s. XIV.
Mailand: Ambros. A 156 Sup.; s. XVI. f. 264.
Paris:
Parisin.
2165; s. XVI. f. 192 (»praenotiones«).
2269; s. XV. f. 145v.
2283*; s. XVI. (Exc. ex »προγνωστικ. ὑπομνήματ.«).
Suppl. 35; s. XV—XVI. f. 144.
Rom: Vatic.
283; s. XIV. f. 12v.

1063; s. XIII. f. 109.

Venedig:

Marcian. 281; s. XV. f. 81^{v} (Π. τοῦ προγινώσκειν).

App. cl. V, 5; s. XV. f. 330^{v}.

Πρόγνωσις πεπειραμένη καὶ παναληθής.

Praesagitio omnino vera expertaque.

K. XIX 512—518.

Inc. Τὸν θέλοντα προγινώσκειν οὐ μόνον τὴν ἡμέραν.

Expl. καὶ ὑγρασίαν πλείω σημαίνει.

Modena: Mutinens. 61 (III B 9); s. XV. f. 17^{v} (Inc. ἔτι τὸν θέλοντα).

Paris: Parisin. 2269; s. XV. f. 114.

Rom: Palat. 143; s. XV. f. 167.

Περὶ φλεβοτομίας.

De venae sectione.

K. XIX 519—528.

Inc. Ἐν πάσῃ ἡμέρᾳ καὶ νυκτὸς ὥρᾳ.

Expl. εὐβοηθητότερον γάρ ἐστι.

Berlin: Phillipps. 1571; s. XVI. f. 3 (Initium opusc. = K. XIX 519—521, 15).

Florenz: Laurent. plut. 74, 22; s. XIV. p. 9b (des. imperf.).

Leyden: Voss. 4° 45; s. XIV.

Paris: Parisin. 2228; s. XIV—XI. f. 45.

Περὶ κατακλίσεως νοσούντων προγνωστικὰ ἐκ τῆς μαθηματικῆς ἐπιστήμης.

Prognostica de decubitu ex mathematica scientia.

K. XIX 529—573.

Inc. Περὶ μὲν τοῦ ὑπαρκτικὴν εἶναι.

Expl. ἀδιάπτωτος ἔσῃ ἐν ἅπασι.

Florenz: Laurent. plut.
28, 14; s. XIV ex. f. 154v.
28, 34; s. XI. *hinter* f. 5.
Madrid: Matrit. bibl. nac. 4783 (ol. O 67); s. XVI. f. 30.
München: Monacens. 105; s. XVI. f. 218 (fine mutil. K. XIX 529—545).
Paris: Parisin.
1991; s. XV. f. 29 (*Abschrift des* Laurent. 28, 34). [Diels I.113]
[2139 (?)]
Rom:
Barberin. I 127; s. XVI. f. 189v.
Vatic.
1066; s. XVI. f. 78.
1444; s. XVI. f. 22v. (K. XIX p. 529—571).
1692 B; s. XV. f. 7.
Venedig: Marcian. 336; s. XV—XVI. f. 251v (Expl. ἀναιρεθήσονται γάρ).

Περὶ οὔρων.
De urinis.

K. XIX 574—601.

Inc. Τῶν οὔρων αἱ διαφοραὶ πολλαί μὲν κατὰ μέρος.
Expl. καὶ δῆξιν χολῆς ἤδη σεσηπυίας.

Paris: Parisin.
2165; s. XVI. f. 181v.
2308; s. XV. f. 115.
3035; s. XIV. f. 219v.
Rom:
Palat. 143; s. XV. f. 173.
Reg. Suec. 181; a. 1364. f. 285.
Vatic. 280; s. XV. f. 158 (?).
Venedig: Marcian. App. cl. V 5; s. XV. f. 428.

Περὶ οὔρων ἐν συντόμῳ.
De urinis compendium.

K. XIX 602—608.

Inc. Τῶν οὔρων, ὡς προείρηται.
Expl. διαγνώσεως καὶ προρρήσεως καὶ θεωρίας.

Escurial: Scorial. Φ. III. 11; s. XIV—XV. f. 40 (fine mutil.; *vgl.* f. 47).
Paris:
Parisin. 2316; s. XV. f. 191.
Suppl.
634; s. XIV. f. 112.
446; s. X. f. 92.

Περὶ οὔρων ἐκ τῶν Ἱπποκράτους καὶ Γαληνοῦ καὶ ἄλλων τινῶν.
De urinis ex Hippocrate, Galeno aliisque quibusdam.

K. XIX 609—628.

Inc. Οὖρον δὲ ἄριστόν ἐστιν, ὅταν λευκή τε.
Expl. ὅσῳπερ ἂν ὑφιζάνῃ κάτω, τοσούτῳ βελτίω γίνεται.

[**Paris:** Parisin. 2269 (?)].

Περὶ σφυγμῶν πρὸς Ἀντώνιον.
De pulsibus ad Antonium.

K. XIX 121 629—642.

Inc. Σκοπὸν ἔχομεν ἐν τῷ παρόντι συγγράμματι.
Expl. ὁμοίως καὶ τῶν ἑτέρων χυμῶν.

Berlin: Phillipps. 1566 (ol. Meerm. 269); s. XVI. f. 19 (in fine pauca omissa sunt).
Bologna: Bonon. 3632*; s. XV. f. 63^{v}.
Oxford: Clarkian. 16 (18378); s. XIV. f. 74b (Expl. καὶ μάλιστα ἐπὶ τῶν ἀκμαζόντων = K. XIX 641, 3).

Paris:

Parisin.

1630*; s. XIV. f. 19 (*Krolls Collation in Kalbfleischs Besitz; vgl.* Rhein. Mus. 47 S. 456[3]).

2315; s. XV. f. 393ᵛ—400.

Suppl. 446; s. X. f. 33ᵛ (Inscr. Ἑρμηνεία π. σφυγμῶν καὶ θεωρία. Inc. Ὁπόταν ἰατρὸς ἐπ' ἀρρώστῳ κληθῇ = K. XIX 633, 10. Expl. *wie im* Clarkian. Subscr. ζήτει πρ. Ἀντώνιον φιλομαθῇ).

Venedig: Venet. Bibl. Josephi de Aromatariis (*Verbleib unbekannt*).

Περὶ τῆς τῶν ἐν νεφροῖς παθῶν διαγνώσεως καὶ θεραπείας.
De affectuum renibus insidentium dignotione et curatione liber.

K. XIX 643—698.

Inc. Περὶ οὐσίας νεφρῶν. ἡ οὐσία τῶν νεφρῶν ἰδία.
Expl. καὶ αἴτιον καὶ νόσον καὶ σύμπτωμα εἶναι.

Paris: Parisin. Suppl. 35; s. XV—XVI. f. 61.
Venedig: Marcian. 282; s. XV.

Περὶ μελαγχολίας ἐκ τῶν Γαληνοῦ καὶ Ῥούφου καὶ Ποσειδωνίου καὶ Μαρκέλλου Σικαμίου τοῦ Ἀετίου βιβλίον. [Diels I.114]
De melancholia ex Galeno, Rufo, Posidonio et Marcello Sicamii Aetii libellus.

K. XIX 699—720.

Inc. Ὥσπερ ἐν τοῖς φαινομένοις μέλεσι τοῦ σώματος.
Expl. ἐνίοτε δὲ καὶ ποτίζειν τινὰ τῶν ὑπνωτικῶν.

Rom: Urbin. 70; s. XV. f. 107.
Venedig: Marcian.

[276 (*Verwechselung mit* Π. μελ. χολῆς = K. V 104—148)].

279; s. XV. f. 269ᵛ—271.

[282 (*Verwechselung wie bei* nr. 276).

284 (*Verwechselung wie bei* nr. 276)].

Περὶ ἀντεμβαλλομένων.
De succedaneis liber.

K. XIX 721—747.

Inc. Ἐπειδὴ περὶ τῶν ἀντεμβαλλομένων λόγον ἐνεστήσαντο.
Expl. ἀντὶ ᾠῶν πυρρῶν μέλι ἢ ἕψημα.

Bologna: Bonon. 3632; s. XV. f. 260.
Escurial: Scorial. Υ. III 14; s. XV. f. 238 (Expl. ἀντὶ χολῆς ἔχεος).
Florenz: Laurent. plut. 75, 10; s. XV. p. 1 (Lexicon ordine litterarum compositum, cap. VI tractatus medici anon.).
London: Addit. (Brit. Mus.) 10, 058; s. XV. f. 58ᵛ (Inc. Ἀντὶ ἀκανθίου = K. XIX 723. Expl. Ἀντὶ βαλσαμελαίου κτλ. deest ap. K.).
Paris:
Coislin. 335; s. XV. f. 69 (Inc. *wie im* Lond. Addit.).
Parisin.
1883; s. XIV. f. 785ᵛ.
[2208 (?)].
2238; s. XV. f. 593.
2294; s. XV. f. 101.
2312; s. XV. f. 422.
2315; s. XV. f. 64ᵛ (Pauli Aeginetae frgm. ex Galeno de succ.).
2318; s. XV. f. 72 (*Wie im* Parisin. 2315).
[2319 (?)].
2510; a. 1384. f. 61.
Suppl.
682; s. XI. f. 130.
1193*; s. XVI. f. 17.
1297; s. XI.
Rom:
Palat. 279; s. XIV—XV. f. 266 (Inc. *wie im* Lond. Addit.)
Vatic.
279; s. —. f. 237 (Π. ἀντ. καὶ ἐκ τῶν λέξεων βοταν. *Verbleib unbekannt*).
296; s. XV. f. 476.
1595*; s. IX. f. 200 (*Vgl.* H. Schoene, Mitteilungen zur Geschichte der Medizin 1902, 141).
1898; s. —. f. 67.
2256; s. XIV. f. 33.
Venedig: Marcian. 295; s. XIV. f. 179—186ᵛ (Expl. ἰμίσυος κυπρίου).

Wien: Vindob.
20; s. XV. f. 484 (*Wie im* Parisin. 2315).
26; s. XV. f. 303 (*Wie im* Parisin. 2315).
[28 (?)].
32*; s. XVI. f. 31 (Inc. Ἀντὶ ἀμυγδάλου πικρὸν ἀψίνθιον. Expl. ἀντὶ ὠκίμου ἡδέος μονάγριον).

Περὶ μέτρων καὶ σταθμῶν. [Diels I.115]
De ponderibus et mensuris.

K. XIX 748—781.

Inc. Τί ὁ σταθμός, τί τὸ μέτρον καὶ ἀμφοτέρων διαφοραί.
Expl. πλάγιον δὲ | ἢ S, ὀβολόν. / ∞ ∞.

Bologna: Bonon.
1808; s. XV. f. 64 (Inc. Ὁ σταθμὸς βάρει. Expl. τὴν ῥοπὴν διαφορᾶ).
3632*; s. XV. f. 261.
Carpentras: nr. 1774 (P. V.); s. XVII. f. 313.
Florenz: Laurent. plut. 57 (?), 19; s. XIV. p. 224b.
London: Medical Society H Hi 17 = We 30; s. XV in. f. 56 (Inscr. Περὶ σταθμῶν Γαληνοῦ. Inc. Ὁ σταθμὸς βάρει μετρούμενος. Expl. ἄποιόν ἐστι κατὰ τὴν διαφοράν).
Oxford: Laudian. C 57 (nunc 58; Bodl. 709); s. XV in.
Paris: Parisin. 2149*; s. XVI. f. 159 (ex Oribasio et Gal.).
Rom:
Reg. Suec. 172; s. XIV. f. 229 (Sine auctoris nomine).
Vatic.
269; s. XV. f. 476.
1898; s. —. f. 65. 66. 67.
Venedig: Marcian. 288; s. X.

Dazu: [Britannic. 3637; s. —].

[Περὶ αἰσθήσεων].
De quinque sensibus.

Venedig: Bibl. Josephi de Aromatariis. (*Verbleib unbekannt*).

Περὶ ἀλειμμάτων.
De unguentis.

Jerusalem: Bibl. patriarch. 148; s. XVI. f. 40 (Π. ἀλ. ἐκ τοῦ Ἱππ. καὶ Γαλ. καὶ ἑτέρων φιλοσ. κ. ἰατρ.).

Περὶ ἀνατομῆς.
De anatomia.

Modena: Mutin. 226 (II H 11); s. XVI. f. 271 (De anat. internar. et extern. partium).
Venedig: Marc. App. cl. V 4; s. XV (Π. ἀνατ. τῶν ἐντὸς καὶ ἐκτός).

Dazu: Car. Theyer. 6603 (lat. ?).

[Diels I.116] Περὶ τῆς ἀνατομῆς ἐπὶ τῶν ζώντων.
De anatomia vivorum.

Inc. Medicorum anathomicos necesse est praecognoscere.
Expl. diversitas inter Gal. et Aristotelem.

[Cod. Mich. Cantacuzeni]?

Περὶ ἀνέμων, περὶ πυρός,
περὶ ὕδατος ὀμβρίου καὶ ὕδατος ποταμοῦ καὶ ὕδατος θαλασσίου
καὶ ὕδατος λίμνης καὶ ὕδατος φρέατος,
ἔτι καὶ γῆς λευκῆς καὶ κοκκίνης.
De ventis, igne, aquis, terra.

Cod. Mich. Cantacuzeni (*bei* Foerster de antiquit. et libr. mss. Constantinopol. p. 27 *und* Costomiris Rev. des ét. gr. II p. 382/383 no. ΛΔ').

Περὶ ἀνεντάτων.
De non intentis.

Rom: Angelic. 17 (C. 5. 4); s. XIV. f. 9 (Inc. Ἀνέντατον ποιῆσαι καὶ συνουσίας).

Περὶ ἀνθράκων.
De carbunculis.

Bologna: Bonon. 1808; s. XV. f. 116.

Περὶ ἀπεψίας. [Diels I.117]
De cruditate.

Inc. Σημεῖον ἐσχάτης ἀπεψίας τοῦ φλεβώδους γένους.
Expl. ἔτι δὲ ἧττον τὸ μελανθὲν κατὰ τὴν νεφέλην.

Paris: Parisin. 2256; s. XV. f. 535v—538v.

Περὶ ἀποδείξεων.
De demonstrationibus.

Paris: Parisin. 2320; s. XVI. f. 1 (Ἱππ. καὶ Γαλ. καὶ ἑτέρων φιλοσόφων ... περὶ θεωρημάτων τε καὶ ἐπιστάσεων ἀληθοῦς ἀποδείξεως. Inc. Ὁ νόμος μὲν πάντα κρατύνει. *Vgl.* Costomiris Rev. des ét. gr. II 378—380).
Rodosto: nr. — (Γαλ. περὶ ἀποδείξεων ἰατρῶν. *Vgl.* Foerster de antiqu. et libris mss. Constantinopol. *und* Costomiris *a. a. O.* p. 383).

Λεξικὸν βοτανικόν.
Lexicon botanicum.

Athos: Athous Βιβλ. μον. Ἰβήρων 4271. 151; s. XV. f. 224 (Inc. Ἄρκευστον ἢ καντζάρου ἢ κέδρος. Expl. Σισύμβριον τὸ βάρσαμον).
Berlin: Phillipps. 1570; s. XVI. f. 63 (Inc. Ἀκταία· ἡ κουφοξυλαία. Expl. ὤκιμον τὸ βασιλικόν).
Escurial: Scorial. Σ. III. 17; s. XVI. f. 114v (Inc. *wie im* Athous. Expl. ἡ ῥίζα ὡς ἂν κρομιδίου).
Florenz: Laurent. plut. 75, 10; s. XV. p. 1 (Cap. V tractatus medici anon.).
London: Harleian. (Brit. Mus.) 6305; s. XVI (?). f. 153 (Inc. *und* Expl. *wie im* Berolin.).
Mailand: Arch. del Capitolo Metropol. 2; s. XV. f. 132v—135 (Inc. *und* Expl. *wie im* Berol.).
Modena: Mutinens. 61 (III B 9); s. XV. f. 17v (Inc. *und* Expl. *wie im* Berol.).
[**Oxford:** Bodleian. Cat. mss. Angl. n. 2062].

Paris:

Coislin. 335; s. XV. f. 63 (Inc. *wie im* Athous).

Parisin. 2151*; s. XVI. f. 97.

Imprimés, Réserve Te 138, 27; s. XV. f. 31ᵛ.

Rom:

Barberin. I 127; s. XVI. f. 207 (Inc. Ἀβρότονον. Expl. ὑπάρχει δυνάμεως).

Vatic.

279*; s. —. f. 237 (*Verbleib unbekannt*).

294; s. —. f. 265 (Inc. Ἀείζωον τὸ ἀμάραντον).

Upsala: Upsal. 8 (e don. Jo. Gabr. Sparfvenfeld. 49); s. —. (*Ob von Galen, ist fraglich*).

Wien: Vindob. med. 1*; s. V—VI. f. 1.

Περὶ γάλακτος.
De lacte.

Bologna: Bonon. 3632; s. XV. f. 265.

[**Florenz:** Laurent. ap. Bandini III 122 (De sero lactis)] (*nicht von Galen*).

Περὶ γενέσεως.
De generatione.

Paris: Parisin. Suppl. 681; s. XIII—XVI. f. 6.

Περὶ γονορροίας.
De nimia seminis profusione.

Bologna: Bonon. 1808; s. XV. f. 270ᵛ.

[Diels I.118] Περὶ γυναικείων.
De gynaeceis i. e. de passionibus mulierum.

Paris: Parisin.

2153; s. XV. f. 218 (de morbis mulierum).

2270; s. XV—XVI. f. 177.

Rom: Barberin. I 127; s. XVI. f. 255 (Inc. Μήτρα λέγεται καὶ ὑστέρα. Expl. in cap. περὶ τῶν δίμηνα καὶ τρίμηνα φθειρουσῶν· πρὸς τὰς μὴ συλλαμβανούσας.

Διαίρεσις.
Distinctio.

Inc. Τὰ κατὰ φύσιν ἢ στοιχεῖά εἰσιν ἢ μόρια ἢ χυμοὶ ἢ δυνάμεις ἢ ἐνέργειαι ἢ ὧραι.
Expl. ἐσθιώμενος.

Mailand: Trivultian. 685; s. XV (XIV). f. 83—86 (*Vgl.* Schoene, Sitz.-Ber. d. Berl. Akad. 1901 p. 1256).

Περὶ διαίτης.
De victus ratione.

London: Harleian. (Brit. Mus.) 5626; s. XV—XVI (?). f. 53 (Διαιτητικὸν ὑγιεινῶν παραγγελμάτων).

Dazu:
[R. Burscough 7621 *und* 7673 (Isag. ad regimen Galeni)].
Mich. Cantacuzeni (*bei* Foerster de antiquit. et libr. mss. Constantinopol. p. 27 *und* Costomiris Rev. des ét. gr. II p. 382/383 no. ΛΑ'. Γαλ. περὶ διαίτης τοῦ ἀνθρώπου καὶ π. ἀνθρώπων ἐκδεδιῃτημένων).

Περὶ διαίτης καὶ θεραπειῶν πρὸς ἀντικένσορα πατρίκιον.
De diaeta et morbis curandis.

Inc. Ἐπειδὴ θεραπεῦσαι λόγῳ ὀρθῷ οὐκ ἐγχωρεῖ.
Expl. ἢ τρία ἐδέσματα καὶ πινέτω πλείονα.

Cambridge: Cantabrig. bibl. univ. FF 3, 30; s. XVI. no. 5.
Paris: Parisin. 2230; s. XIV. f. 120.

Εἰσαγωγὴ διαλεκτική. [Diels I.119]
Institutio logica.

Ed. M. Mynas, Paris 1844.
C. Kalbfleisch, 283 Lips. 1896.

Inc. (Τῶν φαινομένων τὰ μὲν αἰσθήσει γιγνώ)σκομεν ἅπαντες ἄνθρωποι.
Expl. μεθοδικοῦ λόγου συλλογιστέον.

Paris: Parisin. Suppl. 635; s. XIII. f. 3v.

Περὶ τῶν ἑαυτῷ δοκούντων.
De propriis placitis.

Ed. Helmreich, Philol. 52 266 [1893] p. 431; 59 [1900] p. 316.
vgl. Kalbfleisch, Philol. 55 [1896] p. 689.
Frgm. dieser Schrift ist Π. οὐσ. τῶν φυσ. δυνάμ. = K. IV 757—766, *s. o.* S. 72.

Mailand: Ambros. Q 3 Sup.*; s. XV—XVI. f. 185 (frgm. —. *Kalbfleischs Collation in dessen Besitz*).
Paris:
Parisin. 2332*; s. XV (XIV). f. 199ᵛ (Inc. Ἐδείχθη. Expl. νομίζουσιν).
Suppl. 634*; s. XIV. f. 23ᵛ. 26ᵛ.
Wien: Vindob. med. 15*; s. —. f. 138 (Inc. *und* Expl. *wie im* Parisin. 2332).

Περὶ ἐγκεφάλου καὶ μηνίγγων.
De cerebro eiusque tunicis.

Inc. Γυμνώσα ἐπιτηδείως τὸν ἐγκέφαλον ὄψει.

London: Burneian. (Brit. Mus.) 94; s. XV (XVI). f. 170.

Περὶ ἐθῶν.
De consuetudinibus.

Ed. R. Dietz Lips. 1832.
Iw. Müller Erlang. 1879.
Gal. scr. min. II 9—31.

Inc. Τῶν θεραπευτικῶν σκοπῶν ἕνα.
Expl. καὶ πλῆθος ἀθροίζουσιν.

Florenz: Laurent. plut. 75, 7; s. XIV. p. 237b.
Padua: Bibl. Joannis Rhodii. (*Verbleib unbekannt*).
Venedig: Bibl. Josephi de Aromatariis; s. — (de moribus. *Verbleib unbekannt*).

[Περὶ ἐκτρώσεως (?)]. [Diels I.120]
De abortivo foetu.

[**Cambridge:** Cantabr. Caius Coll.]
[946; s. —.]
[6605; s. —.]
[**Leyden:** Vossian.]

Περὶ ἑλκῶν.
De vulneribus.

Bologna: Bonon. 1808; s. XV. f. 301ᵛ. (Π. ἑλκῶν τῶν μὴ κακοήθων οὐλῆς δεομένων).

Περὶ τῆς ἰατρικῆς ἐμπειρίας
= »*Sermo adversus empiricos medicos*«.

Ed. gr. cum lat. Gadaldini versione H. Schoene, Sitz. d. Kgl. Pr. Ak. d. W. 1901 p. 1255—1263.
Galeni de optimo docendi genere liber, adnotabant et emendabant seminarii philologorum Bonnensis sodales; accedit libri adversus empiricos fragmentum. Bonnae 1906.

Mailand: Trivult. 685; s. XV. f. 120ᵛ—122 (Frgm. Inc... τὸν ς' ἔτι θεάσασθαι περιμενεῖς. Expl. ἢ οὐκ ἂν αὐτοσχεδίως ...).
Venedig: Marcian. App. cl. V, 9; s. XV. f. 508 (Inc. ἢ σπανίως ἢ ἀμφιδόξως = p. 1263, 2 Sch. Expl. *wie im* Trivult.).

Πρὸς Γαῦρον περὶ τοῦ πῶς ἐμψυχοῦται τὰ ἔμβρυα.
Ad Gaurum quomodo animetur fetus.

Ed. K. Kalbfleisch, Abh. d. Kgl. Pr. Ak. d. W. 1895.

Inc. Τὸ περὶ τῆς εἰς τὰ σώματα.
Expl. ἄνθρακος φλόγα· πολλοῖς γὰρ ...

Paris: Parisin. Suppl.
635; s. XIII. f. 12—23ᵛ.
727; s. XIX. f. 21—49.

Περὶ ἐνυπνίων.
De insomniis.

Paris: Parisin. 2308; s. XV. f. 249.

[Περὶ Ἐπικτήτου].
Galeni et Simplicii testimonia de Epicteto.

Inc. Ὁ Περγαμηνός.
Expl. περισώζεται.

Florenz: Laurent. Conventi soppressi 163; s. XVI. f. 5.

[Diels I.121] Περὶ ἑπταμήνων βρεφῶν.
De septimestri partu.

Ed. R. Dietz, Severi de clysteribus liber [Regimontii 1836] append. p. 45—46.
Cf. Athenaeus ap. Oribas. t. III p. 78 Dbg.-Bu.

Florenz: Laurent. plut.
74, 2*; s. XI. p. 281b (Inc. Τῆς κυήσεως οὐχ εἷς ὡρισμένος)
74, 3; s. XII. p. 98.
[**Leyden:** Vossian. 2324].
Paris: Parisin. 2210; a. 1357. f. —.
Rom: Barberin.
I 80 (= 273); s. —. f. 42.
I 152; s. XVI. f. 39.
Venedig: Marcian. App. cl. V, 4; s. XV. no. 11.

Περὶ ἐρυσιπέλατος.
De erysipelate.

Bologna: Bonon. 1808; s. XV. f. 118.

Περὶ ζωῆς καὶ θανάτου.
De vita et morte.

Florenz: Laurent. plut. 75, 19; s. XIV. p. 193.
Oxford: Baroccian. 88; s. XV—XVI. f. 48b (Expl. ἢ καὶ τοῦ θανάτου).
Paris: Parisin. 2320; s. XVI. f. 23 (*Wie im* Baroccian.).

Περὶ ζῴων.
De animalibus.

Paris: Parisin. 2510; a. 1384. f. 80 (de animalibus marinis et terrestribus ad morbos curandos idoneis).
[**Rom:** Vatic. ap. Montfaucon p. 34 (de motu animalium)].

Dazu: Mich. Cantacuzeni (*bei* R. Foerster de antiquit. et libr. mss. Constantinopol. p. 27 *und* Costomiris Rev. des ét. gr. II p. 382/83. no. ΛΒ'. Γαλ. π. ζῴων μορίων καὶ τῆς αὐτῶν σημειώσεως).

Περὶ ζῴων φθαρτικῶν.
De animalibus noxiis.

Athen: nr. 1493; s. XII ex. no. 3—5 (3. Θεραπεία πρὸς τὰς ἀπὸ τῶν ἰοβόλων ἑρπετῶν ἱπταμένων καὶ ἐνύδρων θηρίων πληγάς. 4. Περὶ ζῴων φθαρτικῶν καὶ αἵματος, σπερμάτων τε καὶ ῥιζῶν καὶ μεταλλικῶν καὶ λοιπῶν θανατηφόρων καὶ τῆς τούτων θεραπείας. 5. Περὶ ζῴων φθαρτικῶν).
Athos: Athous Βιβλ. μον. Ἰβήρων 4271. 151; s. XV. f. 71 A. 74 A. 80 A (= Athen. no. 3—5; f. 71 A Inc. Σφηκῶν καὶ μελισσῶν ἁρμόζει. f. 74 Inc. Ζῷα μὲν οὖν ἐστι φθαρτικά. f. 80 Inc. Περὶ βοτανῶν. Βοτάνη ἀγριοπήγανον. Αὕτη ποιεῖ πρὸς τὰς ἐμπνευματώσεις).

Περὶ ἥπατος. [Diels I.122]
De iecore.

Florenz: Laurent. App. 2; s. XV. f. 344.

Περὶ θηριακῆς.
De theriaca.

Madrid: Matrit. Bibl. reg. 44 (ol. 23); s. XV. f. 180ᵛ (π. τῆς μεγάλης θηριακῆς τῆς δι' ἐχιδνῶν. Inc. Πολλῆς οὔσης διαφωνίας περὶ τὰς γραφικὰς ἀποδείξεις. Expl. δεῖ δὲ σαρκῶν μὲν δύο μέρη βάλλεσθαι, ἄρτων δὲ ἕν).
Paris: Parisin. 2183; s. XV. f. 164ᵛ (Formulae theriacae).

Περὶ θλάσματος.
De contusionibus.

Bologna: Bonon. 1808; s. XV. f. 213.

[Περὶ τῶν ΙΒ' θυρῶν (πυλῶν ?)].
De XII portis.

Cambridge: Cantabrig. Caius Coll. 47; s. XV. no. IV (Frgm. Inc. in porta XVII καὶ βλάβης εἶδον. Expl. in porta XIX ἰατροὶ τοῦ κόπτειν τὴν αἴεραν).
Oxford: [Ashmol. mss. Angl.]
[7638 (Gal. liber de XII portis)].
[7787 (Gal. liber de XII portis)].

[Περὶ ἰατρικῆς τέχνης].
[*De arte medica*].

[Cod. Frc. Bernardi 3651 (Theoria et practica medicinae)].

[Diels I.123] Ἰατροσόφια.
Iatrosophia.

Athen: Atheniens. 1479; s. XIX (Ἰατροσ. ἀπηνθισμένον ἀπὸ τοῦ Γαλ., Παύλου τοῦ Αἰγ., etc.).
Athos: Athous
Βιβλ. μον. Ἰβήρων
4294. 174; s. XVII. f. 463 (Ἰ. ἐκλελεγμένον ὑπὸ πολλῶν ἰατρικῶν βιβλίων Γαλ. Ἱππ. καὶ ἄλλων πολλῶν σοφῶν ἰατρῶν).
4655. 535; s. XVI. (Ἰ... Γαλ. Ἱππ. καὶ Μελετίου. Inc. Ὅτι ὁ κόσμος).

Παντελεήμονος 5769. 262; s. XVIII. f. 15 A (Ἰ. ... Γαλ. Ἱππ. Μελετ. καὶ Παύλ. τοῦ Αἰγιν.).
Castellorizo (Μεγίστη): nr. — (Ἰ. ... Γαλ. Ἱππ. καὶ Μελετ.; *vgl. den* Athous 4655).
Florenz: Laurent. App. 2; s. XV. f. 222 (Ἰατρικὸν Ἱππ. καὶ Γαλ. ἰατρεῖαι διάφοροι).
Jerusalem: Bibl. Mar-Saba 432; a. 1662. f. 1 (Ἰ. ... Γαλ. Ἱππ. καὶ Μελ. ...).
London:
Harleian. (Brit. Mus.) 5626; s. XV (XVI). f. 2. (Ἰατροσόφ. ... Ἱππ. Γαλ. Ἀρχιγ. etc.).
Addit. (Brit. Mus.) 28, 830; s. XVII. f. 15 (Ἰ. ... ἐκ τῶν βιβλίων τοῦ Ἱππ. καὶ Γαλ.).
Palermo: Panormit. bibl. naz. XIII C 3; s. xvi. f. 1—44ᵛ (Ἰ. Ἱππ. καὶ Γαλ. καὶ ἑτέρων φιλοσ. καὶ ἰατρῶν. Inc. Περὶ ἤθους ἰατρῶν. Ποδαπὸν δεῖ εἶναι τὸν ἰητρόν. Expl. ἐν οὔρῳ, ἐν πτύσμασιν, ἐν ἱδρῶτι) *und* f. 121—238 (Ἀνθολόγιον ἰατροσοφικὸν τοῦ Ἱππ. τοῦ Κῴου καὶ Γαλ. ... καὶ ἑτέρ. ἰατρῶν).
Paris:
Coislin.
300; a. 1318. f. 214ᵛ.
335; s. XV. f. 21—60. *und* f. 75 (Jatros. Gal. Hipp. Melet. cap. DCIV).
Parisin. 2324; s. XVI. f. 1.
Suppl. 684; s. XV—XVIII. f. 211—266ᵛ (Ἰ. ἐκλελεγμ. ἐκ τοῦ Γαλ. καὶ Ἱππ. καὶ ἄλλ. τινῶν. Inc. Ἐγὼ Γαληνὸς πεπειραμένος. Expl. μετὰ ὄξους ὀλίγον καὶ ὠφελεῖται. *Vgl.* Costomiris, Rev. des ét. gr. II [1889] p. 378).
Petersburg: Petropolit. 116; a. 1318. f. 214ᵛ (Ἰ. ἐκ τῶν Γαλ. εἰς πᾶν εἶδος ὠφέλιμον).
Rom: Barberin. III 63 (= 245); s. XVI. f. 394 (Ἰ. ἐκλελεγμ. Γαλ. Ἱππ. καὶ Μελετίου περὶ γυναικός).
Wien: Vindob.
med. 47; s. XVI. f. 9 (Ἰ. ... Γαλ. περὶ πάντων νοσημάτων).
[Vindob. Lambec. ed. Kollar I p. 272 (Ἰ. Γαληνοῦ καθ' Ἱπποκράτους)] (*vgl.* R. Foerster de antiquit. et libris mss. Constantinopol. p. 20 *und* 28b. Costomiris Rev. des ét. gr. II p. 381 sq.).

Dazu: cod. Mich. Cantacuzeni *bei* Foerster *a. a. O.* p. 27 (MB'. Ἰ. ... Ἱππ. Γαλ. καὶ Μελετίου).

Περὶ ἰατρῶν.
De medicis.

Cod. Mich. Cantacuzeni (*bei* Foerster de antiquit. et libr. mss. Constantinopol. p. 27 *und* Costomiris Rev. des ét. gr. II p. 382/3 no. ΛΓ'. Γαλ. π. ἰατρῶν διδασκάλων καὶ μαθητῶν).

Ἱππιατροσόφιον.
Hippiatrosophium.

[**Leyden:** Vossian. Cat. bibl. Lugd. Bat. p. 398 n. 50].

Dazu: cod. Mich. Cantacuzeni (*vgl.* R. Foerster de antiqu. et libr. Constantin. Rostochii 1877 p. 27 no. KH'. Costomiris Rev. des ét. gr. II 382 s.).

[Diels I.124] Τοῦ Ἱπποκράτους εἰς τὰ ἀναλυτικὰ βιβλία ΙΔ', καὶ ἐξηγεῖται αὐτὰ ὁ Γαληνός.
Hippocratis liber resolutionis, quem Galenus explicat.

[**Konstantinopel:** Constantinopol. apud Verdier].
[**Wien:** Vindob. ap. Lambec.—Kollar I p. 273].

[Εἰς Ἱπποκράτους περὶ ἡλικιῶν νοσημάτων].
In libr[um] Hippocratis de aetatum aegritudinibus.

[**Venedig:** Marcian.].

Scholion in Hippocratis παραγγελίας.

Ed. Daremberg, Not. et Extr. des mscrts. méd. I [Paris 1853] p. 200—202.

Inc. Ἐκ τῶν Γαληνοῦ. Ὅσα μὲν εἴωθε.
Expl. διόπερ καὶ ὡρμήμεθα γράψαι.

Rom: Urbin. 68; s. XIV. f. 26v.

Περὶ προσοχῆς καὶ προγνώσεως τῶν μελλόντων καθαίρεσθαι.
De dignotione hominum purgandorum.

Inc. Προσέχειν οὖν χρὴ καὶ τοὺς παχεῖς.
Expl. καὶ βράσον ὀλίγον καὶ χῦσον αὐτό.

London: Addit. (Brit. Mus.) 10, 058; s. XV. f. 127.

Πῶς χρὴ ἐπιβοηθεῖν τοῖς ποιοῦσι (leg. πιοῦσι) φάρμακον καὶ μὴ καθαιρομένοις.
Qua ratione adiuvandi ii sint, qui remedio hausto non purgantur.

Rom: Palat. 143; s. XV. f. 175ᵛ.

Διαθήκη περὶ τῆς τοῦ ἀνθρωπείου σώματος κατασκευῆς.
De hominis natura testamentum.
Περὶ τῆς τεσσάρων τῶν ὡρῶν τε καὶ ιβ' μηνῶν διαίτης.
De victu singulis mensibus servando.

Athos: Athous
Βιβλ. μον. Διονυσίου 3701. 167; s. XV. (Inc. Ἐγὼ Γαληνὸς πεπειραμένος πάνυ τοῦ τῶν ἀνθρώπων ἤθους).
Ἰβήρων 5034. 914; s. XVII. (Inc. *wie im* Athous μον. Διονυσίου. Expl. πρὸς ὑγείαν τοῦ σώματος τοῖς καλῶς χρωμένοις).
Ξηροποταμοῦ 2432. 99; s. XVII. (Διαθ. ... Γαλ. Ἱππ. καὶ Μελετίου π. κατασκ. ἀνθρ. κτλ.).
Berlin:
Phillipps.
1462; s. XV/XVI. f. 410 (Inc. *und* Expl. *wie im* Athous μον. Ἰβήρων).
1566; s. XVI. f. 6 (*Wie im* Phillipps. 1462).
Berol. qu. 5 (304); s. XV/XVI. f. 53ᵛ (*Wie im* Athous Ξηροποταμοῦ).
Florenz: Laurent. plut. 74, 10*; s. XIV. p. 13b (Inc. Οὐ μικρόν μοί ἐστι καταφρονῆσαι). [Diels I.125]
Jerusalem:
Bibl. d. hl. Grabes
199; s. —. f. 64ᴬ (Δίαιτα ἀκριβὴς π. τῶν τεσσάρ. στοιχείων τοῦ χρόνου καὶ περὶ καταστάσεως ὑγιεινῆς τοῦ ἀνθρώπου καὶ τῆς κατασκευῆς αὐτοῦ).
363; a. 1596. f. 211 B (*Wie* nr. 199).
Bibl. d. hl. Kreuzes 68; s. —. no. 2 (*Wie im* Athous Διονυσ.).
London: Addit. (Brit. Mus.) 10, 058; s. XV. f. 71ᵛ (*Wie im* Athous Ἰβήρων. Expl. καλῶς χρωμένοις, καὶ παραφυλάττουσι ταῦτα).
Mailand: Ambros. O 117 Sup.; s. —. f. 89 (*Wie im* Hierosol. Bibl. d. hl. Grabes 199).
Paris: Parisin.
2091*; s. XV. f. 8.
2316; s. XV. f. 439ᵛ (Liber de iis quae singulis mensibus servanda sunt).
Rom:
Palat. 279; s. XIV—XV. f. 311 (Inc. *wie im* Athous Διονυσίου).
Vatic. 1700; s. XIV. f. 27ᵛ (Δίαιτα ἀκριβὴς π. καταστάσεως ὑγιεινῆς τοῦ ἀνθρώπου καὶ τῆς κατασκευῆς αὐτοῦ).
Venedig: Bibl. Josephi de Aromatariis (de hominis structura. *Verbleib unbekannt*).

Wien: Vindob. med.
32; s. XVI. f. 11 (Διαθ. Γαλ. διδάσκουσα ἡμᾶς ἅπαντα κατ' ἀνθρωπίνου σώματος).
53; s. XVI. f. 8v—10v (*Wie im* Athous Ξηροποτ.).

Περὶ κεφαλαλγίας.
De dolore capitis.

Athos: Βιβλ. μον. Ξηροποταμοῦ 2342. 99; s. XVII. (Περὶ πόνου κεφαλῆς).
Oxford: Canonician. 1; s. XVI. f. 128b (Γαλ. θεραπεία εἰς κεφαλαλγίαν).

Περὶ κλοκίων.
De ... (*De excrementis* [N.38])

Inc. Ἔπαρον τὸ κλόκιον.
Expl. καὶ κατάλυσιν τῆς σαρκός.

London: Medical Society H Hi 17 = We 30; s. XV in. no. 33 Dbg. (Expl. τὸ ἧπορ αὐτοῦ βεβλαμμένον).
Oxford: Roe 15 (Bodl. 261); s. XV ex. f. 102v.
Paris: Parisin. 2224; s. XV. f. 44.

Περὶ κυνάγχης.
De angina.

Florenz: Laurent. App. 2; s. XV. f. —.

Περὶ λεπτυνούσης διαίτης.
De victu attenuante.

Ed. K. Kalbfleisch, 281a; cf. 64 Lips. 1898.

Inc. Ἐπειδὴ τὰ πλεῖστα τῶν χρονίων ἀρρωστημάτων.
Expl. ἄλλα πάντα φυλάττεσθαι προσήκει.

Paris: Parisin. Suppl. 634; s. XIV. f. 133—140.

Περὶ λεύκης. [Diels I.126]
De lepra alba.

Bologna: Bonon. 1808; s. XV. f. 293ᵛ.

Περὶ λίθων.
De lapidibus.

Madrid: Matrit. bibl. nac. 4631 (ol. N 110)*; a. 1474. f. 155 (Inscr. Π. λίθων Διοσκορίδου. »Hic commentarius apud Iriarte impressus ex Dioscuride Aëtio Galeno aliis consutus est«).

Περὶ μετάλλων.
De metallis.

Paris: Parisin. 1310; s. XV. f. 444 (Aristotelis et Gal. frgta. de metallis quae reperiuntur in Cypro insula. *Vgl.* Galenus XII 214. 219. 226. 239 K.).

Περὶ μηχανημάτων.
De machinamentis.

Florenz: Laurent. plut. 74, 7*; s. IX. p. 154 (Inc. Μόνον μὲν ἱκανόν ἐστι).

Περὶ σώματος μορίων.
De corporis partibus.

Rom: Palat. 295; s. XV—XVI. f. 187 (Frgm. Galeni; Inc. Ὁ δὲ γαργαρεὼν ὃν καὶ σταφύλην καλέουσι).

Περὶ νόσων.
De morbis Excerpta.

Jerusalem: Bibl. d. hl. Grabes 179; s. XV. f. 202 (Σύντομος διδασκαλία Γαλ. τοῦ σπεύσαντος γράψαι εἰς τὰ τῶν μορίων πάθη κτλ.).
Mailand: Ambros. A 95 Sup.; s. XV. f. 78.
München: Monacens. 39; s. XVI (»fort. Galeni«).

Oxford: Baroccian.

[88; s. XV (XVI). (Ex Gal. et aliis de morbis et medicamentis variis)]. (*Vgl. unter* π. οὔρων *und* π. σφυγμῶν).

131; s. XIV in. f. 341 (Προθεωρία τῆς περὶ αἰτίας περὶ διαφορᾶς νοσημάτων. Inc. Ἀρχὴ οὖν καὶ κρηπίς. Expl. ὑποκειμένου χειρήσομεν).

Paris:

[Coislin. apud Montfauc. II 448 (Exc. ex Hipp. Gal. Meletio)]. (*Wohl* Coislin. 335; *vgl. unter* Ἰατροσόφια).

Parisin.

2156; s. XV. f. 47 (de morborum curatione. Init. deest).

2158; s. XV. f. 47 (*Wie im* Paris. 2156).

2178; s. XV. f. 42 (Exc. de morbis hominum et remediis).

[2230; s. XIV (De variis morborum generibus remediisque ad illorum curam maxime idoneis)]. (*Es ist wohl* f. 120: De diaeta et morbis curandis *gemeint*).

Turin: Taurinens. 6b IV 6; s. XVI. (»fort. Galeni«).

[**Wien:** Vindob. 131 (Frgm. protheoriae de causis variorum morborum)].

[Diels I.127]

Ὅρος, τί ἐστι φάρυγξ.
Fauces definiuntur.

Florenz: Laurent. App. 2; s. XV. f. 359.

Περὶ οὔρων.
De urinis.

Bologna: Bonon. 3636; s. XIV—XV. f. 125—126 (Inc. Ἄριστον οὖρόν ἐστι. Expl. τότε καὶ συνίσταται τὸ οὖρον).

Escurial: Scorial.

Σ. III. 17; s. XVI. f. 110 (Inc. Τὸ φυσικὸν οὖρον ἔνε ξανθόν. Expl. πάσχει τὰ νεῦρα σημαίνει).

Υ. III. 14; s. XV. f. 49ᵛ (Inc. Οὖρον ἄριστον μέν ἐστι πρῶτον μὲν ὁποῖον τὸ κατὰ φύσιν).

Φ. III. 12; s. XV. f. 8ᵛ (Inc. Σημεῖον ἐσχάτης ἀπεψίας. Expl. καὶ ἀσθένειαν ἐκ χρονίου νοσήματος).

Florenz:

Laurent. plut.

74, 31; s. XIV. p. 22b (Inc. Τὴν περὶ τῆς τῶν οὔρων διαφορᾶς).

75, 19; s. XIV. p. 12.

Magliabecch. 1; s. XVI. f. 207ᵛ (Inc. Τί δηλοῖ τὸ λεπτὸν καὶ ὠχρὸν οὖρον. Expl. τοῦ μελαγχολικοῦ χυμοῦ).

Gallipoli: Ἐκκλησ. ἁγίου Νικολάου 38; s. XIV. f. 52 (Γαλ. π. οὔρων) *und* 57ᵛ (τοῦ αὐτοῦ· ποῖον οὖρον ἄριστόν ἐστιν ἐπὶ τῶν νοσούντων).

[**Leyden**]:

[Voss. 31; s. —].

[Warnerian. 53; s. —].

London:

Addit. (Brit. Mus.) 17, 900; s. XVII. f. 93 (Inc. Οὖρον λευκόν).

Medical Society H Hi 17 = W 30; s. XV in. no. 27 Dbg. [Diels I.128]

Modena: Mutinens. 115 (II D 16); s. XV. f. 9.

Neapel: Bibl. dei Gerolamini XXII. I; s. XV. f. 167ᵛ—170 (Inc. *wie im* Scorial. Φ. III. 12. Expl. πολυειδῆ καὶ ἄπεπτα).

Oxford:

Baroccian. 88; s. XV—XVI. f. 47b (Inc. Ἐὰν ἔστι κλόκιον. Expl. καὶ οὐ σύντομον θάνατον).

Laudian. 58 (nunc 59; Bodl. 708); s. XV. f. 374 (Inc. *wie im* Lond. Addit. 17, 900. Expl. μαρασμὸν σημαίνει).

Roe 15 (Bodl. 260 [261 *bei* Ackermann]); s. XV ex. f. 89b (Inc. *und* Expl. *wie im* Laudian.)

Palermo: Panormit. bibl. naz. XIII C 3; s. XVI. f. 84ᵛ—85 (Inc. *und* Expl. *wie im* Laudian.).

Paris:

[Coislin. ap. Montf. II 447]. (*Es ist wohl* Coislin. 335; s. XV. f. 198ᵛ *gemeint; vgl. unter Excerpta varia*).

Parisin.

2224; s. XV. f. 42 (Ex Gal. Hipp. etc. de urinis).

2228; s. XIV—XI. f. 63 (de urinis ex Gal. Philagr. etc.).

2260; s. XVI. f. 33.

2269; s. XV. f. 128 (De praesagitione ex urinis).

2294; s. XV. f. 68ᵛ.

2309; s. XVI. f. 49.

2330; s. XVI. f. 16ᵛ *und* 23ᵛ.

Suppl.

446; s. X. f. 91 (Π. τῶν κατὰ φύσιν οὔρων. Inc. Ἐπὶ τῶν πυρεκτικῶν μάλιστα νοσημάτων. Expl. θάνατον σημαίνουσιν · εἰ δὲ καὶ περὶ ...).

634; s. XIV. f. 103 (De urinis ex Hippocrate et Galeno. *Abschrift besitzt Helmreich.* »Ist mit K. XIX 609 ff. nicht identisch.« Helmreich).

Rom:

Barberin. I 127; s. XVI. f. 262. Inc. *wie im* Lond. Addit. 17, 900. Expl. κατάλυσιν τῆς σαρκός).

Palat. 428; S. XV—XVI. f. 1 (Inc. Πλεῖον κουφίζει εἰς τόν).
Vatic.
280; s. XV. f. 158ᵛ (Περὶ οὔρων πονηρῶν. Τί δηλοῦσιν αἱ πιτυρώδεις στάσεις. Inc. Ὅταν δὲ δαπανήσει) *und* f. 159 (Π. τῶν κατὰ φύσιν οὔρων. Inc. *wie im* Scorial. Υ. III. 14).
2256; s. XIV. f. 78ᵛ (Inc. *und* Expl. *wie im* Laudian.).

Venedig: Marcian. App. cl. V, 5; s. XV. f. 431 (Π. διαφορᾶς οὔρων. Inc. Ἐπὶ τῶν πυρετικῶν μάλιστα. Expl. προβαίνειν τὴν νόσον).

Wien: Vindob.
med.
[19 (?)].
47; s. XVI. (Expl. *wie im* Laudian.).
phil. 178; s. XV. f. 25ᵛ (Π. οὔρων διὰ στοιχείων. Inc. α. ὑελίον βορβορῶδες. Expl. δηλοῖ τὴν ῥύσιν).

Dazu: [August. cat. p. 27 (ex Gal. et Theoph. Protosp.)].

[Diels I.129]

Περὶ ὀφθαλμῶν.
De oculis.

Venedig: Marcian. 276*; s. c. XII. f. 268 (Γαλ. περὶ τῶν ἐν τοῖς ὀφθαλμοῖς παθῶν διάγνωσις. Inc. Ὀφθαλμοὶ νοσοῦσιν. »Nur 6 Zeilen, die aber mitsamt dem Titel von derselben Hand wieder durchgestrichen worden sind« Schoene).

[Περὶ τῶν παροξυσμῶν χρόνων ?].
De paroxysmorum temporibus.

Paris: Parisin.
2269; s. XV. f. 151ᵛ.
2270; s. XV—XIV. f. 53.

Περὶ ἀρίστης πέψεως τῆς γαστρός.
De optima ventris concoctione.

Inc. Νήστεσιν ἔτι οὖσιν ἡμῖν.
Expl. τὸν οἰκεῖον ἀπολαβόντα κόσμον.

Bologna: Bonon. 3636; s. XIV—XV. f. 120.

Πρὸς Πατρόφιλον περὶ πλευρίτιδος.
De laterum morbo ad Patrophilum.

Inc. Ἔστι δήποτε τὸ πάθος ἡ φλεγμονή.
Expl. Εὔδηλον εἶναι νομίζω, κἂν ἐγὼ μὴ λέγω.

Paris: Parisin. 2228; s. XIV—XI. f. 48v (Expl. κἂν ἐγὼ μὴ λέγω).
Wien: Vindob. med. 30; s. XV. f. 475—477 (Expl. δίδου μεσονύκτιος μετὰ σαχάρου).

Περὶ τῶν ἐν τῷ Πλάτωνος Τιμαίῳ ἰατρικῶς εἰρημένων.
De iis, quae medice scripta sunt in Platonis Timaeo, fragmentum.

Ed. Daremberg, Paris 1848.

Inc. comm. mutil. προτεταγμένοις μορίοις, τὸ δέρμα.
Expl. τὸ κενούμενον αὐτῆς ἐπισπᾶται.

Paris: Parisin. 2383; s. XVI. f. 27—34v (Sine auctoris nomine. *Kalbfleischs Collation in dessen Besitz*).

Περὶ ποδάγρας. [Diels I.130]
De podagra.

Oxford: Canonician. 1; s. XVI. f. 98 (Ἑρμηνεία περὶ τῆς ποδαλγίας τοῦ σοφωτάτ. Γαλ. προοίμιον. Inc. Ἐπεὶ ὥρισεν. Expl. παραδηλώσω περὶ τῆς ποδαλγικῆς νόσου).
Paris: Parisin. 1630; s. XIV. f. 216 (Frgm. de podagra. Inc. Ἐκ τοῦ γένους. Cf. K. XIII 334).

Προγνωστικά.
Prognostica.

Florenz: Laur. plut. 74, 10; s. XIV. (Σημεῖα ἰατρικά etc.).
München: Monacens.
276; s. XIV. f. 5 (Προγνωστικὰ ἀρρώστων Ἱππ. καὶ Γαλ. καὶ Πλάτ. etc.).
278; s. XII (*Wie im* Monac. 276).
Oxford: Baroccian. 88; s. XV—XVI. f. 47 (Ἱππ. καὶ Γαλ. καὶ Παύλ. Ἰτάλου καὶ etc. διάγνωσις περὶ ... ἀρρώστων καὶ τελευτῆς ἀνθρώπου. Inc. Τὸ α' ἄσπρον. Expl. σημαίνει θάνατον).

Paris: Parisin.

2283; s. XVI. (Προγνωστ. ὑπομνήμ.).

2494; s. XV. f. 258—260ᵛ (Προγνωστικὸν περὶ ἀνθρώπου. Inc. Συνέστηκεν ὁ κόσμος ἐκ δ' στοιχείων. Expl. εἰς τὰ μέλη ὅλου τοῦ σώματος. *Vgl.* Costomiris, Rev. des ét. gr. II [1889] p. 308 sq.).

Venedig: Marcian. App. cl. V 5; s. XV. f. 145 (Prologus de prognosticis in morbis acutis. Inc. Σκοπός ἐστιν ἐνταῦθα τῷ).

Περὶ πυρετῶν.
De febribus.

Bologna: Bonon. 3632; s. XV. f. 132 (De febrium differentiis).

Modena: Mutin. 237 (III G 18); s. XVI. f. 368 (Inc. Ἔοικεν ὁ ἑκτικὸς πυρετός. Expl. ὁμοίαν ποιησάμενοι τοῖς ἐφημέροις. *Ob von* Galen?).

Paris:

Coislin. 334; s. XV. f. 10.

Parisin.

2167; s. XVI. f. 202 (De febrium causis).

2269; s. XV. f. 163 (De febri semitertiana anon.).

Suppl. 446; s. X. f. 31ᵛ (Ἀποσημείωσις πυρεκτικιούντων. Inc. Κατεκλίθη ὁ νοσῶν ἐν ἀρχῇ τῆς α' ἡμέρας. Expl. ἡνίκα πυρετοὶ ὦσιν ἐπὶ τῷ κάμνοντι).

Rom: Palat.

157; s. XIV. f. 1.

297; s. XV—XVI. (De febrium substantia et differentiis. Inc. Σκοπὸν οὖν ἔχομεν. *Vgl.* Palladius *bei* Ideler, Phys. et med. I p. 107).

400; s. xv. f. 7 (Inc. Ἱπποκράτης ὁ διδάσκαλος ἡμῶν).

[Diels I.131] Περὶ σπέρματος.
De spermate.

Oxford: Bodl. Miscell. 20; s. XIV. f. 375 (De spermate ex Aristotele et Galeno. Inc. Καὶ τὸ γεννητικόν).

Περὶ στοιχείων.
De elementis.

Paris: Parisin.

1883*; s. XIV. f. 35ᵛ.

2317*; s. XVI. f. 21ᵛ *und* 43ᵛ.

Περὶ στομάχου.
De stomacho.

Bologna: Bonon. 1808; s. XV. f. 143 (Περὶ ἀτονίας στομάχου καὶ ὑπτιασμοῦ καὶ ἀνατροπῆς).

Περὶ σφυγμῶν.
De pulsibus.

Gallipoli: Ἐκκλησ. ἁγίου Νικολάου 38; s. XIV. *hinter* f. 39. 41v.
London: Medical Society
H Hi 17 = We 30; s. XV in. no. 37 Dbg. (Inc. Ὁ σφυγμὸς κίνησίς ἐστιν. Expl. εἰς τὸ βάθος τοῦ σώματος, ὕστερον δέ. Daremberg, Mscrts. méd. de l'Angleterre I 162: »apocryphe«).
H Hi 21. 22 = We 28. 29; s. XV ex. f. 333v (Inc. Αἴσθησιν ἐναρμονίῳ τινὶ κινήσει. Expl. βραδὺς πυκνὸς ἀραιὸς καὶ ἀνώμαλος) *und* f. 341 (Inc. *wie im* H Hi 17. Expl. ἐπεὶ πολλάκις καὶ παραυτίκα τελευτᾷ).
Neapel: Oratorian. 152; s. XIV—XV.
Oxford: Baroccian. 88; s. XV—XVI. f. 48b (Γνωρίσματα σφυγμῶν περὶ τε ζωῆς καὶ θανάτου ἀνθρώπων. Inc. Κράτει σφυγμός. Expl. ἢ καὶ τοῦ θανάτου).
Paris:
Parisin.
2155*; s. XIV. f. 315v—319v. (*Abschrift besitzt Hr. cand. phil. Gossen, Berlin*).
2178; s. XV. f. 1 (Exc. de pulsibus).
2229*; s. XIII. f. 43v.
2320; s. XVI. f. 23 (*Wie im* Baroccian.).
2332*; s. XV (XIV). f. 130 (?).
3035*; s. XIV. f. 209—219.
Suppl. 629*; s. XIX. f. 59—65.
Rom: Barberin. I 127; s. XVI. f. 1v (Inc. *wie im* Lond. Medical Society H Hi 17. Expl. οὐ χαλεπῶς εὑρήσετε) *und* f. 251 (Inc. *wie im* Lond. Medical Society H Hi 17. Expl. ἐν τοῖς καρποῖς παρείς) *und* f. 278v (Inc. Πῶς ἐνεστῶσαν κρίσιν. Expl. ὄγκοι γίγνοιντο. Sine auctoris nomine).

Περὶ ὑαλίων. [Diels I.132]
De vasis vitreis.

Paris: Parisin. 2320; s. XVI. f. 20v (Μέθοδος τῶν ὑαλίων).
Turin: Taurinens. 17 B VII 22 (B I 12); s. XVI. XVIII. f. 48v. (*Verbrannt*).

Περὶ ὑδάτων.
De aquis.

E. 107 Mailand: Ambros. B 157 Sup.; s. XV—XVI. f. 133 (Inc. καὶ λάπαρα τῶν ἄλλων ἀπάντων ὑδάτων. Galeni esse frgm. putat Schoene).

Dazu vgl.: Oribas. ad Eunap. I c. 14 (Περὶ ὑδάτων ἐκ Γαληνοῦ Ὀριβασίου Ῥούφου etc.).

Περὶ ὕλης ἰατρικῆς.
De materia medica.

Cod. Mich. Cantacuzeni (*bei* Foerster de antiquit. et libr. mss. Constantinopol. p. 27 *und* Costomiris Rev. des ét. gr. II p. 382/383. no. Λ'.

Φάρμακα.
Remedia.

Athos: Athous Βιβλ. μον. Ἰβήρων
4271. 151; s. XV. f. 176 A (Ζουλαπίου σύνθεσις. Inc. Ζουλάπιον εἰς βῆχα).
4339. 219; s. XVIII (Περὶ ἐλαίων).
4508. 388; s. XVI (Κοκκία καθαρτικὰ στομάχου καὶ κεφαλῆς).
Bologna: Bonon.
1808; s. XV. f. 123ᵛ (Ἡ διὰ πτέργης [sic!]· μάλαγμα πηγανηρόν) *und* f. 299ᵛ (Ξηρὰ ἀνακαθαρτικὰ καὶ σαρκωτικὰ κεφαλικὰ λεγόμενα).
3632; s. XV. f. 205 (Περὶ τῶν ἱερῶν καὶ πικρῶν ἀντιδότων cap. ιθ').
Escurial: Scorial. III. R. 3; s. XI. f. 138 (Ἀντίδοτον ὠφελοῦν εἰς τὴν μέλαιναν χολὴν καὶ εἰς τὴν ξανθήν. Expl. ἔχει καὶ θέλης· ἐστὶν γὰρ ὠφελιμώτατον).
Florenz: Laurent. plut.
74, 10; s. XIV. p. 82b (Varia medicamentorum genera. Inc. Ἐπιμελούμενον τῆς σῆς; *vgl.* Hipp. Ep. ad Ptol.).
75, 17; s. XIV. p. 1 (Quaedam remedia evacuantia. Inc. Τοῖς ἀποδακρυτικοῖς χρώμεθα).
London:
Addit. (Brit. Mus.) 10, 058; s. XV. f. 65 (Σκευασία τῆς ἱερᾶς). f. 74 (Δυναμερόν. Inc. Ὁ περὶ τῶν ἀντιδότων καὶ ἐλαίων. Expl. καρποβαλσάμου κόκκους κ', νάμ$^{\alpha}$ [sic!] ταύρων). f. 106ᵛ (Περὶ ἐλαίων καὶ μύρων. Inc. Ὀμφάκινον ἔλαιον γίνεται. Expl. [Diels I.133] καὶ βράσας ἕως συστάσεως ἔχει πολυτίμως). f. 115ᵛ (Περὶ ἁπλῶν διδομένων φαρμάκων. Inc. Ἐλατήριον· καθαίρει φλέγμα καὶ χολὴν ὅσον. Expl. καὶ ὀλίγον οἶνον ὕδωρ ἄγει). f. 123 (Sine auctoris nomine. Περὶ συνθέτων φαρμάκων καὶ τίσι ταῦτα δοτέον. Inc. Τὸ διακιτρίου [sic!] καθαίρει μὲν φλέγμα. Expl. πρόσβαλλε

δακρύ^δ κεράτια δ'). f. 128 (Περὶ δυνάμεων ἐμπλάστρων. Inc. Ἡ διάμπαρος τονοῖ καταπαν^τ [sic]. Expl. [?] βράσας τὸ ἀφέψημα ἄντλιε).

Medical Society H Hi 17 = We 30; s. XV.

Modena: Mutinens. 216 (II H 1); s. XVI. f. 36ᵛ (Frgm. ex l. de simplicibus, calefaciunt et refrigerant. Inc. Ὅσα ἐστὶ μέσα τῶν θερμαινόντων ... χρησιμώτατόν ἐστι ...).

Neapel: Oratorian. 152; s. XIV—XV (Quaenam medicamenta quibus infirmitatibus prosint).

Oxford:

Baroccian. 150; s. XV in. f. 6 (Σκευασία τῆς πικρᾶς; *vgl. den* Lond. Addit. 10, 058. f. 65).

Clarkian. 16 (18378); s. XIV. f. 95 (Περὶ ἐβένου. Inc. Ἔβενος τῶν εἰς χυλὸν ἀναλυομένων ἐστὶ ξύλων. Expl. καὶ ῥεύματα καὶ φλυκταίνας ἁρμόττουσιν).

[Laudian. cat. mss. Angl. n. 877].

Paris:

Coislin. 335; s. XV. f. 21. 69. 75 (*bei* Montfauc. II p. 448).

Parisin.

2164; s. XVI. f. 213 (De salibus).

[2230; s. XIV.] (*Es ist* f. 37 Anonymi collectio medica ex variis Gal. operibus *gemeint*; *vgl.* Costomiris, Rev. des ét. gr. II [1889] p. 377).

2260; s. XVI. f. 196 (De simplicibus medicamentis).

2286; s. XIV. f. 89 (Remedia ad dentium dolores sedandos) *und* f. 103 (Remedia varia).

2294; s. XV. f. 73ᵛ.

2313; s. XIV. f. 1.

2510; a. 1348. f. 108 *und* 133ᵛ.

Suppl. 634; s. XIV. f. 64 (Περὶ καταπλασμάτων. Inc. Τῶν καταπλασμάτων τὰ μέν ἐστιν ἑψητά. Expl. ἄλφιτα τῷ λινοσπέρμῳ. Ed. Costomiris, Rev. des ét. gr. II [1889] p. 371).

Rom:

Angelican. 17 (C. 5. 4); s. XIV. f. 51ᵛ (κατ' ἀλφαβήτου. σπε'. ἀλφοὺς μέλανας ἀποκαθαίρει).

Palat.

143; s. XV. f. 176 (Helleborus quibusnam sit dandus) *und* f. 177 (Inc. Ἀγάλλοχον τὸ μὲν σῶμα).

279; s. XIV—XV. f. 277 (de medicamentis stomacho idoneis. Inc. Ἅπερ ἀεὶ λέγω).

400; s. XV. f. 399 (de prophylacticis adversus arthricos affectus).

Vatic. 2256; s. XIV. f. 79ᵛ (πρὸς δυσεντερικούς).

Venedig: Bibl. Josephi de Aromatariis (de medicamentis purgantibus quaecumque bilem ducunt rubram. *Verbleib unbekannt*).

Wien: Vindob. med. 20; s. XV. f. 486ᵛ—488 (Ἱερὰ Γαληνοῦ. Inc. Ἡ σύνθεσις ἔχει οὕτως. Expl. πίνειν μαλάχης σπέρματος ∠β' [sic!]).

Dazu:
[Ms. Fr. Bernardi catal. mss. Angl. n. 3632] *und* [Ms. a Geo. de Honestis citat., quod Galeni esse negat Silvius ad Mesuen libr. III.]

[Diels I.134]

Περὶ εἰδῶν φιλοσοφίας.
De partibus philosophiae.

Ed. E. Wellmann, Berol. 1882, Progr. d. Koenigst. Gymn..

Inc. Εἰς θεωρητικὸν καὶ πρακτικόν τῆς φιλοσοφίας διαιρουμένης.
Expl. mutil. δι' οὗ ἐμέτρουν τὴν γῆν καὶ ἐ...

Florenz: Laurent. plut. 56, 15; s. XV. p. 206b (Desin. imperf.).
Padua: Bibl. Ioann. Rhodii (Inscr. De philosophia. *Verbleib unbekannt*).
Paris: Parisin. 2176; s. XVI. f. 4.

Περὶ φλεβοτομίας.
De venae sectione.

London: Addit. (Brit. Mus.) 17, 900; s. XVII. f. 204v (Inc. Οἱ πρῶτοι καὶ κυριώτατοι σκοποί. Expl. καὶ ταῦτα μὲν ἐπιεικεῖ [?] φάρμακον) *und* f. 272 (Inc. *wie auf* f. 204v. Expl. εἰ γὰρ πλησιάσει τούτῳ).
München: Monacens. 39; s. XVI. f. 81 (Inc. Ὅτι τοῖς τὰ συνήθη πράττουσι. *Vgl.* Orib. Coll. med. VII 2).
Neapel: Oratorian. 152; s. XIV—XV.
Oxford: Baroccian. 224; s. XV. f. 1 (*Wie im* Monacens. Expl. ἀλλὰ τηρεῖν καὶ αὖθις ἐπαφαιρεῖν).
Paris: Parisin.
2269; s. XV. f. 118.
2320; s. XVI. f. 9v.
Rom:
Palat.
279; s. XIV—XV. f. 212v (Inc. *wie im* Lond. Add.) *und* f. 213v (Inc. Διηγήσατό ποτε).
400; s. XV. f. 68.
Vatic. 279; s. — f. 213 (*Verbleib unbekannt*).
Turin: Taurin.
6b IV 6 (B I 6); s. XVI. f. 185 (Inc. *wie im* Monacens.).
17 B VII 22 (B I 12)*; s. XVI. XVIII. f. 30v (Ex Hipp. Gal. Malet. *etc. Verbrannt.*

Venedig: Marcian. App. cl. II 171; s. XV. (Π. φλεβοτομίας. Inc. Ἀπὸ μὲν τῶν ὁμοιομερῶν. Expl. τμητικοῖς ἰώμεθα *und* Τίς καιρὸς φλεβοτομίας).
Wien: Vindob. med.
28; s. XV. f. 186ᵛ (Inc. *wie im* Lond. Add. Expl. καὶ τῶν ἀλλοτρίων ἀποκριτικήν).
29; s. XV. f. 12 (Inc. *wie im* Lond. Add. Expl. καθαρισμὸν τοῦ ἐγκεφάλου ἐξάγον).

[Περὶ φύσεως ἀνθρώπου]. [Diels I.135]
[*De hominis natura.*]

München: Monacens. 39; s. XVI. f. 80 (Frgm. fort. Galeni. Inc. Θαυμαστὸν γὰρ οὕτως ἀληθῶς τὸ ἀνθρώπινον σύγκραμα).
Rom: Vatic. 695; s. XIV—XV. f. 226 (Περὶ τῆς συστάσεως τοῦ ἀνθρώπου).
[Vatic. apud Montfauc. p. 28 (Gal. de natura hominis)].

Dazu: [Rob. Burscough 7675].

Περὶ χειρουργησιῶν καὶ περὶ κατακλίσεως νοσούντων.
De chirurgorum operationibus et de decubitu infirmorum

Nicht = K. XIX 529 sqq.; *vgl.* Costomiris Rev. des ét. gr. II [1889] p. 377.

Inc. Νομὰς καὶ ὄγκους οἱ ἰατροὶ χειρουργήτωσαν.
Expl. τοῖς καθαιρομένοις στρόφους ποιεῖ.

Florenz: Laurent. plut. 28, 34; s. XI. f. 5 (Expl. αἴτια τῶν νόσων ἐντεῦθεν γνωρίζεται).
Paris: Parisin. 1991; s. XV. f. 29ᵛ—42.
Rom: Vatic. 1444; s. XV. f. 223.

[Περὶ χειρουργίας].
De chirurgia.

[**Oxford:** Bodleian. bibl. Brit. n. 3500].

[Diels I.136]

Περὶ χυμῶν.
De humoribus.

Bologna: Bonon. 3636; s. XIV—XV. f. 126 (Σημεῖα κράσεως χυμῶν. Inc. Σκεπτέον ἐπὶ πάντων. Expl. κατὰ φύσιν οὐδέν τι τούτων ποιήσει).
Jerusalem: Bibl. patriarch. 148; s. XVI. f. 4 (Π. στοιχ. κ. χυμ. Inc. Ὁ κόσμος οὗτος).
Paris:
Coislin. 335; s. XV. f. 198ᵛ (*bei* Montf. II 448).
Parisin. 2317; s. XVI. f. 43ᵛ (Exc. de elementis et humoribus).
Wien: Vindob. med. 28; s. XV. f. 184—185ᵛ (Inc. Ὁ κόσμος ἐκ δ' στοιχείων. Expl. καὶ ἡ διὰ τοῦ γάλακτος).

Περὶ ὡρῶν καὶ ἔτους.
De anni temporibus.

Athos: Athous. Βιβλ. μον. Ἰβήρων
4789. 669; s. XVIII. (Ἑρμηνεία περὶ τῶν ὡρῶν καὶ ἔτους).
5437. 1317; s. XVIII. (Ἰατροσόφιον Γαλ. ἰατροῦ Ἑρμηνεία. Inc. Τὸ ἔαρ ἄρχεται ἀπὸ τῆς κε' τοῦ μηνός).
München: Monac. 525; *vor* a. 1336. f. 160 (Γαλ. ἡ τῆς τῶν ὡρῶν τάξις ... τοῦ ἔαρος).

[Diels I.148]

Excerpta varia.

Athos: Athous
Βιβλ. μον. Ἰβήρων 4310. 190; s. XIII. f. 115 A.
Παντελεήμονος 5578. 72; s. XV. f. 458a (Γαλ. γνώμη. Inc. Ὃ γὰρ οὐκ ἐβούλετο, τοῦτο οὐκ ᾤετο).
Παντοκράτορος 1268. 234; s. XIII (Inc. ...κάστου ἐξ$^{α'}$ γ' κιναμώμου. Expl. εὑρίσκονται καὶ θερμά).
[**Corbie:** Bibl. S. Petri Corbeiens. Montf. p. 1407].
[**Dubin:** Bibl. Narcissi 1218].
Jerusalem: Bibl. d. hl. Kreuzes 85; s. XVI. f. 165 (Πῶς γράφονται αἱ εἰκόνες Ὁμήρου ... Γαληνοῦ ...).
[**Konstantinopel:** Constantinop. ap. Verdier II 57].
Kopenhagen: Hauniens. Bibl. reg. ant. fund. 225; s. XVI (Frgm. Inc. μηδ' ὅλως δάκνοντα. Expl. ῥοδόσταγμα καὶ οἶνος).
Leipzig: Lipsiens. 57; s. XVIII—XIX (Jo. Scaligeri emendatt. in Gal. ex exemplo Guelferbyt. I—IV).
Lesbos: Bibl. τῆς τοῦ Λειμῶνος μονῆς 175; s. XVII.

Messina: Messanens. bibl. univ. 84 (Cf. Rühl Philol. N. F. I 577—588).
Modena: Mutinens.
61 (III B 9); s. XV. f. 31.
151 (II E 18); s. XV. f. 1.
München: [Monacens. (Compendium ex. Gal.)] lat. 807; s. XV. f. 72. [Diels I.149]
Oxford: Bibl. Aed. Christi 34; s. XI. f. 131.
Paris:
Coislin. 335; s. XV. f. 17 *und* 198ᵛ—227.
Parisin.
1831; s. XVI. f. 119 (Frgm. Inc. θυμοῦσιν οὐκέτι ὁμοίως).
1865; s. XV. f. 129.
2149; s. XVI. f. 201.
2155; s. XIV. f. 292.
2210; a. 1357. f. 368.
2237; s. XIV. f. 165ᵛ.
2510; a. 1348. f. 108.
Suppl.
292; s. XVII. f.
292; s. XVII. f. 269.
683; s. XVIII. f. 1ᵛ.
764; s. XIV. f. 1.
1194; s. XV. f. 1.
1202; s. XIII—XVI. f. 16.
Rom: Palat.
143; s. XV. f. 178ᵛ (Inc. Περὶ δὲ τῶν τεκμηρίων).
199; s. XIII. f. 2ᵛ.
297; s. XV—XVI.
Turin: Taurin. 17 B VII 22 (B I 12); s. —. f. 48ᵛ (*Verbrannt*).
Venedig:
Marcian. 509; s. XV.
App. cl.
V 10; s. XVI. f. 39.
V 13; s. XIV—XVI. f. 119.
V 18—22; s. — (Ed. Aldina Gal., cuius in margine notae scriptae sunt).
Wien: Vindob.
med.
13; s. —.
15; s. —.
37; s. —.
53; s. XVI. f. 11—59.
[Vindob. Lambec. VI p. 93].

[Lambec. VI p. 100].
[Lambec. VI p. 151 (Anon. tabulae divisionum in plusculis libris Gal.)].
[Lambec. VI p. 153]
[Lambec. ed. Kollar I p. 275 (Videtur fuisse Mich. Cantacuzeni)].

[Diels I.150] *Indices in Galenum.*

London: Medical Society (»nicht aufzufinden«. Kalbfl. *Vgl.* Costomiris Revue des études grecques II [1889] p. 381. Index auctorum a Gal. citatorum).
Paris:
Bibl. Facult. Medic. nr. ? (Lexicon Gal.).
Parisin. Suppl. 793; s. XVII. (Lud. Kusteri index in Gal.).
Rom: Palat. 428; s. XV—XVI. (Index in Gal., Alex. Aphr. et Hipp. aliquot opuscula).

Scholia in Galenum.

Paris:
Parisin.
2147; s. XVI. (»Probe bei Daremberg, Gal. in Timaeum«).
2383; s. XVI.
Suppl. 634; s. XIV. f. 19—26v (*Vgl.* Kalbfleisch, de victu atten. p. VIII).

Addenda.

S. 41 zum 1. Brief an Ptolem.: Parisin. Suppl. 446; s. X. f. 69ᵛ (Expl. διὸ χρῶ τοῖς περιπάτοις καὶ ...). [Diels I.151]

S. 46 zu **Escurial:** Scorial. Φ. I. 10; s. XVI. f. 196ᵛ (*Wie im* Neapolit.).

S. 59 zu K. I 40—52 *hinter dem Titel:* Galeni de optimo docendi genere liber, adnotabant et emendabant seminarii philologorum Bonnensis sodales; accedit libri adversus empiricos fragmentum. Bonnae 1906.

S. 60 zu K. I 224—304: *Ein Teil dieser Schrift, nämlich* = K. I 289—304, *ist das Fragment* Περὶ προγνώσεως K. XIX 497—511.

S. 89 zu K. IX 431—549: Expl. *im* Laurent. *wie im* Ambros. D 293 Inf. —. *Eine Prüfung der Pariser Handschriften an Ort und Stelle hat ergeben, daß* nr. 2315 *und* Suppl. 446 *zu* Π. σφυγμῶν πρ. Ἀντώνιον *zu stellen sind (s. also S. 113), und daß* nr. 2155, 2332, 3035, Suppl. 629 *z. T. innerhalb anonymer Traktate Fragmente verschiedener Galenischer Schriften über Pulse enthalten (s. also den allgem. Artikel* Περὶ σφυγμῶν *S. 131). Der Inhalt von* 2229; s. XIII. f. 43ᵛ *ist noch unbekannt.*

S. 113 zu K. XIX 609—628: **Königsberg (Pr.):** Regimont. S. 35; s. XV. f. 273ᵛ (Frgm. Expl. καθ' ἑαυτὴν = K. XIX 611, 7).

II.

The Other Physicians

Under the title **Zeichenerklärung** (*Table of Symbols*), Diels' catalogue includes some abbreviations and *sigla*, the list of which appears on page 2 of the first issue of the catalogue (1905). Those abbreviations, utilized precisely in the present reproduction of Diels are the following with their respective explicitation:

*	=	die Hds. enthält nur Exzerpte.
[ ]	=	die Hds. ist nur aus Ackermann's *Hist. litteraria Hippocratis* (Kühn Med. Gr. Opp. XXI, 1 ff.) und *Hist. litt. Cl. Galeni* (Kühn M. G. O. I, XVII ff.) oder aus Littré (Œuvr. compl. d'Hippocr. Par. 1839—61. 10 Bde.) bekannt.
J.	=	Galenus, editio Iuntina 1528 (Exemplar der Vatikanischen Handbibliothek).
K.	=	Kühn.
L.	=	Littré.

*	=	the manuscript contains only extracts.
[ ]	=	the manuscript is known only through Ackermann's *Hist. litteraria Hippocratis* (Kühn Med. Gr. Opp. XXI, 1 sq.) and *Hist. litt. Cl. Galeni* (Kühn M. G. O. I, XVII ff.) or Littré (Œuvr. compl. d'Hippocr. Par. 1839—61. 10 vols).
J.	=	Galen, Iuntina 1528 edition (copy of the Vatican Library).
K.	=	Kühn.
L.	=	Littré.

Abraham.

[Diels II.3]

Excerpta varia.

Escurial: Scorial. Ω. I. 8; s. XIV. f. 78v (Στήλη ἐκλίγματος· ἐξελέξατο αὐτὴν ἀβραὰμ ὁ τοῦ Σολομῶντος τῷ ἔχοντι βῆχας κτλ.).
Florenz: Laurent. App. 2; s. XV. f. 353v (Τοῦ Σαρακηνοῦ τοῦ Ἀβράμη καὶ Ἀκταρίου τῶν Μαγγάνων καὶ βασιλικοῦ ἀρχιατροῦ βοήθημα καθαρτικὸν ἐπί τε ἡπατικῶν ἰκτερικῶν καὶ σπληνικῶν καὶ ἰσχιαδικῶν. Inc. Ἀλι λέκχ· ἤγουν χρυσοβάλανον).

Adamantius.

Περὶ ἀνέμων.
De ventis.

Ed. V. Rose, Anecd. gr. I p. 29—48.

Inc. ... συμβαίνοντες ὄνειροι τῇ ἀναθυμιάσει τῶν πνευμάτων.
Expl. περὶ ὀνείρων γενέσεως ἄρξομαι γράμματος .

Florenz: Laurent. plut.
28, 44; s. XV. p. 2b (Inc. Ἐπειδὴ ἐκ τῶν τῆς γῆς ἀναθυμιάσεων. Expl. καὶ οἰκειότεροι μᾶλλον τοῖς σώμασιν ἡμῶν).
56, 1; s. XIII—XIV. f. 284.
Paris: Parisin. 2381; s. XV. f. 80v.

Περὶ παλμῶν.
De palpitationibus. (*Ob echt?*)

Inc. Περὶ παλμῶν μαντικὴ πρὸς βασιλέα Πτολεμαῖον.
Expl. τέλος τῶν παλμῶν.

Athos: Βιβλ. μον. Ἰβήρων 4301. 181; s. XVI. f. 2.

Excerpta varia.

Carpentras: nr. 1774 (P., V); s. XVII. f. 165 (De ponderibus et mensuris).

London: Harleian. (Brit. Mus.) 5626; s. XV—XVI. f. 2 (Ἰατροσόφιον ποιηθὲν ὑπὸ διαφόρων φιλοσόφων … Ἀδαμαντίου …).
Paris: Parisin.
2208; s. XIV. f. 385 (Oribasii et Adam. fragmenta de ponderibus et mensuris. *Gedruckt* Orib. V 85).
2217; s. XI—XV. f. 285ᵛ (Opuscula).

[Diels II.4]

Aelianus.

Epistula anepigrapha.

Inc. Ὁ φυσικός σου κόσμος παρώχηκεν.

Oxford: Baroccian. 50; s. XI. f. 386b (»An Aeliani?« Coxe).

Aelius Promotus.

Δυναμερόν.
Dynameron.

Vgl. E. Rohde, Kl. Schr. I 380 ff.

Inc. Ἐπειδὴ πολλοῖς ἐγγεγυμνασμένος.
Expl. ἐλαίου μυρσίνου τὸ ἀρκοῦν.

Escurial: Scorial. Φ. I. 2; s. XVI. f. 139 (*Apographon des* Marcian.).
Venedig: Marcian. 295; s. XIV. f. 191ᵛ—274ᵛ (*Abschrift besitzt E. O. Winstedt, Oxford. Teilweise Abschrift in Wellmanns Besitz*).

Φυσικὰ καὶ ἀντιπαθητικά.
Physica et Antipathetica.

Vgl. E. Rohde a. a. O.

Leyden: Vossian. 29; s. —.
Mailand: Ambros. S 3 Sup.; s. XV/XVI. f. 114.
Rom: Vatic. 299; s. XV. f. 494—495ᵛ. (*Abschrift besitzt E. O. Winstedt, Oxford. Rohdes Abschrift in Wellmanns Besitz*).

Ἰατρικά. Τὰ λείποντα ἀπὸ τοῦ νηκ, $^{\overline{\epsilon\epsilon 3}}$, ἐκ τοῦ βιβλίου τοῦ Προμώτου.
Iatrica.

Mailand: Ambros. S 3 Sup.; s. XV/XVI. f. 21 (Inc. Ἄλλο βαπτικὸν κικίδια).

Περὶ ἰοβόλων καὶ δηλητηρίων φαρμάκων.
De animalibus virus eiaculantibus et de venenis.

Vgl. E. Rohde a. a. O.

Mailand: Ambros. S 3 Sup.; s. XV/XVI. f. 69—112^{v} (*Collation im Berol. fol. 39 [275]*).
Rom: Vatic. 299; s. XV. f. 473—493^{v} (*Abschrift im Berol. 39 [275]. Rohdes Abschrift mit der Collation des* Ambros. *in Wellmanns Besitz).*

Aëtius Amidenus. [Diels II.5]

Ἰατρικῶν λόγοι ΙΣΤ'.
Iatricorum libri XVI.

L. I—VIII
ed. Aldus Venet. 1534.
L. VII (*Augenheilkunde*)
ed. I. Hirschberg Leipzig. 1899.
L. IX part.
edd. Mustoxydes et Schinas Venet. 1816.
L. XI
ed. Daremberg, Rufus p. 85—126. 557—567. 568—581.
L. XII
ed. Costomiris Paris. 1892.
L. XVI
ed. Zervos Lips. 1901.
L. I—XVI lat.
ed. Cornarius Lugd. 1549.

Inc. Περὶ δυνάμεως τῶν ἁπλῶν φαρμάκων. Αἱ διαφοραὶ τῶν κατὰ μέρος.
Expl. ἀπὸ βαλσάμου Γο γ' ἤτοι οὐγγίας τρεῖς.

Athos:
Βιβλ. μον. Βατοπεδίου Α 29; s. —.

Ἐσφιγμένου 41*; s. XV (*vgl.* Costomiris, Rev. des ét. gr. III p. 177).

Λαύρας

Ω 70; s. —.

Ω 72; s. —.

(*Außer* Ω *70 und 72 noch 4 weitere Hdss. bei* Costomiris Rev. des ét. gr. III p. 166 *und* 127.)

Berlin:

Phillipps. 1534 (Meerm. 229); s. XVI ex. (*Abschrift von Buch XIII in Wellmanns Besitz.*)

Berol. fol.

37 (273); s. XVI. f. 1.

38 (274); s. —. f. 1 (L. IX—XVI. Apogr. cod. olim Boerhaaviani, nunc Lipsiensis).

Bologna: Bonon.

1808*; s. XV. f. 6 (L. II 15—20. 22. 24—26. 30—39. 196 usque ad p. 41, 17 Ald. et L. I p. 7, 17—10, 17), f. 35v (L. III 114. 115. 116. 93), f. 43v (L. III 19 p. 50v usque ad διαίρεσις; subicitur καὶ ἔρινον μαλακὸν βεβρεγμένον — οὕτως σαρκοῖ ἄριστα), f. 44v (Ex l. III 22 et l. I litt. Δ et E), f. 80 (L. III 57—64. 66—69. 70. 71. 74—79. L. V 133—137. 140), f. 159 (L. I p. 3—7, 49; subiciuntur f. 169v ταύτην ἱερὰν καλοῦσι — ἀπαρβάτως), f. 170v (Ex l. III 110—113. 138. 139. 141. 143), f. 175. 182v (Ex l. VI 24. VI 23. 28). f. 201 (Ex l. IV 3—20. VII 98—101), f. 225 (L. IV 21—26. VI 66—79. 80. 81. 83—86. 88. 93—95. VIII 12. 13— 15. 9. 16. 17. 19. 20. 22—24), f. 253v (Ex l. VIII 40—42), f. 262v (Ex l. VI 50—53).

3632*; s. XV. f. 59 (Ex l. V 28—44 p. 80—81 Ald.), f. 62v (Ex l. V 45), f. 67v (L. V 26), f. 71 (Ex l. I), f. 92 (L. II 13—36), f. 97v (L. II 4—82 p. 16v—31), f. 125 (L. II 198—204. 208. 209— 214 p. 41—42), f. 127 (L. II 220. 228. 230. 235. 236. 239. 241—245. 254—257. 260. 263. 269. L. III 138—140. 142. II 223. 226. III 143. 148. 149. 150. 158. III 160—163. 166. 170), f. 236 (L. IV 101—104. 108); (*Olivieris Collation der Bücher I. II. XVI und Bruchstücke in dessen Besitz*).

Escurial: Scorial.

Σ. III. 17*; s. XVI. f. 102 (Frgm. l. I inc. αἱ διαφοραὶ τῶν κατὰ μέρος ἐνεργειῶν. expl. στρόφους πραΰνει).

Τ. II. 14; s. XVI. f. 199v (L. IV et V).

Φ. I. 6; s. XVI. f. 1 = 153 (L. IX—XVI).

Φ. II. 15; s. XIV. f. 1 (Frgm. l. XVI 72 π. μύλης), f. 7 (Frgm. l. XIII 63—70), f. 8 (L. XII 37 προσαγέσθω —XVI).

Υ. IV. 14; s. XV (L. I—VI).

Ω. I. 8*; s. XIV. f. — (Π. κατάρρου καὶ κορύζης = l. VIII 57, f. 167 Ald. et π. βηχὸς = l. VIII f. 169 Ald.), f. 22v (Π. ὀρθοπνοικῶν ἀσθματικῶν τῶν λεγομένων δυσπνοικῶν, ἐκ τῶν Γαλ.), f. 31 (Π. τῶν ἐν καρδίᾳ παλμῶν, ἐκ τῶν Γαλ. = l. VIII 64), f. 34ᵛ (Π. αἵματος ἀναγωγῆς, ἐκ τῶν Γαλ.), f. 55 (Π. τῶν ἐν τῇ τραχείᾳ ἀρτηρίᾳ ἑλκῶν), f. 55ᵛ (Π. ἐμπυηματικῶν), f. 58 (Π. ἐμπύων καὶ φισιάσεως [sic!]).

R. I. 12; s. XV. f. 1 (L. IX—XII) *und* f. 135ᵛ (L. XIII—XVI).

Florenz: Laurent. plut.

75, 2; s. XIV. p. 1 (L. IX—XV. *Olivieris Abschrift von Buch IX. X. XIII—XV und Collation von Buch XI und XII in dessen Besitz.*).

75, 5; s. XIV. p. 1 (L. VI—VIII. *Olivieris Collation in dessen Besitz; vgl.* Olivieri, L' oftalmologia di Aetios nel cod. Laur. 75, 5 in: Studi italiani XII p. 261 ff.) *und* p. 151b (Ex l. II et III).

75, 7; s. XIV. p. 1 (L. XIII—XVI).

75, 10; s. XIII. p. 55 (L. IX cap. extr.—XII 69). [Diels II.6]

75, 12; s. XV. p. 1 (L. I—III).

75, 13; s. XV. p. 1 (L. XIV—XVI).

75, 18 s. XIV. p. 1 (L. IX—XIII).

75, 20; s. XIV. p. 1 (L. I—V).

75, 21; s. XIII. p. 1 (L. IX—XVI).

Holkham: nr. 283; s. XVI. f. 1 (L. I—VIII).

Leipzig:

Bibl. senat. 391 (Repos. I fol. 36 a. a); s. XVIII (L. IX—XVI).

Bibl. univ. 65; s. XIX. p. 1 (L. IX. X).

Leyden:

B. P. 6; s. XIV (Libri IV).

Voss. fol. 58*; s. XV (Ex l. I. III. IV. V. VII. VIII).

London:

Harleian. (Brit. Mus.) 5626; s. XV (XVI?). f. 1 (L. III).

Sloan. (Brit. Mus.) 2434*; s. XVII (?). f. 1. 19ᵛ. 51. 104.

Medical Society Wf 7; s. XVI (L. IX—XV).

Messina: Bibl. S. Salvatoris 84; s. X—XI. (L. I—III p. 63 ed. Ald. *Vgl.* Rühl, Philol. nov. ser. I 581. Olivieri, Studi ital. IX 299—367. *Olivieris Collation in dessen Besitz*).

Oxford:

Baroccian. 88; s. XVI. f. — (L. I. II 12. 82. 84 ss. 193 alia) *und* f. 109ᵛ (L. V praeter capp. 121—131. L. VI praeter capp. 1—3 partim, quorum loco capp. l. III praeter 1—9. 162—170. 174. 175. 179—185).

Canonic. 109; s. XV ex. (L. IX—XVI 17).

Laud. C 60 (Bodl. 749); s. XVI. f. 1 (L. IX—XII 49 τικτῶν).

Miscell. 189*; s. XV. f. 1 (Tabula capp. l. IX cum prioribus versib. capitis 1).

Roe 14; s. XV. f. 86 (L. V 140 inc. Ὀξύμελι. expl. κεκτημένων) *und* f. 282 (L. XII).

Padua: Bibl. S. Ioann. in Virid. ad dextr. plut. 16 (*Verbleib unbekannt*).

Palermo: Bibl. naz. XIII C 3*; s. XVI. f. 940—951^{v} (Inscr. Ἐκ τῶν Γαλ. προοίμιον περὶ τῶν δ' τάξεων ἑκάστου γένους τῶν ἁπλῶν φαρμάκων) *und* f. 956—1047 (De plantis ord. alph. Inc. Ἀκαλήφη. Expl. ἀδίκτος ἐστίν).

Paris:

Faculté de médecine 76; s. XVI—XVII. f. 1 (L. IX—XVI).

Parisin.

1883; s. XIV. f. 180^{v}. (*Coll. mit der Ald. im Berol. fol. 39 [275]*).

2191; s. XIV. f. 1. (*Coll. mit der Ald. im Berol. fol. 39 [275]*).

2192; s. XV. f. 3.

2193; s. XV. f. 1.

2194; s. XV. f. 3 (L. V—XIV).

2195; s. XIII. f. 1 (L. V—VIII).

2196; s. XI (L. IX—XII).

2197; s. XVI (L. XIII—XVI).

2198; a. 1522. f. 1.

2199; s. XVI (L. V. VI 1—55. IX—XV).

2228; s. XI. f. 150 (L. V. VI praeter capp. 97 dimid. et 98. VII. VIII partim. X).

2230; s. XIV. f. 156 (L. V) *und* f. 195 (L. VIII).

2237*; s. XIV. f. 163 (L. IV—X).

2256; s. XV. f. 34 (L. I. II).

2270; s. XIV—XV. f. 177 (L. XVI inscr. Γαλ. περὶ γυναικειων παθῶν).

Suppl.

630—632; s. XIV. XI. XIX (L. I. VI—XII. XIII—XVI).

1240; s. XI (L. I—VI a fine mutil. *Coll. im Berol. 39 [275].*).

Bibl. de la ville de Paris 58; s. XVI—XVII (L. IX—XVI).

Patmos: nr. 277; s. XVII (L. IV).

Raudnitz:

Bibl. ducis Lobcovic. VI F c 37; s. XIV—XV (L. VIII—XIV).

Raudnitiens. 11; s. —.

Rom:

Ottobon. 311; s. XV—XVI. f. 95^{v} (L. II).

Palat. 199; s. XIII. f. 101 (Libri IX, omisso l. VII, de ocularibus morbis).

Vatic.

282; s. XVI. f. 146 (L. VI—XVI).

297; s. XIV. f. 1.

298; a. 1387. f. 5.

1904; a. 1306. f. 130 (L. I).

1911; s. XIII. f. 1 (L. I. II).

2202; s. XIV—XV. f. 3—318 (L. I—IV).

Toledo: Bibl. del cab. de la igl. catedr. 101, 15*; s. XV. p. 296 (Ex l. XIII 86).

Venedig: Marcian.
289; s. XV (L. I—VII).
290; s. XV (L. VIII—XVI).
291; s. XV (*Coll. mit der Ald. p. 1—98 von Weigel im Berol. fol. 39 [275]*).
596; s. XV (L. I—VIII).

Wien: Vindob.
med.
6; s. XV. f. 3 (Expl. καὶ ὠφελεῖ τοὺς ἐμέτους. *Coll. mit der Ald. von Weigel im Berol. fol. 39 [275]*).
12; s. XV. f. 1—269ᵛ (Expl. τεθαμβημέναν ὄκνον πρὸς ... *Coll. mit der Ald. von Weigel im Berol. 39 [275]*).
28*; s. XV. f. 118—139ᵛ (Ex l. II 3. 75 etc.).
51; s. — (*L. VIII coll. von Weigel im Berol. 39 [275]*).
52; s. — (*L. VIII coll. von Weigel a. a. O.*).
Suppl.
8; s. XVII (L. VIII—XVI. Inc. Προείρηται μὲν περὶ τούτου).
81; s. XVI. f. 1—307ᵛ (L. VIII—XIII (Inc. Ἀσκληπιάδου τροχίσκος. Expl. ἐκ προδήλου αἰτίας).

Excerpta varia. [Diels II.7]

Athos: Βιβλ. μον. Ἰβήρων 4340. 220; s. XVII (Π. φλεβοτομίας).

Berlin:
Phillipps. 1583; s. XV. f. 101 (Π. οὔρων, π. σφυγμῶν).
fol. 39 (275); s. XIX (De alimentorum facultatibus, *Abschrift des Parisin. 1883. — Verzeichnis der Hdss. des A. in d. Vaticana*).

Bologna: Bonon. 3632; s. XV. f. 114ᵛ (Capita Aëtio tributa), f. 132 (De febrium differentiis), f. 143 (Π. συνουσίας ἀμέτρου καὶ ἐμμέτρου. Inc. Φυσικῶν ἔργων), f. 172—181 (Περὶ γυναικῶν παθῶν μητρικῶν καὶ τῶν ὁμοίων), f. 233ᵛ (*Olivieris Collation der Bücher I. II. XVI und Bruchstücke in dessen Besitz*).

Erlangen: nr. 90; s. XVI. f. 1 (Σύνοψις τῶν τρίτων βιβλίων Ὀριβασίου τοῦ πρὸς Ἰουλ. καὶ τοῦ πρὸς Εὐστάθ. ... Γαλ. καὶ Ἀρχιγ. καὶ Ῥούφου κτλ. »Cod. descriptus est ex Ald. a. 1534«).

Escurial: Scorial. Σ. III. 17*; s. XVI. f. 1 (Synopsis simpl. Gal. medicamentorum liber II) *und* f. 9. 220 (Libri I excerpt.).

Florenz: Laur. plut. 75, 8; s. XV. p. 1 (Διάγνωσις οὔρου), p. 3 (Ἀκριβεστάτη σύνοψις περὶ οὔρων ἐκ τῆς ἰατρικῆς τέχνης τῶν Περσῶν. Inc. Τὸ οὖρον μέχρι καὶ τῆς), p. 3b (Περὶ τῆς ἐκ σφυγμῶν σημειώσεως excerptum brevissimum).

Gallipoli: Ἐκκλησ. ἁγ. Νικολάου 38; s. XIV. f. 81 (Π. τῆς ἐκ σφυγμῶν σησειώσεως. Inc. Προσδοκωμένης ἤδη τῆς κράσεως. Expl. δεῖ προσδοκᾶν ἔσεσθαι).

Jerusalem: Bibl. patriarch. 273; s. XVIII. f. 1 (Χολῆς ξανθῆς καθαρτικόν. Inc. Ἀλόη τὸ μὲν ὅλον).

Leyden: Voss. 8° 18; s. XVI.

London:

Addit. (Brit. Mus.)10, 058; s. XV. f. 101ᵛ.

Harleian. (Brit. Mus.) 6305; s. XVI. f. 3 (?). (Inc. Ἐγὼ δὲ διὰ παντὸς τῷ διὰ τῶν κωδίων χρῶμαι).

Medical Society

H Hi 17 = We 30; s. XV in. no. 21 Dbg. (Remedia).

H Hi 21. 22 = We 28. 29; s. XV ex. f. 346 (*Wie im* cod. Gallipoli 38. Expl. τάσιν τινὰ τῆς ἀρτηρίας βραχεῖαν).

Madrid: Matrit. bibl. nac. 4631 (ol. N 110); a. 1474. f. 155 (Inscr. Π. λίθων Διοσκορίδου. impress. Iriarte).

Mailand: Ambros. A 157 Sup.; s. X (XI?). (*Schoenes Collation in Olivieris Besitz.*)

Modena: Mutinens. 61 (III B 9); s. XV. f. 29ᵛ (Frgm. inc. Ἕπονται δὲ καὶ τοῖς πυρετοῖς ἱδρῶτες. Expl. στοχάσασθαι τοῖς ἀτμοῖς ἐν λουτροῖς).

Moskau: Mosquens. 468; s. XVI. f. 152 (Π. βοτανῶν κατὰ στοιχεῖον Inc. Ἀργεμὸν βοτάνη ῥίζαν ἔχει).

Neapel: Bibl. dei Gerolamini XXII. I; s. XV. f. 176 (Ποδαγρικαὶ θεραπεῖαι πρόχειροι. Inc. Κένωσις διὰ φλεβοτομίας. Expl. ἐπίθες).

Oxford: Canonic. 1; s. XVI. f. 70 (Π. τροφῶν δυνάμεων. Inc. Χρὴ δὲ ὥσπερ τι καὶ ἄλλον. Expl. πρὸς εἴκοντας εὔχυμον γενά [?]).

Paris:

Parisin.

2153; s. XV. f. 218—289 (*Vgl.* Rose, Soranus p. 412 ss).

2237; s. XIV. f. 165ᵛ (Ex Gal. Orib. Aët.).

2256; s. XV. f. 34 (Synopsis simplic. Gal. medicamentorum; libri II. *Vgl. den* Scorial. Σ. III. 17).

2847; s. XVI. f. 139.

Suppl.

637; s. XV. f. 67ᵛ (De cephalalgia).

683; s. XVIII. f. 1ᵛ (Fragmenta) *und* s. XVI. f. 55ᵛ (De symptomatibus urinarum).

Rom:

Barberin. I 49; s. XV. f. 1—165.

Palat.

279; s. XIV—XV. f. 312ᵛ (De febrium diagnosi et curatione).

358; s. XV—XVI. f. 230 (De capillorum defluvio. Inc. Περὶ τὸ μὴ ἀπορρεῖν τρίχας).

Urbin. 70; s. XV. f. 107 (Π. μελαγχολίας ἐκ τῶν Γαλ. καὶ Ῥουφ. καὶ Ποσειδ.).

Vatic.

299; s. XV. f. 156 (Κόμητος τοῦ ὀψικίου ἐκ τῶν ἁπλῶν Γαλ. Inc. Ἀδιάφοροι τῶν κατὰ μέρος. Expl. καὶ μάλιστα νήπια).

2304 (ol. 2217); s. XV. f. 8. 17—19 (Πρόλογος περί τε δυνάμεων φυσικῶν ἐπὶ σωμάτων = Lib. I init. magni operis), f. 9—16ᵛ (Inc. Καὶ διὰ ῥινῶν μετὰ γάλακτος. Expl. ἧπαρ ἐκκαθαίρει μὲν καὶ ῥύπτει = pars συντάγματος κατὰ στοιχεῖον π. βοτανῶν, i. e. libri I), f. 19 (Inc. Τὸ δὲ ἀβρότονον θερμόν ἐστι. Expl. ἐν αὐτῷ τῷ ἐγκεφάλῳ ἐνισταμένης. Προεργά = pars prior libri I).

Venedig:

Marcian. 279; s. XV. f. 269ᵛ (*Wie im* Urbin.).

App. cl.

V 13; s. XIV—XV. f. 136 (Π. βοτανῶν κατὰ στοιχεῖον).

V 16; s. XVI. f. 42ᵛ (Π. τροφῶν δυνάμεων frgm.).

Africanus.

[Diels II.8]

Ἐκ τῶν Ἀφρικανοῦ Κεστῶν ὅπερ ἐστὶν κεστὸν [sic!] ΙΓ', κεφ. κβ': Καθαρτικὰ ἁπλᾶ.
Ex Africani Cestis cestum XIII cap. 22: *De purgantibus simplicibus.*

Florenz: Laurent. plut. 74, 23; s. XIV. p. 204 (Inc. Κυκλωμένου χυλῷ. Expl. μιχθεὶς καὶ ποθείς).

Oxford: Baroccian. 224; s. XV in. f. 50ᵛ (Inc. Κυκλαμίνου χυλός. Expl. μυχθεὶς καὶ ποθείς).

Περὶ σταθμῶν καὶ μέτρων.
De ponderibus et mensuris.

Berlin: Berol. fol. 37 (273); s. XVI. f. 501ᵛ.

Escurial: Scorial. Φ. I. 2; s. XVI. f. 72.

Paris:

Parisin.

2191; s. XIV. f. 344.

2192; s. XV. f. 316ᵛ (*Abschrift von 2191*; *vgl.* Costomiris Rev. des ét. gr. III 167).

2193; s. XV. f. 402.

Bibl. de la ville de Paris 58; s. XVI—XVII. f. 609.

Rom: Vatic.

298; a. 1387. f. 591.

1949; s. —. f. 198ᵛ.

Venedig: Marcian. 291; s. XV. f. 449 (Inc. Ἐπειδὴ πολλαχοῦ σταθμῶν).

Aglaias.

Πρὸς τὰς ἀρχομένας ὑποχύσεις Ἀγλαΐου, εὐγενεστάτου Βυζαντίων, ἐξ Ἡρακλέους τὸ γένος κατάγοντος, Ἀλεξάνδρου μαθητοῦ, συμμαθητοῦ δὲ Δημοσθένους καὶ φίλου, στίχοι ἡρωελεγεῖοι.
Ad suffusiones incipientes Aglaiae ..., Alexandri discipuli, condiscipuli Demosthenis et amici, versus heroelegi

Ed. Sichel, Rev. de philologie II [1847] p. 17—19.
Bussemaker, Poet. buc. et did. Paris 1851 p. 97.

Inc. Ἀγλαΐας τόδε σοι Βυζάντιος ἐσθλὸν ἰάλλω.
Expl. Τημελέως τ' ἀπόθου τεῦχος ἐς ἀργύρεον.

Paris: Parisin. 2726; s. XV.
Venedig: Marcian. 480; s. —. f. 169.

Alexander.

Ἱπποκράτους ἢ Ἀλεξάνδρου ἐπιστολὴ πρὸς Πτολεμαῖον βασιλέα.
Hippocratis vel Alexandri epistula ad Ptolemaeum regem.

Paris: Parisin. 2240; s. XVI. f. 156ᵛ.

[Diels II.9]

Alexander Aphrodisiensis.

Ἰατρικὰ ἀπορήματα καὶ φυσικὰ προβλήματα.
Problematum physicorum et medicorum eclogae. Libri V.

L. I et II ed. Ideler, Phys. et Med. I p. 3—80.

Inc. Τῶν προβλημάτων τὰ μὲν αὐτόθεν.
Expl. ἐξυδαρωθῆναι καὶ ἐμπνευματωθῆναι.

Berlin: Phillipps. 1558*; s. XVI. f. 25 (Excerpta ex Alex. Aphr. naturalibus et moralibus ed. L. Spengel Monachii 1842).
Bologna: Bonon. 3635; s. XIV. f. 1 (Libri I et II) *und* f. 51ᵛ (Excerpta. Inc. Οἱ μὲν πλεῖστοι τῶν παλαιοτέρων ἰατρῶν. Expl. ἐξευρεῖν τὴν γονήν).
Cambridge: Cantabr. bibl. univ. F. F. 3. 30; s. XVI. no. 6.

Escurial: Scorial. Υ. I. 9; s. XVI. f. 55 (Frgm. libri II).
Florenz: Laurent. plut. 75, 13; s. XV. p. 121 (L. I et II).
Jerusalem: Bibl. patriarch. 108*; s. XIII. f. 80 B.
London: Harleian. (Brit. Mus.) 6295; s. XV (XIV sec. catal.). f. 1 (Expl. ἐνδιδόναι τῆς οἰκείας ὁρμῆς καὶ φορᾶς) *und* f. 25 (L. IV et V).
Madrid: Matrit. bibl. nac. 4616 (N 84); s. XV. f. 46ᵛ. 54ᵛ.
Modena: Mutin.
109 (II D 10); s. XIV—XV. f. 3 (L. I et II; Idel. 6, 1—80, 36) *und* f. 24ᵛ (L. III).
135 (II E 2); s. XV. f. 118 (Inc. Διὰ τί τοὺς ἀνθρώπους. Expl. ὁμοίως δὲ καὶ ἐπὶ νεφελῶν).
145 (II E 12); s. XV. f. 52 (L. I et II).
210 (III G 6); s. XVI. f. 299ᵛ (L. I et II).
Oxford: Baroccian. 131*; s. XIV. f. 404b—405.
Palermo: Panorm. bibl. naz. IV H 8; s. XV. f. 85ᵛ—125.
Paris:
Coislin. 332; s. XV. f. 32ᵛ (Capita 291).
Parisin.
1883; s. XIV. f. 1.
1884; a. 1503. f. 1.
1893; s. XVI. f. 153 (Libri II).
2047*; s. XV. f. 6.
2047 A; s. XIV. f. 1 (Libri II, initio mutili).
2048; s. XV. f. 1 (Libri II).
2230; s. XIV. f. 123ᵛ (Problemata physica 150).
2381; s. XV. f. 93 (Problemata physica).
3044; s. XV. f. 69 (Problemata).
Rom: Palat. 199; s. XIII. f. 18.
Venedig: Marcian. 257; s. XII (L. III et IV).

Ἀπορίαι καὶ λύσεις διάφοροι.
Quarundam difficultatum solutiones.

Bologna: Bonon. 2294; s. XVI. f. 61 (Quaestionum libri IV).
Modena: Mutin.
145 (II E 12); s. XV. f. 65 (Περὶ τετραπόδων ἀπορίαι καὶ λύσεις διάφοροι. Τόμος ε', probl. Α'—ΞΓ').
210; (III G 6); s. XVI. f. 178 (*Wie im* Bonon.).
Oxford: Baroccian. 131; s. XIV in. f. 62b.
Paris:
Coislin. 332; s. XV. f. 1.

Parisin.
1268; s. XII. f. 295v.
1630; s. XIV. f. 181.
Rom: Vatic. 1614; s. XVI. f. 1 (Σχολίων ἀποριῶν καὶ λύσεων κεφάλαια τοῦ Α' λόγου).
Venedig: Marcian. App. cl.
V 10; s. XV. f. 1 (*Wie im* Bonon.).
V 16; s. XVI. f. 167 (Ἐπί τισιν ἀπορίαις λύσεις. Inc. Διὰ τί τῶν ἀλόγων ζώων).
Wien: Vindob. med. 44; s. XV—XVI. f. 231 (Inc. *wie im* Marc. App. V 16. Expl. καὶ βλέφαρα οἰδαλέα καὶ ἀπλότριχα καὶ πολιώδη).

Περὶ κράσεως καὶ αὐξήσεως.
De nutritione et augmento.

Inc. Πῶς δ' ἂν παραδέξαιτό τις.
Expl. τοῦ παραδόξου τε καὶ θαυμαστοῦ δόγματος.

Escurial: Scorial. X. I. 11; s. XVI. f. 64.
Paris: Parisin. 2028; s. XV—XVI. f. 107.

[Diels II.10] Περὶ κράσεως καὶ μίξεως.
De mixtione.

Paris: Parisin.
1848; s. XV. f. 136.
2540; s. XVI. f. 93.
Venedig: Marcian. 257; s. XII.

Περὶ πυρετῶν.
De febribus.

Ed. Fr. Passow, Bresl. 1822.
Ideler, Phys. et Med. I 81—106.

Inc. Ἤιτησας ἡμᾶς, Ἀσκληπιαδῶν ἄριστε.
Expl. σαφῶς ἐδήλωσα λέγων.

Florenz: Laurent. plut. 75, 14; s. XV. p. 1.
Paris: Parisin. Suppl. 836; s. XVII. f. 91.

Wien: Vindob. med.
10; s. XVI. f. 1.
[15; s. —] (*Abschrift im Berol. fol. 39 [275]*).

Excerpta varia.

Berlin: Berol. fol. 39 (275) — (*Collationen kleinerer Stücke*).
Paris: Parisin. 1865; s. XV. f. 8ᵛ.
Rom:
Palat. 428; s. XV—XVI. f. 1 (Index in Galeni, Alexandri Aphr. et Hippocratis aliquot opuscula).
Vatic. 1692 B; s. XV. f. 34ᵛ (Περὶ τῆς ἡρακλείας λίθου καὶ διὰ τί ἕλκει τὸν σίδηρον. Inc. Ἐμπεδοκλῆς ταῖς ἀποῤῥοίαις. Expl. τῶν ἀψύχων ἔχει. Ex libro II quaest. naturalium?).

Alexander Rex.

Περὶ τῆς τῶν ζ' βοτανῶν δυνάμεως.
De Septem herbarum facultate.

Vgl. Costomiris, Rev. des ét. gr. IV [1891] p. 98 sq.

Inc. Πρώτη βοτάνη ἡ λεγομένη ἀσφόδελος.
Expl. καὶ χρῶ ἐναργῶς.

London: Addit. (Brit. Mus.) 17, 900; s. XVII. f. 89ᵛ.
Oxford: Roe 15 (Bodl. 261); s. XV ex. f. 103.
Rom: Barberin. I 127; s. XVI. f. 249ᵛ.

Alexander Sophista. [Diels II.11]

Βίβλος τὰς τῶν ἱερῶν βοτανῶν περιέχουσα κράσεις.
De sacrarum herbarum temperamentis.

Vgl. Costomiris, Rev. des ét. gr. IV [1891] p. 98.

Inc. Περὶ ἀμπέλου βοτάνης τῆς καὶ βρυωνίας.
Expl. ὤκιμον λεῖον σὺν ὕδατι πινόμενον.

Oxford: Baroccian. 150; s. XV in. f. 67v.

Dazu: Cod. Joh. Sambuci.

Περὶ γενέσεως ἀνθρώπου.
De hominis generatione.

Vgl. Costomiris, Rev. des ét. gr. IV [1891] p. 98.

Inc. Ἀλλὰ μηδεὶς ὑπολαμβανέτω ἄψυχον εἶναι.
Expl. ἐκ τῶν θ' μηνῶν ἀποπνιήκεται (sic!).

Paris: Parisin. Suppl. 165; s. XV. f. 116 (*Abschrift besitzt Mr. E. O. Winstedt in Oxford*).

Alexander Trallianus.

Θεραπευτικά.
Therapeutica. Libri XII.

Ed. Puschmann, Wien 1878—79.

Inc. Περὶ ἀλωπεκίας. Ἡ ἀλωπεκία πάθος ἐστὶ τριχῶν.
Expl. περὶ τῶν πυρετῶν εἰς θεραπείαν ἡγούμεθα.

Berlin: Phillipps. 1535 (ol. Meerm. 229); s. XV ex.
Cambridge: Cantabr. Caius Coll. 77; s. XV—XVI. f. 1 (*Coll. im Leydens. Periz 4° 2/9 fasc. 2*).
Escurial: Scorial. Φ. I. 2*; s. XVI. f. 196 *und* 308 (*Apographon des* Marcian. 295).
Florenz:
Laurent. plut. 74, 10; s. XIV. p. 86.
Riccard. 10 (K. I. 12); a. 1583. f. 67.
Moskau: Mosquens. 446; s. XV. f. 5.
Paris:
Parisin.
2200; s. XV. f. 1.
2201; s. XV. f. 1.
2202; s. XVI. f. 1.
2203; s. XVI (L. I et II fine mutil.).

2204; s. XVI. f. 7 (fine mutil.).
Suppl.
764*; s. XIV. f. 12 (Ex libro XI. Sine auctoris nomine. Inscr. Εἰδήσεις ἰατρικαὶ διάφοροι).
1297*; s. XI. f. 1 (*Vorlage des* Marcian. 295).

Rom:
Ottobon. 89; s. XVI. f. 1.
Vallicell. 15 (B. 70); s. XIV (XV). f. — (L. I usque ad τὸ ἰνίον ὀδύνωνται πολλάκις · ἐὰν δὲ ...).

Venedig:
Marcian. 295*; a. 1470. f. 1 (Ex libris XII. *Apographon des* Paris. Suppl. 1297).
App. cl. V, 9; s. XV.

Ἐπιστολὴ περὶ ἑλμίνθων. [Diels II.12]
Epistula de lumbricis.

Ed. Ideler, Phys. et Med. I 305—311.
Puschmann II p. 586—599.

Inc. Γέγραφάς μοι, φίλτατε Θεόδωρε, περὶ τοῦ σοῦ παιδὸς ἀπολέσθαι κινδυνεύσαντος.
Expl. εἰ καλῶς προσέχεις καὶ ἀκριβῶς ποιήσεις.

Escurial: Scorial. — (Puschm. I p. 90. *Verbleib unbekannt*).
Florenz: Laurent. App. 2; s. XV. f. 323.
Mailand: Ambros. S 3 Sup.; s. XVI. f. 170.
Oxford: Bodleian. — (Puschm. I p. 90).
Rom: Vatic. — (Puschm. I p. 89).

Περὶ ὀφθαλμῶν.
De oculis. Libri III.

Ed. Puschmann, Berl. Stud. V 2 [1886] p. 134—179.

Inc. Ἅπαντα μὲν ἰατρὸς ἄριστος ἰᾶσθαι τὰ πάθη.
Expl. (lib. II): μάλιστα εὐδοκιμεῖν δυναμένων.

Escurial: Scorial. Φ. I. 2 (?); s. XVI. f. 191 (*vgl.* Puschm. I p. 90).
Venedig: Marcian. App. cl. V 9; s. XV. f. 265—274 (L. I et II).

[Diels II.13]

Alexander (Trallianus?).

Περὶ διαγνώσεως σφυγμῶν ἐπὶ τῶν πυρεσσώντων [sic!]
καὶ περὶ οὔρων ἀφορισμοί.
Opusculum de pulsuum dignotione in febricitantibus et aphorismi de urinis.

Vgl. Puschmann I p. 88.

Paris: Parisin. 2316; s. XV. f. 207^{v}.

Alexander Trallianus.

Excerpta varia.

Berlin: Berol. fol. 39 (275) — (*Varianten in einer Ausg. des Alex. Trall. von Gampylius in der Bibl. der Minerva zu Rom*).
Bologna: Bonon. 3632; s. XV. f. 207 (Ἱερὰ ἀντίδοτος).
Escurial: Scorial.
Ω. I. 8; s. XIV. f. 1. 15. 20. 22. 48^{v} *u. öfter.*
III. R. 3; s. XI. f. 141^{v} (Medicamina sine auctoris nomine; *vgl.* Dioscuridis de mat. med. libri V ed. M. Wellmann, vol. II p. XII. *Teilweise Abschrift in Wellmanns Besitz*).
Florenz: Laurent. App. 2; s. XV. f. 328^{v}. 332. 338. 345^{v}. 346.
Paris: Parisin. 2178; s. XV. f. 11^{v} (De febrium differentiis) *und* f. 42 (De morbis hominum et remediis).

[Diels II.14]

Andreas Caesareae in Cappadocia Archiepiscop[us].

[Ἀπορίαι καὶ λύσεις ἐκ τοῦ Θεραπευτικῶν λόγου Β'.]
Interrogationes et responsiones ex libro II. therapeuticae.

Paris: Parisin. 2314; s. XIV—XV. f. 345^{v}.

Andreiomenus.

Ἰατρικαὶ παρασημειώσεις ἀναγκαῖαι.
Notae medicae.

Inc. Εἰς συνουσίαν.

Athos: Βιβλ. μον. Ἰβήρων 4271. 151; s. XV. f. 228.

Andromachus.

Θηριακὴ δι' ἐχιδνῶν ἡ καλουμένη Γαλήνη.
Theriaca ex anguibus, Tranquillitas dicta.

Ideler, Phys. et Med. I 138—143.
Bussemaker, Poëmat. rell. p. 94—97.
Vgl. Galen. XIV p. 32 sq. K.

Inc. Κλῦθι πολυθρονίου βριαρὸν σθένος ἀντιδότοιο.
Expl. Ἱλάσεται τὴν σὴν αἰὲν ἀνωδυνίην.

London: Addit. (Brit. Mus.) 10, 058; s. XV. f. 161v (manu recentiore).
Venedig: Marcian. 281; s. XV. f. 96.

Excerpta.

Florenz: Laurent. App. 2; s. XV. f. 273v (Commemoratur Andreas).
Paris: Parisin. 1630; s. XIV. f. 217 (Remedia in podagram).

Antonius Pyropulus. [Diels II.15]

Excerpta varia.

Paris: Coislin. 335; s. XV. f. 1 (Remedium pro tussi).
Rom: Angelic. 4 (C 4. 16); s. XVI in. f. 294 (Ἑρμηνία).

Antyllus.

Excerpta varia.

Berlin: Berol. fol. 39 (275) — (*Coll. kleinerer Stücke*).
Florenz: Laurent. plut.
74, 7; s. IX. p. 115 (Περὶ ὑδροκεφάλων. Inc. Τὸ ὑδροκέφαλον. Ex Orib. IV 200).
75, 7; s. XIV. p. 224 (Διαιτητικά. Ex libro II. de victus ratione. Inc. Τῶν καθαιρόντων τὰ μέν. Ed. C. F. Wolz, Antylli veteris chirurgi quae ap. Orib. libro 44. 45 et 50 leguntur. Diss. inaug. Jen. 1842) *und* p. 225 (Περὶ κλυσμῶν, ὅτι διὰ τρεῖς αἰτίας παραλαμβάνονται. Inc. Παραλαμβάνονται οἱ κλυσμοί. »Antyllo tribuit Bandini III p. 151«).
London: Harleian. (Brit. Mus.) 5626; s. XV—XVI. f. 2 (Ἰατροσόφιον ποιηθὲν ὑπὸ διαφόρων φιλοσόφων ... Ἀντίλλου ...).
Rom:
Barberin. I 127; s. XVI. f. 205ᵛ (Περὶ ἑψήσεως τῶν ἐμβαλλομένων εἰς τὰς ἐμπλάστρους φαρμάκων. Inc. Λιθαργυρ ... ἐν ταῖς ἕψησι. Expl. καταχέονται τὰ τηκτά).
Vatic. 295; s. XV. f. — (Περὶ πεσσῶν).
Venedig: Marcian. App. cl. II 171; s. XV (Ὡς φλεβοτομητέον *und* Περὶ καθάρσεως).
Wien: Vindob. med. 8; s. XV. f. 278ᵛ (*Wie im* Barberin.).

Apollonius Citiensis.

Εἰς Ἱπποκράτους περὶ ἄρθρων πραγματεία, βιβλ.Γ'.
Commentarius in Hipp[ocratis] de articulis, libri III.

Ed. H. Schoene Lips. 1895.

Inc. Θεωρῶν φιλιάτρως διακείμενόν σε, βασιλεῦ Πτολεμαῖε.
Expl. τῆς ἐνδεχομένης διαστολῆς τεύξεται.

Berlin: Phillipps. 1533; s. XVII. f. 90 (Liber III), f. 121 (L. I), f. 135 (L. II).
Bologna: Bonon. 3632*; s. XVI. f. 419—434 (Imagines).
Florenz: Laurent. plut. 74, 7; s. IX. p. 179b.
Leipzig: Lipsiens.
59; s. XIX. no. 2 (conscr. a Fr. del Furia Florentino et a K. G. Kuehnio).
64; s. XVIII. p. 1.
Paris:
Faculté de Méd. (*vgl.* Dietz, Schol. in Hipp. et Gal. I prf. p. XI).

Parisin.
2247; s. XVI.
2248; s. XVI.
Suppl. 270; s. XVII. f. 351.

Archelaus.

[Diels II.16]

Fragmentum.

Inc. Ἐστὶ τῆς ἰατρικῆς τέχνης σκοπὸς μὲν ὑγίεια, τέλος δὲ ἡ κτῆσις αὐτῆς (*vgl.* Galenus I p. 64 K.).
Expl. καὶ τἄλλα πάντα χρῶ καὶ ὁ θεὸς βοηθο (sic).

Bologna: Bonon. 3632; s. XV. f. 43.

Archigenes.

Excerpta varia.

Berlin: Berol. fol. 39 (275) — (*Coll. kleinerer Stücke*).
Florenz: Laurent. plut. 74, 7; s. IX. p. 113 (Περὶ ὑποδραμόντος αἵματος. Inc. Ὑποδρομὴ δὲ αἵματος. Ex Orib. IV 193), p. 114 (Περὶ τῆς τῶν ῥαφῶν διαστάσεως. Inc. Τοὺς δὲ περισωθησομένους. Ex Orib. IV 197), p. 127 (Περὶ τῶν ἀφαιρεθησομένων μερῶν. Ex Orib. IV 244. *Vgl.* Harles, Anall. histor.-medica de Archigene et de Apolloniis medicis etc. Lips. 1816).
London: Harleian. (Brit. Mus.) 5626; s. XV—XVI. f. 2 (Ἰατροσόφιον ποιηθὲν ὑπὸ διαφόρων φιλοσόφων ... Ἀρχιγένους ...). [Diels II.17]
Oxford: Baroccian. 150; s. XV in. f. 3b (Ἀντίδοτος ἱερά) *und* f. 77 (Pauca de simplicibus ex ... et Archigene).
Paris:
Parisin.
2276; s. XVI. f. 217 (Archigenis et Philagrii opusculum de renum calculis, ex Aëtio).
2286; s. XIV. f. 89 (Remedia ad sedandos dentium dolores ex ... Archigene).
3076; a. 1616. f. 56 (De nephritide).
Suppl. 1202; s. XIII. f. 16 (Excerpta varia ex Diosc., Oribasio ... Archigene).
Rom: Vatic. 178; s. XIV. f. 142^{v} (Περὶ συναπισμοῦ. Inc. Τὸ ἀπὸ νάπυος. Expl. καταχύσει παρηγορητέον).

Aretaeus.

Περὶ αἰτίων καὶ σημείων ὀξέων παθῶν Α' Β'.
De causis et signis acutorum morborum libri II.

K. 1—66.

Inc. (lib. 1) [περὶ παροξυσμοῦ ἐπιληπτικῶν.] ... ἀμβλύτητες, ἴλιγγοι, τενόντων βάρεα.
Expl. (lib. 2) οὕνεκεν οὐκ ἴσχει ὑστέρην ἀνήρ.

Berlin:
Berol. fol. 39 (275). (*Varianten aus* Vatic. 286. *Probecoll. von Hdss. der* Marciana).
Phillipps.
1531 (Meerm. 223); s. XVI. f. 1 (Inc. περὶ τετάνου. σπασμοὶ οἱ τέτανοι).
1532 (Meerm. 225); s. XVI. f. 77.
Escurial: Scorial. y. I. 8; s. XVI. f. 162 (initio mutil. Inc. *wie im* Phillipps. 1531 l. I 8).
Florenz: Laurent. plut. 75, 15; s. XV. p. 1 (L. I c. 1—4 perierunt).
Leipzig: Lipsiens. 63 (ol. 1109?) s. XVI. f. 1.
London:
Harleian. (Brit. Mus.) 6326; s. XVI ex. f. 2.
Medical Society H Hi 23 = We 32a; s. XVI in.
Mailand: Ambros. B 157 Sup.; s. XV—XVI. f. 1 (Inc. a l. I c. 6).
München: Monac.
70; s. XVI. f. 254 (Inc. *wie im* Phillipps. 1531).
72; s. XVI. f. 113 (L. I c. 1—6 desunt).
Neapel: Neapol. 305 III D 21; s. XIV.
Oxford: Bibl. Aed. Christi 81; s. XVII.
Padua:
[Bibl. Cathedr. P 129; s. —].
Bibl. Tomasini (Desunt l. I. c. 1—6. *Verbleib unbekannt*).
Paris:
Parisin.
2186; s. XVI. f. 1.
2187; s. XVI. f. 1v.
2202; s. XVI. f. 147.
2220; s. XVI.
2288; s. XVI. f. 1.
2289; s. XVI. f. 1.
2334; s. XVI. f. 1.
[2682 (?)].
Suppl.
445; s. XIX. (Opp. c. mss. bibl. reg. a M. Myna collata).

633; s. XIX. (Var. lectt. e codd. Paris. 2186. 2187. 2202. 2220. 2288. 2289 2334.).

Rom: Vatic. 286; s. XV. f. 1 (ab initio mutil.).

Venedig:

Bibl. Josephi de Aromatariis; s. — (*Verbleib unbekannt*).

Marcian. 270; s. XV (Inc. a l. I c. 6. *Coll. im Berol. fol. 39 [275]*).

Dazu: [Claromontan.; duo Menteliani; Sarrazianus].

Περὶ αἰτίων καὶ σημείων χρονίων παθῶν Α' Β'.

De causis et signis diuturnorum morborum libri II.

K. 67—184.

Inc. (lib. 1) [Περὶ χρονίων παθῶν]. Χρονίων νούσων πόνος μὲν πολύς.

Expl. (lib. 2) ἀνανεῶσαι τὸν ἄνθρωπον οὐκ ἄπιστον ἐς τέρατος ἰδέην.

Berlin:

Berol. fol. 39 (275). (*Varianten aus* Vatic. 286. *Probecoll. von Hdss. der* Marciana).

Phillipps.

1531; s. XVI. f. 16ᵛ.

1532; s. XVI. f. —.

Escurial: Scorial. y. I. 8; s. XVI. f. 181ᵛ.

Florenz: Laurent. plut. 75, 15; s. XVI. p. 15.

Leipzig: Lipsiens. 63 (ol. 1109?); s. XVI. f. 14. [Diels II.18]

London:

Harleian. (Brit. Mus.) 6326; s. XVI ex. f. 48ᵛ.

Medical Society H Hi 23 = We 32a; s. XVI in.

Mailand: Ambros. B 157 Sup.; s. XV—XVI. f. 24ᵛ.

München: Monac.

70; s. XVI. f. 272.

72; s. XVI. f. 129.

Neapel: Neapolit. 305 III D 21; s. XIV.

Oxford: Bibl. Aed. Christi 81; s. XVII.

Padua:

[Bibl. Cathedr. P 129].

Bibl. Tomasini (*Verbleib unbekannt*).

Paris:

Parisin.

2186; s. XVI. f. 1.

2187; s. XVI. f. 1v.
2202; s. XVI. f. 154v.
2288; s. XVI. f. 1.
2289; s. XVI. f. 1.
2334; s. XVI. f. 1.
[2682 (?)].
Suppl. 445; s. XIX. (Opp. c. mss. bibl. reg. a M. Myna collata).
Rom: Vatic. 286; s. XV. f. 32v.
Venedig:
Bibl. Josephi de Aromatariis (*Verbleib unbekannt*).
Marcian. 270; s. XV (*Coll. im Berol. fol. 39 [275]*).

Dazu: [Claromontanus; Menteliani duo].

Ὀξέων νούσων θεραπευτικόν Α' β'.
De curatione acutorum morborum libri II.

K. 185—291.

Inc. (lib. 1) [Προοίμιον]. Ὀξέων νούσων ἄκεα ξυναφέα.
Expl. (lib. 2) τοῖσι γεγραμμένοισι καὶ μούνοισι ἢ ἅπασι χρέεσθαι.

Berlin:
Berol. fol. 39 (275). (*Varianten aus* Vatic. 286. *Probecoll. von Hdss. der* Marciana).
Phillipps.
1531; s. XVI. f. 48v.
1532; s. XVI. f. —.
Escurial: Scorial. y. I. 8; s. XVI. f. 218.
Florenz: Laurent. plut. 75, 15; s. XVI. p. 40.
Leipzig: Lipsiens. 63 (ol. 1109?); s. XVI. f. 38.
London:
Harleian. (Brit. Mus.) 6326; s. XVI ex. f. 118.
Medical Society H Hi 23 = We 32a; s. XVI in.
Mailand: Ambros. B 157 Sup.; s. XV—XVI. f. 70.
München: Monac.
70; s. XVI. f. 305.
72; s. XVI. f. 162.
Neapel: Neapol. 305 III D 21; s. XIV.
Oxford: Bibl. Aed. Christi 81; s. XVII.

Padua:
[Bibl. Cathedr. P 129].
Bibl. Tomasini (*Verbleib unbekannt*).
Paris:
Parisin.
2186; s. XVI. f. 50v.
2187; s. XVI. f. 68.
2202; s. XVI. f. 175v.
2220; s. XVI. f. 76 (L. I).
2288; s. XVI. f. 89.
2289; s. XVI. f. 88.
2334; s. XVI. f. 219.
[2682 (?)].
Suppl. 445; s. XIV. (Opp. c. mss. bibl. reg. collata).
Rom: Vatic. 286; s. XV. f. 92.
Venedig:
Bibl. Josephi de Aromatariis (*Verbleib unbekannt*).
Marcian. 270; s. XV (*Coll. im Berol. fol. 39 [275]*).

Dazu: [Claromontanus; Menteliani duo].

Χρονίων νούσων θεραπευτικόν Α' Β'.
De curatione diuturnorum morborum libri II.

K. 292—346.

Inc. (lib. 1) [Προοίμιον]. Ἐν τῇσι χρονίῃσι νούσοισι ἡ ἀμβολή.
Expl. (lib. 2) ἐξ ἀχροίης δὲ εὐχροίην καὶ ἀπὸ σκελετίης εὐσαρκίην.

Berlin:
Berol. fol. 39 (275). (*Varianten aus* Vatic. 286. *Probecoll. von Hdss. der* Marciana).
Phillipps.
1531; s. XVI. f. 81v (Expl. σχεδὸν τὰ = K. 322, 4).
1532; s. XVI. f. — (Expl. *wie* 1531).
Escurial: Scorial. y. I. 8; s. XVI. f. 252v (scatet lacunis).
Florenz: Laurent. plut. 75, 15; s. XVI. p. 63.
Leipzig: Lipsiens. 63 (ol. 1109?); s. XVI. f. 61 (Expl. *wie im* Phillipps. 1531).
London:
Harleian. (Brit. Mus.) 6326; s. XVI ex. f. 183v (Lib. I usque ad c. 13 γάλακτι).
Medical Society H Hi 23 = We 32a; s. XVI in. (L. II c. 2. 23. 5—7).

[Diels II.19] **Mailand:** Ambros. B 157 Sup.; s. XV—XVI. f. 111ᵛ (non pauca desunt).
München: Monac. 72; s. XVI. f. 193.
Neapel: Neapolit. 305 III D 21; s. XIV.
Oxford: Bibl. Aed. Christi 81; s. XVII. (fine mut.).
Padua:
[Bibl. Cathedr. P 129].
Bibl. Tomasini (*Verbleib unbekannt*).
Paris:
Parisin.
2186; s. XVI. f. 50ᵛ.
2187; s. XVI. f. 68.
2202; s. XVI. f. 141 (init. et fine mutil.).
2288; s. XVI. f. 89 (in fine mut.).
2334; s. XVI. f. 219.
[2682 (?)].
Suppl. 445; s. XIX. (Opp. c. mss. bibl. reg. collata).
Rom: Vatic. 286; s. XV. f. 145 (Expl. in med. c. 5).
Venedig:
Bibl. Jos. de Aromatariis (*Verbleib unbekannt*).
Marcian. 270; s. XV (*Coll. im Berol. fol. 39 [275]*).

Dazu: [Claromontanus; Menteliani duo].

Artemidorus.

Περὶ οὔρων.
De urinis.

Inc. Περὶ τοῦ ὑδατώδους οὔρου.
Expl. μελανώδη μακρονοσίαν σημαίνει καὶ θάνατον.

London: Regius (Brit. Mus.) 16 C XVI; s. XVI. f. 8 (»mit lat. Interlinearübersetzung.« Kalbfleisch).

Asclepiades. [Diels II.20]

Ὑγιεινὰ παραγγέλματα.
Praecepta salubria.

Ed. Ideler, Phys. et Med. I p. 202.
Bussemaker, Poët. de re phys. et medica rell. p. 132—134.

Inc. Εὐεξίας τράπεζαν, εἰ θέλεις, μάθε.
Expl. καὶ σανδαράχῃ τὰ ὅμοι' οἶδε πράττειν.

Florenz: Laurent. plut.
57, 50; s. XVI. p. 577b (Sine auctoris nomine. Expl. ἐκφυγεὶς νόσους).
59, 17; s. XV. p. 74 (Sine auctoris nomine).
87, 16; s. XIII. p. 14 (Sine auctoris nomine. Expl. λατρόφωνος εὑρέθη).
Lesbos: Βιβλ. τῆς τοῦ Λειμῶνος μονῆς 268; a. 1552. no. 24.
Moskau: Mosquensis (*vgl.* Bussemaker *a. a. O. p. 75*).
München: Monacensis (*vgl.* Bussemaker *a. a. O.*).
Rom:
Ottobon. 441; a. 1477. f. 476.
Vatic. 1343; s. XV. f. 2 (Expl. καύματος χρόνῳ).
Wien: Vindob.
hist. 94; s. XVI. f. 61v (Sine auctoris nomine. Expl. σύκοις δὲ συχνοῖς καὶ σταφυλαῖς ἐκτρέφου).
phil. 178; s. XV. f. 35 (Ὑγ. π. σύντομα Ἀσκλ. ταῦτα καὶ Διοσκορίδους).

Excerpta varia.

Vgl. Gumpert, Asclepiadis Bith. fragmenta. Weimar 1794.

Berlin: Berol. fol. 39 (275) — (*Collationen kleinerer Stücke*).
Bologna: Bonon.
1808; s. XV. f. 128 (Inc. Ὁ δὲ Ἀσκληπιάδης σκευάζεσθαι κελεύει τὴν πικρὰν ὡς Θεμίσων).
3632; s. XV. f. 233v (Καθαρτικῶν συγγραφή).
Escurial: Scorial. Ω. I. 8; s. XIV. f. 24 (Ἀσθματικόν. Inc. Ἀριστολοχία στρογγύλη. Ex Aetio.).
Florenz: Laurent. plut. 74, 7; s. IX. f. 127 (Ὅτι καὶ διὰ νόσον χρονίαν ἔξαρθροί τινες γίγνονται. Quod diuturno morbo quibusdam articuli prolabuntur. Inc. Ὅτι χωρὶς φανερᾶς. Ex Oribas. IV 243).

Oxford: Baroccian. 88; s. XV—XVI. f. 164b (Ἐκ τῶν Ἀσκληπιάδου καὶ Διοσκορίδου περὶ ἀναπνοῆς).
Paris: Parisin. 2286; s. XIV. f. 89 (Remedia ad sedandos dentium dolores, ex Asclepiade ...).

Athenaeus.

Περὶ οὔρων σύνοψις.
Synopsis de urinis.

Inc. Ἐάν ἐστι τὸ οὖρον καθαρόν.
Expl. ἡ νόσος ἀπηλεῖ.

Berlin: Phillipps. 1571; s. XVI. f. 9 (Sine auctoris nomine).
Oxford:
Baroccian. 88; s. XVI (»Attribuitur Simeoni Setho codd. medd. 25 § 4 et 40 § 6 bibl. Vindob. Cf. cod. Laud. 58, cod. Mediom. 1537, cod. ol. Regius 2239, cod. Vat. 300. Cf. praeterea cod. Escorial. III 14 f. 197 et Paris. gr. 2260 f. 13«. *Vgl.* Daremberg Not. et Extr. I 17).
Laud. 58 (nunc 59; Bodl. 708); s. XV (»Σημειώσεις οὔρων. Inc. iisdem fere verbis atque opus Barocc. 88 traditum. Des. πλευρῖτιν σημαίνει. Est pars operis sub Athenaei nomine traditi [v. Barocc. 88 § 4]; exstat etiam Paris. gr. 2239. f. 160«. *Vgl.* Daremberg Not. et Extr. I 62).
Paris: Parisin. 2320; s. XVI. f. 18v (Expl. εἰς θάνατον ὤποια [sic!]. *Abschrift in Wellmanns Besitz*).

[Diels II.21] Βίβλος περιέχουσα φαρμάκων ἐμπειρίας κατ᾽ ἀλφάβητον σαφῶς ἐκτεθεῖσα.
De remediis ordine alphabetico.

Inc. Ἀποφλεγματισμὸς κεφαλῆς.
Expl. ἐψημένον καὶ χριόμενον.

Oxford: Baroccian. 150; s. XV in. f. 48v (»Non pauca congruunt cum remediorum collectione sub Dioscoridis et Stephani nomine tradita«. Daremberg, Not. et Extr. I 37).

Excerpta.

Oxford: Baroccian. 88; s. XV (XVI). f. 47 (Ἱπποκράτους διδασκάλου καὶ Γαληνοῦ σοφοῦ καὶ Παύλου Ἰτάλου καὶ Ἀθηναίου ῥήτορος καὶ Ἰωάννου Τζέτζου διάγνωσις περὶ ἰαλίων [sic!] ἀρρώστων καὶ τελευτῆς ἀνθρώπων. Inc. τὸ α΄. ἄσπρον. Expl. σημαίνει καὶ θάνατον).

S[anctus] Basilius.

Περὶ γενέσεως ἀνθρώπου.
De hominis generatione. Libri III.

Vgl. Meletius Exc. Ed. Garnier, t. I p. 324.

Bologna: Bonon. 2911; s. XVI. f. 73 (*Vgl.* Krumbacher, Sitz.-Ber. d. bayr. Akademie 1892 II p. 342 sqq.).
Oxford: Miscell. 20; s. XIV. f. 302.
Paris: Parisin.
478; s. XV. f. 105v.
500; s. XI. f. 184v.
2299; s. XV. f. 191.

[Πρὸς Εὐστάθιον τὸν ἰατρὸν περὶ τῆς τῶν αἱρετικῶν ἀντιλογιῶν λύσεως.]
Ad Eustathium medicum de obiectionum haereticorum solutione.

Paris: Parisin. 912; s. XIV. f. 519.

Beniaminus. [Diels II.22]

Γαληνοῦ καὶ Ἱπποκράτους περὶ βετονίκης
= *Medicinae variae Beniamini Iudaei.*

Inc. Αὕτη ἡ βοτάνη φύεται.
Expl. καὶ ἰᾶται συντόμως.

Venedig: Marcian. App. cl. V, 8; s. XIV. f. 171 (»Γαλ. καὶ Ἱππ. περὶ βετονίκης in codice legitur; cui opusculo catalogus attribuit titulum Beniamini Iudaei Medicinae variae«).

Φάρμακα ἐκκαθαίροντα ἅπαν περίττωμα τοῦ τε ἐγκεφάλου καὶ τοῦ στομάχου.
Medicamenta purgantia omne cerebri ac stomachi excrementum.

Florenz: Laurent. plut. 75, 16; s. XV. p. 3.

Excerpta.

Florenz: Laurent. App. 2; s. XV. f. 272ᵛ (»Commemoratur Iudaeus B.«).

Cassius Iatrosophista.

Ἰατρικαὶ ἀπορίαι καὶ προβλήματα φυσικά.
Quaestiones medicae et problemata physica.

Ed. Ideler, Phys. et Med. I p. 144—167.

Inc. Διὰ τί τὰ στρογγύλα ἕλκη.
Expl. ἄνευ τραυμάτων καταγμάτων.

Berlin: Berol. fol. 39 (275) —. (»Abschrift von Cassius ἰατρ. ἀπ. κ. πρ. φυσ. von der Hand Bernards mit Anmerkungen und zum Teil mit lat. Übs. von demselben«).
Bologna: Bonon. 3635; s. XIV. f. 79.
Madrid: Matrit. bibl. nac. 4616 (N 84)*; s. XV. f. 55 (Ex Cassii probl. XII. XX. XXIII. XXXV. LXIII. LXIV. *Collation in Wellmanns Besitz*).
Modena: Mutin.
109 (II D 10); s. XIV—XV. f. 79ᵛ (Ideler I 144, 1—152, 4).
145 (II E 12); s. XV. f. 70 (Ideler I 144—151, 37).
210 (III G 6); s. XVI. f. 371.
Paris: Parisin.
1943; s. XVI. f. 43ᵛ (Quaestt. medicae de animalibus et quadrupediis).
2047 A; s. XIV. p. 51.
Rom: Vatic. 1614; s. XVI. f. 153 (*Coll. mit der Pariser Ausgabe 1541 im Berol. fol. 39 [275]*).
Venedig: Marcian. 257; s. XII.

Cornelius Celsus.

[Diels II.23]

Περὶ ἰατρικῆς *fragmentum.*

Paris: Parisin. Suppl. 755; s. XIX. f. 123.

Chariton.

[Φάρμακα].
De pastillis, pillulis, zulapiis et clysteribus.

Paris: Parisin. 2240; s. XVI. f. 1.

Chrysostomius (?).

Ἀπόδειξις περὶ τῆς κατασκευῆς τοῦ ἀνθρωπείου σώματος.
De corporis humani constitutione demonstratio.

Inc. Ὑπόκειται μὲν ὁ πνεύμων.

Mailand: Ambros. Q 94 Sup.; s. —. f. 364v (»In margine χρυσο$\overline{\text{σμι}}$.«).

Cleopatra.

Περὶ μέτρων καὶ σταθμῶν. [Diels II.24]
De mensuris et ponderibus.

Ed. Hultsch, Metrol. script. I 233—236.
Vgl. Galen. XIX 767—771 K.

Inc. Ἡ μνᾶ ὄνομα σταθμοῦ ἔχει οὐγγίας ις'.
Expl. ὁ δὲ κύαθος κοτύλης τὸ ς''.

Berlin: Phillipps.
1538; s. X. f. 390v (Ἐκ τῶν Κλεοπ. Κοσμιτικῶν π. στ. κ. μέτρ.).
1540; s. XVI. f. 11v med.
Bologna: Bonon. 457 vol. XXIV no. 1; s. XVII. f. 2 (Inc. Ἡ μνᾶ ὄνομα ἔχει).

Carpentras: nr. 1774 (P., V); s. XVII. f. 139.
Escurial: Scorial.
Φ. I. 11; s. XVI. f. 15ᵛ.
Ψ. I. 13; s. XVI. f. 116ᵛ.
Leipzig: Lipsiens. 66; s. XVII. f. 112.
Paris: Parisin.
2275; a. 1465. f. 1.
2320; s. XVII. f. 216ᵛ.
2327; a. 1478. f. 15.
Rom: Vatic.
1174; s. XIV—XV. f. 134ᵛ.
2259; s. —. f. 132.

Excerpta varia.

Escurial: Scorial. Υ. III. 17; s. XVI. f. 209 (Ξηρίον τὸ μέγα ποιοῦν πρὸς ὑποφορὰς τριχιάσεις μυοκεφάλους).

Coeranus.

Ἀποθεραπευτικά.
De arte recuratoria.

Florenz: Laurent. plut. 75, 19*; s. XIV. p. 5.

Constantinus Melitiniota.

[Περὶ ἀντιδότων.]
Antidotarium e persica lingua in graecam a Constantino Melitiniota versum.

Paris: Parisin. 2194; s. XV. f. 400ᵛ.

Crateuas.

[Diels II.25]

Ῥιζοτομικόν.
De herbis.

Vgl. Costomiris, Rev. des ét. gr. II [1889] p. 358—363.
M. Wellmann, Crateuas. Abhdl. der Ges. d. Wiss. zu Göttingen. Bd. 2. S. 3 ff.

Paris: Parisin.
2183*; s. XV (Codex Dioscuridis interpolati).
2286*; s. XIV. f. 1—54v (Excerpta continentur opere Dioscuridis περὶ ῥιζῶν κτλ.).
Venedig: Marcian.
92*; s. XIII. f. 92v (»Fragmenta continet e Vindob. med. 1 desumpta.« Wellmann).
271*; s. XV (Codex Dioscuridis interpolati).
Wien: Vindob. med.
1*; s. V—VI. f. 18v.
5*; s. XVI (»E Vindob. med. 1.« Wellmann).
6*; s. —.

Craton.

Προγνωστικὰ ἀρρώστων ζωῆς καὶ θανάτου.
Prognostica de infirmorum vita et morte.

Rom: Vatic. 1470; s. XIII. f. 158.

Cyrillus Alexandrinus.

Περὶ μέτρων καὶ σταθμῶν.
De mensuris et ponderibus.

Paris: Parisin. 1389; s. XVI. f. 387v.

Excerpta.

Paris: Coislin. 335; s. XV. f. 1 (Formulae remediorum variae, inter quas ... Cyrilli Alexandr. fragmentum).

Damascenus.

Excerpta.

Bologna: Bonon. 3632; s. XV. f. 189v (Περὶ τῶν ἀντιδότων. Στήλη τῆς ἱερᾶς Δαμασκηνοῦ).

[Diels II.26]

Damascius.

Ἑρμηνεία εἰς τοὺς ἀφορισμοὺς Ἱπποκράτους.
Expositio in aphorismos Hippocratis. Sectiones VII.

Ed. Dietz, Scholia in Hipp. et Gal. II p. 238–544.
Vgl. Costomiris, Rev. des ét. gr. II [1889] p. 357 sq.

Inc. Ὁ βίος βραχύς.

München: Monac. 227; s. XVI. f. 1.
Paris:
Parisin. 2150; a. 1584.
Suppl. 682; s. X—XIX. f. 85 (Apogr. codicis 2150).

Ἐξήγησις εἰς τὸ Προγνωστικὸν τοῦ Ἱπποκράτους.
Expositio in Prognostica Hippocratis. Sectiones II.

Rom: Vatic. 2154; s. XVI. f. 3.
Zaragoza: Bibl. d. cat. d. Pilar 1115 (olim 1427); s. XVI. f. 1.

Damnastes.

Περὶ κυουσῶν καὶ βρεφῶν θεραπείας.
De curatione puerperarum et infantium.

Inc. Τὸ ἑπταμηνιαῖον ἀφροῦται μέν.

Florenz: Laurent. plut. 74, 2*; s. XI. f. 281v (*Abschrift besitzt Mr. E. O. Winstedt, Oxford*).

Excerpta.

Paris: Parisin. 2210; a. 1357. f. 368.

Democritus.

Περὶ συμπαθειῶν καὶ ἀντιπαθειῶν.
De sympathicis et antipathicis.

Ed. Fabricius, Bibl. gr. IV p. 333—338. [ed. I].
Gemoll, Progr. Striegau 1884 p. 3—6.
Vgl. Rohde, Kl. Schr. I p. 383 sq..

Inc. Ἔναγχος ἐμόχθεον ἐρευνήσας τῆς φύσεως.
Expl. ἢ κορῶναι ἡσυχῆ φθεγγόμεναι.

Leyden: Voss. fol. 25; s. XV.
Mailand: Ambros. S 3 Sup. (R 3 Sup. errore Gemoll); s. XV—XVI. f. 122.
Rom: Vatic.
299; s. XV. f. 498.
1902; s. —. f. 268.

Προγνωστικά. [Diels II.27]
Prognostica.

Rom: Vatic. 2304 (ol. 2217); s. XV—XVI. f. 6 (Προγν. περὶ οἰδημάτων. Inc. Οἴδημα ἄπονον περὶ τοῦ προσώπου καὶ τῆς ἀριστερᾶς χειρός. Expl. τῷ αὐτῷ χρόνῳ τελευτᾷ. Fragmentum. *Krolls Abschrift im Besitze der Berl. Akademie.*)

Excerpta varia.

Florenz: Laurent. App. 2; s. XV. f. 340ᵛ (Πρὸς ἔμετον στομάχου), f. 356 (Παύλου γενικοῦ καὶ Δημοκρίτου περὶ πόνων ἰσχίου), f. 359 (Περὶ φλεγμονῆς γαργαρεῶνος. Inc. Γαργαρεών ἐστι ἡ λεγομένη παρά).
Rom: Vatic.
299; s. XV. f. 309—314ᵛ. 329. 366ᵛ. 391 (Varia capita Pseudo-Democritea; *vgl.* E. Rohde, Kl. Schr. I p. 383 adn.).
1174; s. XIV—XV. f. 1 (Ἐκ τῶν Δημοκρίτου φυσικῶν καὶ μυστικῶν) *und* f. 33 (Περὶ πορφύρας φυσικῆς).

Diocles.

Ἐπιστολὴ προφυλακτικὴ πρὸς Ἀντίγονον βασιλέα.
Ad Antigonum regem epistula de tuenda valetudine.

Paulus Aegin. ed. Aldin. a. 1528 f. 13v—14.
Vgl. unten Inc. *und* Expl. *der Epistel des* Diocles *an* Ptolemaeus.

Inc. Διοκλῆς Ἀντιγόνῳ βασιλεῖ. Ἐπειδή σοι συμβαίνει.
Expl. εἰς τροπὰς χειμερινὰς ἡμέραι με'.

Athen: nr.
1236; s. XVIII.
1444; s. XVIII. no. 3.
Athos: Βιβλ. μον. Ἰβήρων 4302. 181; s. XVI. f. 158.
Bologna: Bonon. 3636; s. XIV—XV. f. 127 (Sub nomine Pauli Aegin.)
Cambridge: Cantabr. bibl. univ. F. F. 3. 30; s. XVI. no. 7.
Escurial: Φ. I. 10; s. XVI. f. 197.
Florenz: Laurent. plut. 75, 8; s. XV. p. 454b.
[Diels II.28] **Madrid:** Matrit. bibl. nac. 4759 (ol. N 138); s. XVI. f. 137.
Mailand: Ambros. H 49 Sup.; s. —. f. 16.
Modena: Mutin. 115 (II D 16); s. XV. f. 186.
München: Monac. 70; s. XVI. f. 228.
Neapel:
Bibl. dei Gerolamini XXII. I; s. XV. f. 174.
Oratorian. 152 (Pil. XXII no. 1); s. XIV—XV.
Oxford:
Baroccian. 224; s. XV in. f. 50v.
Miscell. —; s. XV.
Paris:
Coislin. 335; s. XV. f. 10.
Parisin.
396; s. XIII. f. 455.
1631; s. XIV—XVI. f. 168v.
2244; s. XIV—XV. f. 253v.
2847; s. XVI. f. 137.
Parma: Bibl. Palat. Fondo De-Rosssiano 7; s. XV. f. 245.
Rom:
Palat. 428; s. XV—XVI. f. 26.
Vatic. 1904; a. 1306. f. 226.

Upsala: Upsal. bibl. acad. 8 (Sparfwenf. 49); s. XV. f. 119.
Wien: Vindob. med.
11; s. —. f. 56 (Expl. ἐστὶ τὸ ὠάλοιμα ὠφελοῦν εἰς καψίδα ὀφθαλμῶν).
22; s. —. f. 56—60.
27; s. XVI. f. 101.
32; s. XVI. f. 111ᵛ (Expl. περὶ τῶν ἅπασι μάλιστα συνήθων ἡμῶν ὁ λόγος).

Ἐπιστολὴ πρὸς Ἀντίγονον βασιλέα περὶ μέτρων καὶ σταθμῶν.
Ad *Antigonum regem epistula de mensuris et ponderibus.*

Escurial: Scorial. Υ. III. 14; s. XV. f. 236 (Inc. Τὸ γράμμα ἄγει κεράτια ϛ'. Expl. τοῦ ἐλαίου ℔ ιη').

Ἐπιστολὴ Ἱπποκράτους, ἄλλοι δὲ Διοκλέους, πρὸς Πτολεμαῖον βασιλέα Αἰγύπτου.
Hippocratis vel, ut alii volunt, Dioclis epistula ad Ptolemaeum Aegypti regem.

Ed. Fabricius, Bibl. gr. XII [1724] p. 585—592.
Vgl. oben Inc. *und* Expl. *der Epistel des* Diocles *an* Antigonus.

Inc. Ἐπειδή σοι συμβαίνει.
Expl. εἰς τροπὰς χειμερινὰς ἡμέραι με'.

Bologna: Bonon. 3633; s. XV. f. 126.
Paris: Parisin.
2229; s. XIII. f. 25.
2301; s. XII—XIV. f. 124.
Rom: Barberin. I 127; s. XVI. f. 310.
Turin: Taurin. 287 c I 42; s. XV. f. 201 (*Durch Feuer stark beschädigt*).
Venedig: Marcian. App. cl. V 16; s. XVI. f. 146.

Excerpta varia. [Diels II.29]

Paris: Parisin. 2286; s. XIV. f. 89 (Remedia ad sedandos dentium dolores, ex ... Diocle ...).

Diodorus.

Περὶ μέτρων καὶ σταθμῶν.
De mensuris et ponderibus.

Inc. Ἡ ἰταλικὴ μνᾶ λίτραν μίαν θ''. ἡ ἀττικὴ μνᾶ λίτραν μίαν ς''.

Berlin: Phillipps. 1539; s. XVI. f. 3ᵛ.
Florenz: Laurent. plut. 75, 6; s. XIV. f. 127.
London: Addit. (Brit. Mus.) 5108; s. XV ex. f. 4ᵛ.
Rom: Corsinian. 14 (Rossi 358); s. —. f. 11.

Dionysius Simplex.

Περὶ κατασκευῆς ἀνθρώπου.
De fabrica hominis.

Paris: Parisin. 36; s. XIV—XV. f. 164ᵛ.

Dioscurides.

Opera varia.

Athen: nr. 1480; s. XIX (Δ. τὰ ἅπαντα εἰς τὸ κατὰ στοιχεῖον μετακοσμηθέντα ὑπὸ Ἀντωνίου Ποθητοῦ τοῦ Ναξίου).
Padua: Bibl. Ioannis Rhodii (D. graece. *Verbleib unbekannt*).
Paris: Parisin.
2183; s. XV. f. 163ᵛ (Notha).
2185; s. XVI. f. 194ᵛ (Notha).

Περὶ ὕλης ἰατρικῆς Ε'.
De materia medica libri V.

Ed. C. Sprengel, Lipsiae 1829. 1830. I 1—828.
Lib. III. IV ed. M. Wellmann, Berolini 1906.

Inc. (lib. 1) [Προοίμιον]. Πολλῶν οὐ μόνον ἀρχαίων ἀλλὰ καὶ νέων συνταξαμένων.
Κεφ. α' [Περὶ ἴριδος]. Ἶρις [οἱ δὲ ἶρις ἰλλυρική].
Expl. (lib. 5) ὕλης τε καὶ βοηθημάτων ταμιεύσασθαι ἅλις ἔχει.

Athos:

Βιβλ. μον. Ἰβήρων 4336. 216; s. XV. f. 1.

Βιβλ. μον. Λαύρας; s. XII. f. 9 (alphab.).

Berlin: Phillipps. 1530; s. XVI. f. 1 (alphab. Expl. ὑπὸ σκορπίου ἄπονοι διαμένουσιν = Spr. 284, 2).

Bologna: Bonon. 3632*; s. XV. f. 377—378. 385—416ᵛ. 417ᵛ (Imagines plantarum, quae ut in ind. f. 16ᵛ adnotatum est ad D. referenda sunt: Δ. τὰ βότανα ἱστορημένα. Apographon cod. Vindob. med. 1). [Diels II.30]

Cheltenham: Phillipps.

3084; s. XV. f. 1 (Inscr. ⟨περὶ βοτανῶν⟩ καὶ ῥιζῶν καὶ χυλισμάτων καὶ σπερμάτων συνφύλλων ⟨τε καὶ⟩ φαρμάκων, κατὰ στοιχεῖον. Inc. ἀβρότονον τὸ μέγα. Expl. περὶ ὠκίμου ... πληγέντες ὑπὸ σκορπίου, ἄσωστοι διατίθενται; *vgl. den* Berolinens. Phill.).

21975; s. IX. f. 1 (Inc. mutil. καὶ κοιλίαν καὶ ἔμμηνα κινεῖ. alphab.), f. 200—220. 221. 243. 270.

Edschmiadzin (Provinz Ararat): nr. ?; s. VIII (Fragmenta libri III. *H. C. Conybeares Kopie und Photographien in Oxford, Bodl. e 19 [31528]*).

Escurial: Scorial.

Σ. I. 17; s. XV. f. 1 (alphab.).

T. II. 12; s. XVI. f. 4—138 (alphab.).

III. R. 3; s. XI. f. 1 (Exordium ducit ex fragmento cap. 20 [c. 22 editionis] libri II. — Libri VI).

Florenz: Laurent.

plut.

74, 17; s. XII. p. 112 (Liber V qui des. imperfecte. »Hic codex pars est codicis Marc. 273.« Wellmann).

74, 23; s. XIV. p. 1 (Libri IX).

Conventi soppressi 59*; s. XIV. f. 1 (Ex l. II 1—V 103 = Spr. 167, 10—771, 12).

Göttingen: Hist. nat. 90 (impr. a. 1598 c. nott. mss. Ioh. Grammi [1685—1749]).

Leyden: Voss. fol. 58; s. XV (Lib. I).

London: Harleian. (Brit. Mus.) 5679; s. XV. f. 2 (Libri II titul. et prooem. desunt).

Madrid: Matrit. real bibl. 44 (ol. 23); s. XV ex. f. 13.

Mailand:

Ambros.

A 95 Sup.; s. XIV ex. f. 19—49ᵛ. 92—95. 104—150 (alph.).

C 102 Sup.; s. XV. f. 1—29 (Περὶ ἐπιστήμης ἰατρικῆς τὸ περὶ βοτάνων βιβλίον α'. Expl. τὰ πρὸς ὀξυδορκίαν ὀφθαλμικά) *und* f. 30 (»Herbarium D. plantarum figuris exornatum.« M. Wellmann).

C 119 Sup.; s. XV (Libri VII).

Arch. del Capitolo Metrop. 2; s. XV. f. 11—113ᵛ.

Mileae: Mileens. 78; a. 1774 (Libri VIII).

Modena: Mutinens. 115 (II D 16); s. XV. f. 10 *und* 19.
München: Monac. 236; s. XV. f. 83 (Sine titulo. Libri VI—IX).
Padua:
Bibl. Ioannis Rhodii (Variae lectt. in D. de m. m. *Verbleib unbekannt*).
Bibl. Marci Mantuae (Lib. I. *Verbleib unbekannt*).
Paris:
Parisin.
2179; s. IX (Lib. II [101] 202—V 124).
2180*; s. XV. f. 1.
2182; a. 1481. f. 7.
2183; s. XV. f. 1.
2184; s. XVI. f. 1 (alphab.).
2185; s. XVI. f. 1.
2224; s. XV. f. 284 (Libri VIII).
2260; s. XVI. f. 260 (Libri IV fine mutil.).
2287; s. XV—XVI. f. 1 (Libri VI fine mutil.).
Suppl.
493; s. XIX (Variae lectt. e codice Athoo Βιβλ. μον. Λαύρας a Myna collato).
1098; s. XVI (Aldina a. 1518 cum collatt. et nott. mss. Angelii Vergetii et Ranconeti).
1197*; s. XI. f. 120 (Frgm. libri IV).
Rom:
Palat.
48; s. XVI. f. 1 (Lib. II 54—VIII).
77; s. XIV. f. 15 (Lib. I—IX).
Urbin. 66; s. XV. f. 1—120 (Inscr. Περὶ παντὸς εἴδους βοτανῶν καὶ ῥιζῶν καὶ τῶν θεραπειῶν αὐτῶν. alphab.).
Vatic.
284; s. XI—XII (?). f. 252 (Liber VI).
289; s. XIV—XV. f. 5 (Libri VII).
2182; s. XV. f. 58 (Liber III—IV, a cap. σοα' ad φοα').
Venedig:
Marcian.
92; s. XIII. f. 92ᵛ (alphab.).
271; s. XV in.
272; s. XV (alphab.).
273; s. XII (Sine titulo. Ordo et numerus capitum ab editt. discrepat).
597; s. XV (alphab.).
App. cl.
V, 2 (Variae lectt. ex duobus codd. mss. manu saec. XVI. in marg. edit. Cornarii Basil. 1529).

V, 3 (Edit. Paris. apud Petrum Haultinum a. 1549 cum annotatt. manu Melchioris Guilandini).

Wien: Vindob.

med.

1; s. VI in. f. 12ᵛ (Inscr. *wie im* Phillipps. Cheltenham 3084. Inc. Ἀείζων τὸ μέγα. Expl. *wie im* Phil. 3084).

14; s. XVI. f. 1—46ᵛ (Sine titulo. Lib. I *und* II 1—26. Expl. δριμὺ δηκτικὸν εὔτριπτον δια ... *Coll. im Berol. fol. 39 [275]*).

16*; s. XV—XVI. f. 43—48ᵛ (»Fragmentum D. alphab.« M. Wellmann) *und* f. 56 (»D. libris V digestus«. M. Wellmann. Expl. f. 184ᵛ ἐπ' ὠφελείᾳ διδομένῳ [sic] ἕνεκα τῶν ἐπιφερομένων κινδύνων).

28; s. XV. f. 67—115 (Inscr. Βίβλος ἑρμηνεὺς πόων βοτανῶν κτλ. κατὰ στοιχεῖον. Inc. Ἀψίνθιον. Expl. Ὤκιμον).

29; s. XV. f. 22ᵛ—73 (*Wie in nr.* 28. Expl. ἐν τῷ ὑπογαίῳ ἀποθνήσκει).

suppl. 28 (olim Neapolitan.); s. VII. f. 1—172 (Inc. Ἀριστολοχία μακρά. Expl. Χαμαικίσσου ... ἑπτὰ ἡμέρας).

lat. 16; s. VIII—IX (Tab. cod. I p. 2 s). f. 62. 65 rescr. (Lib. III 82. 83. 78. 79 ed. Wellm.).

Περὶ δηλητηρίων φαρμάκων καὶ τῆς αὐτῶν πορφυλακῆς καὶ θεραπείας. [Diels II.31]
De venenis eorumque praecautione et medicatione.

Spr. II 1—41.

Inc. (προοίμιον). Ἀποδόντες ἐν τοῖς προγραφεῖσι βιβλίοις, φίλτατε Ἄρειε.
Expl. παρῃτησάμην ἀναγράφειν ἐνταῦθα.

Athos: Athous Βιβλ. μον. Λαύρας —; s. XII. f. 218 (Inscr. Περὶ τῆς τῶν ὠφελεῖν ἢ βλάπτειν δυναμένων φαρμάκων ἐνεργείας).

Berlin: Phillipps. 1530; s. XVI. f. 219ᵛ.

Cheltenham: Phillipps. 21975; s. IX. f. 306 (Inscr. *wie im* Athous).

Escurial: Scorial.

Σ. I. 17; s. XV. f. 188 (Inscr. *wie im* Athous. *Collation in Wellmanns Besitz*).

III. R. 3; s. XI. f. 129ᵛ (*Collation in Wellmanns Besitz*). [Diels II.32]

Florenz: Laurent. plut. 74, 23; s. XIV. f. 183ᵛ.

London: Harleian. (Brit. Mus.) 5679; s. XV. f. 209 (in tit. om. καὶ θεραπείας).

Madrid: Matrit. real bibl. 44 (ol. 23); s. XV ex. f. 164ᵛ.

Mailand:

Ambros.

A 95 Sup.; s. XIV ex. f. 129ᵛ—133ᵛ.

L 119 Sup.; s. XV. f. 177v.
Arch. del Capitolo Metrop. 2; s. XV. f. 114—119 (in tit. om. καὶ θεραπείας; *vgl. den* Harleian.).
Modena: Mutinens. 115 (II D 16); s. XV. f. 167v.
Paris: Parisin.
2182; s. XV. f. 174v.
2183; s. XV. f. 147.
2184; s. XVI. f. 188.
2185; s. XVI. f. 175.
2224; s. XIV—XV. f. 427v.
Rom:
Palat. 77; s. XIV.
Urbin. 66; s. XV. f. 146—155 (Inscr. *wie im* Athous).
Venedig: Marcian.
92; s. XIII. f. 92 (Inscr. *wie im* Athous).
271; s. XV in. f. 137.
272; s. XV. f. 233.
597; s. XV.

Περὶ ἰοβόλων, ἐν ᾧ καὶ περὶ λυσσῶντος κυνός.
De iis, quae virus eiaculantur, animalibus libellus, in quo et de rabioso cane.

Spr. II 42—91.

Inc. (προοίμιον). Τὸν μὲν περὶ τῶν ἰοβόλων ζῴων καὶ θανασίμων φαρμάκων λόγον.
Expl. ὡσαύτως δὲ καὶ ὁ τῆς μήκωνος ὀπός. Τοιοῦτος μὲν ὁ θηριακὸς τρόπος.

Athos: Athous Βιβλ. μον. Λαύρας; s. XII. f. 227.
Berlin: Phillipps. 1530; s. XVI. f. 230.
Cheltenham: Phillipps. 21975; s. IX. f. 319v.
Escurial: Scorial. Σ. I. 17; s. XV. f. 197v.
Florenz: Laurent. plut. 74, 23; s. XIV. f. 190v (Tribus libris dispos.).
Madrid: Matrit. real bibl. 44 (ol. 23); s. XV ex. f. 171.
Mailand:
Ambros. L 119 Sup.; s. XV. f. 186.
Arch. del Capitolo Metrop. 2; s. XV. f. 119v—126.
Modena: Mutinens. 115 (II D 16); s. XV. f. 175.
Paris: Parisin.
2182; s. XV. f. (148 s) 134.
2183; s. XV. f. 154.

2184; s. XVI. f. 197v.
2185; s. XVI. f. 184.
2224; s. XIV ex. f. 434v.

Rom:

Barberin. II 58; s. XVI. f. 47 (D. liber VII. Expl. ἰατρῶν σωθέντας ἔγνωμεν).
Palat. 77; s. XIV.
Urbin. 66; s. XV. f. 155.
Vatic. 284*; s. XI—XII. f. 265 (Inc. Γνήσιον καὶ ὠφέλιμον ἐφάνη μοι. Expl. ἑξῆς τὰ λοιπά, mutil. in fine).

Venedig: Marcian.

271; s. XV. f. 143.
272; s. XV. f. 244 (Tit. om.).
597; s. XV.

Περὶ εὐπορίστων ἁπλῶν τε καὶ συνθέτων φαρμάκων Α' Β'.
De facile parabilibus tam simplicibus quam compositis medicamentis libri II.

Spr. II 92—338.

Inc. Ἡ τῶν ἁπλῶν φαρμάκων παράδοσις, τιμιώτατε Ἀνδρόμαχε.
Expl. ἐν δυσὶ τόμοις συνειληχότες ἐπεστάλκαμέν σοι.

Athos: Βιβλ. μον. Ἰβήρων 4337. 217; s. XVI. f. 10.

Florenz:

Laurent. plut.
74, 10; s. XIV. p. 27.
74, 20; s. XV. p. 1.
Riccard. 91 (K. II 7); s. XV.

Kopenhagen: Hauniens. bibl. univ. e donatione variorum 4° 277; s. XV—XVI. f. 5.

London: Sloanean. (Brit. Mus.) 804; s. XVI. (?) f. 2 (»Kunststück eines Kalligraphen, dem viell. ein Druck vorgelegen hat, den er nachzuahmen sucht.« Kalbfleisch).

Neapel: Neapolit. 307 III D 23; s. XV. f. 1.

Rom:

Palat. 400*; s. XV. f. 383.
Vatic. 290; s. XVI. f. 1.

[Diels II.33] Βίβλος περιέχουσα περὶ πείρας ἰατρικῆς, περὶ ἁπλῶν τε καὶ συνθέτων φαρμάκων κατὰ ἀλφάβητον ὑποτεταγμένη.
Liber agens de experientia medica, de simplicibus et compositis medicamentis, ordine litterarum digestus.

Inc. Ἄβρωτα διατηρεῖ ἀπὸ μυῶν.
Expl. καὶ σμύρνη ἐνταζόμενον.

Florenz: Laurent. plut. 75, 8; s. XV. p. 4 (Frgm. litteram A non excedens).
Leyden: Voss. fol. 59; s. XIV.
London: Addit. (Brit. Mus.) 17, 900; s. XVII. f. 268ᵛ.
München: Monac. 484 (542) (?); s. —.
Oxford: Baroccian. 150; s. XV in. f. 41ᵛ.
Padua: Bibl. Ioannis Rhodii (D. et Stephani Ath. de pharmacis ordine litterarum. *Verbleib unbekannt*).
Paris: Parisin.
- 2151; s. XVI. f. 65 (*Wie im* cod. Bibl. Io. Rhodii).
- 2181; s. XVI. f. 1 (*Wie im* cod. Bibl. Io. Rhodii).
- 2238; s. XV. f. 539.
- 2243; a. 1339. f. 553.
- 2286; s. XIV. f. 1.

Wien: Vindob.
- 11; s. —.
- 18; s. XV. f. 94 (*Wie im* cod. Bibl. Io. Rhodii. Lectt. specimen *im* Berol. fol. 39 [275]).
- 28; s. —.
- 32; s. XVI. f. 29—30ᵛ (Expl. ὁ τοιοῦτος ἀνέλπιστος).
- 39; s. —.
- 52; s. XV. f. 39—48 (Expl. καὶ διακρατούμενον).

Μετάφρασις εἰς Νικάνδρου θηριακὰ καὶ ἀλεξιφάρμακα.
Metaphrasis in Nicandri Theriaca et Alexipharmaca.

Leyden: Voss. fol. 59; s. XIV.
Paris:
- Bibl. Mazarine 4461; s. XV. f. 104.
- Parisin.
  - 2182; a. 1481. f. 134 *und* 148.
  - 2183; s. XV. f. 147 *und* 155.
  - 2184; s. XVI. f. 188 *und* 197.

2185; s. XVI. f. 175 *und* 184.
Bibl. de la ville de Paris 12; s. XV. f. 104.
Rom: Urbin. 66; s. XV. f. 165v.

Περὶ μέτων καὶ σταθμῶν.
De mensuris et ponderibus.

Hultsch, Metrol. script. I 239—244.

Inc. Ἐγὼ φίλτατε περὶ σταθμῶν καὶ μέτρων.
Expl. πλάγιον δὲ ἢ c ὀβολόν.

Athos: Athous Βιβλ. Μον. Λαύρας, s. XII. f. 6.
Escurial: Scorial. Φ. III. 7*; s. XIV. f. 5v (Inc. Τὸ κεράμιον λίτρας οβ').
Florenz: Laurent. App. 2; s. XV. f. 236v (»Fere eadem quae apud Hu. p. 240, 1—241, 4. 242, 12—244, 8«).
London: Harleian. (Brit. Mus.) 6305; s. XVI (?). f. 157v.
Mailand:
Ambros. A 95 Sup.; s. XV. f. 18.
Arch. del Capitolo Metrop. 2; s. XV. f. 137v—139 (Expl. σταθμοῦ δὲ ὁλκαὶ ρκ').
Modena: Mutinens. 115 (II D 16); s. XV. f. 187.
Oxford: Baroccian. 216; s. —. f. 108b.
Paris: Imprimés, Réserve Te 138, 27*; s. XV. f. 44v.
Rom:
Barberin. I 118; s. IV. f. 293 (Expl. τὸ ἐρυθρὸν τοῦ ξανθοῦ).
Vat.
299*; s. XV. f. 449v (Inc. Τὸ κεράτιον τῷ αὐτῷ. Expl. ὁ κύαθος Γο α' <ε $Γ^{ρ}$ '' α').
1904; a. 1306. f. 227v.

Excerpta. [Diels II.34]

Athen: nr. 1479; s. XIX (Ἰατροσόφιον ἀπηνθισμένον ἀπὸ Γαλ. ... καὶ Δ.).
Athos:
Βιβλ. μον. Ἰβήρων 4337. 217; s. XVI. f. 51 B (Ἑρμηνεία τοῦ Δ. περὶ τοῦ καρωφάλου [sic] καὶ ἄλλων ἑτέρων).
Κουτλουμουσίου 3321. 248; s. XVII (Δ. περὶ ἁπλῶν βοηθημάτων ἐν βίβλῳ ἰατρικῇ Νικολάου Ἱερόπαιδος).
Ξηροποταμοῦ 2432. 99; s. XVII (Διαθήκη τῶν τριῶν ἰατρῶν Γαλ. Ἱππ. καὶ Δ.).
Berlin: Berol. fol. 39 (275); s. — (»Probecollat. von Hdss. des D. in der Marciana«).

Bologna: Bonon.
1808; s. XV. f. 174 (Κοινά βοηθήματα τῶν νηπὰ [sic] περίοδον παροξυνομένων).
3632; s. XV. f. 385—416v.
Cheltenham: Phillipps. 21975; s. IX. f. 332v (Περὶ ἀντιφαρμάκων.).
Escurial: Scorial.
Φ. I. 10; s. XVI. f. 205.
Ω. I. 8; s. XIV. f. 24 (Ἀσθματικόν. Inc. Ἀριστολοχία στρογγύλη).
Florenz: Laurent. plut. 75, 8; s. XV. p. 438 (Quaedam medica βοηθήματα. Inc. Χολιάνδρου κόκκους. Ad D. pertinere susp. Bandini III 153).
Göttingen: Hist. nat. 6; a. 1670 (Simplicium facultates medicae ex antiquis [Dioscoride], opera et stud. G. H. Welsch).
Leyden: Voss. fol. 59; s. XIV (De divisione partium anni et quaenam medicinae singulis conveniant temporibus sec. Aegyptios).
London: Addit. (Brit. Mus.) 8231*; s. XVII. f. 1 (Ὀνομαστικὸν εἰς τὰ τοῦ Δ. π. ὕ. ἰ. Inc. Αἰβαδανέ. Expl. ὤκιμον).
Madrid: Matrit. bibl. nac.
4616 (N 84); s. XV. f. 171 (Περί τινων βοτανῶν δυνάμεως. Inc. Ἀψίνθιον θερμόν ἐστι).
4631 (N 110); a. 1474. f. 89 (Περὶ δυνάμεώς τινων βοτανῶν κατ' ἀλφ. Inc. Ἀλθαία ἣν ἔνιοι) *und* f. 155 (Περὶ λίθων).
Mailand:
Ambros. D 477 Inf.; s. XVI (In partem D. notae M. Ant. Maranthae).
Arch. del Capitolo Metrop. 2; s. XV. f. 139—143v (»Un indice dei nomi delle piante di D. coi relative num. distribuite, almeno in parte, secondo i luoghi nei quali nascono«).
Mitylene: Bibl. gymnas. 33; a. 1774. f. 1—224.
Moskau: Mosquens. 477; a. 1624. f. 8 (Ἀπὸ τὰ ἰατρικὰ βιβλία τοῦ Δ. μερικὰ εἰς κοινὴν μεταγλωττισθέντα. Inc. Περὶ ἴριδος. Expl. Περὶ σελίνου).
Oxford:
Baroccian.
88; s. XV—XVI. f. 164b (Ἐκ τῶν Ἀσκληπιάδου καὶ Δ. περὶ δυ⟨σπνοίας⟩).
150; s. XV in. f. 77 (Pauca de simplicibus).
Is. Casauboni Adversar. 27. f. 145. 146 (Nonnulla ex D. Inc. Ἡ βίβλος περιέχει).
Paris:
Parisin.
1603; s. XVI. f. 178.
2228; s. XIV—XI. f. 92.
2286; s. XIV. f. 124 (Praecepta de sanitate tuenda per XII menses).
2294; s. XV. f. 138 (De plantis et animalibus Exc.).
2313; s. XIV. f. 1 (Remedia varia).
2337; s. XV—XVI. f. 89 (Exc. de simplicibus remediis).

2510; a. 1384. f. 80 (Exc. de animalibus marinis et terrestribus ad morbos curandos idoneis).

Suppl.

3; a. 1616 (Thesaurus Theophrasti et D. auctore Paulo Renealmo Blesensi).

493; s. XIX (Variae lectt. in D.).

1202; s. XIV—XVI. f. 16.

Rom:

Palat. 77; s. XIV. f. 1.

Vatic. 284; s. XI—XII (?). f. 1—251 (Γαλ. τῶν ἁπλῶν βιβλίον ς'—ια' ἔχον ἀπὸ τοῦ Δ. ὅσα Γαληνῷ παραλέλειπται) *und* f. 251ᵛ (Κεφάλαια τῶν ἐν τῷ ς' βιβλίῳ Δ.).

Venedig: Marcian. App. cl. V, 16; s. XVI. f. 154ᵛ (Inc. Μὴν Ἰανουάριος) *und* f. 161 (Inc. μελ' τὸ καλόν).

Wien: Vindob. med. 28; s. XV. f. 67—115 (Βίβλος ἑρμηνεὺς ποῶν βοτανῶν ... κατὰ στοιχεῖον. Inc. Ἀψίνθιον. Expl. ὤκιμον κτλ.).

Zürich: Turicens. C 136; s. XVI. f. 115 (περὶ τοῦ οἴνου) *und* f. 120 (περὶ λυκίου, μυρίκης, σπληνός, λέπρας).

Eleutherus.

[Diels II.35]

Excerpta.

Florenz: Laurent. App. 2; s. XV. f. 358 (Ἐπι ἰσχιαδκικῶν).

Epiphanius.

Φυσιολόγος.
Physiologus.

Athos:

Βιβλ. Μον. Διονυσίου

3766. 232; s. XVII. no. 25.

3778. 244*; s. XVII. no. 2.

3897. 363*; s. XVIII. no. 7.

Ἰβήρων

4272. 152; s. XVI. f. 40.

4310. 190; s. XIII. no. 1.

4325. 205; s. XVII. f. 153.

4450. 330; s. XVIII. no. 11 (Π. φύσεως ἑκάστου).

4468. 348; s. XVI. no. 10.

4497. 377; s. XIV. f. 106.
4720. 600; s. XVII. no. 21.
4788. 668*; s. XVIII. no. 28.
4799. 679; s. XVIII. no. 4.
4815. 695; s. XVI. no. 2.
4925. 805; s. XVII. f. 80.
Κουτλουμουσίου 3260. 2; s. XVI. no. 2.
Παντελεήμονος 5752. 245; s. XVII. no. 5.
Σταυρονικήτα 951. 86; s. XVII. no. 5.
Paris: Parisin.
834; a. 1585. f. 1 (cum lat. versione et notis D. Consali Ponce de Leon Hispalensis).
2027; a. 1449. f. 213.
2426; s. XVI. f. 90.
2509; s. XV. f. 188.
Rom: Vatic. 695; s. XIV—XV (Inc. Ὁ φυσιολόγος ἔλεξε περὶ τοῦ ἐλέφαντος).
Wien: Vindob.
med. 29; s. XV. f. 117 (Inc. Ἀρξώμεθα τοίνυν λαλῆσαι περὶ τοῦ λέοντος βασιλέως. Expl. θηρεύονται παρὰ τοῦ θηρευτεοῦ).
phil. 290; s. —.
theol. 128; s. —.

[Diels II.36] Περὶ μέτρων καὶ σταθμῶν.
De mensuris et ponderibus.

Ed. Dindorf, Lips. 1859.

Inc. Κόρος σίτου μοδίων ν'.
Expl. μετριτὴς ξεστῶν οβ'.

Athos: Βιβλ. μον. Ἰβήρων
4212. 92; s. XVI. f. 28. 31. 4
4871. 751; s. XVII. no. 53.
Cambridge: Cantabr. bibl. univ. Gg I 2*; s. XV. f. 261 (Expl. κουστωδία ἄνδρες ⳁ).
Carpentras: nr. 1774 (P., V)*; s. XVII. f. 144.
Holkham: nr. 289; s. XII. f. 175 (Expl. λίτραν μίαν καὶ ⌈ο ⌈ο η').
Madrid: Matrit. bibl. univ. 30; s. XI. no. III.
Oxford: Miscell.
211; s. XV. f. 73 (Inc. Κόρος σίτου μόδια λ').
212*; s. XVI. f. 87.

Paris: Parisin.
2665; s. XIV—XV. f. 204.
2720; s. XVI. f. 186v.
2731; s. XVI. f. 133v.
2830; a. 1515. f. 232.
Rom: Ottobon. 259; s. XIV—XV. f. 122.

Περὶ τῶν δώδεκα λίθων τῶν ἐν τῷ λογίῳ τοῦ ἱερέως ἐμπεπερονημένων.
De duodecim gemmis panno sacerdotis infibulatis.

Inc. Σάρδιον τὸ βαβυλώνιον καλούμενον.
Expl. εὑρίσκεται δὲ καὶ οὗτος ἐν τῷ ὄρει τῷ αὐτῷ.

Berlin: Berol. 4° 5 (304); s. XV—XVI. f. 70v.
Escurial: Scorial. X. II. 2; s. XVI. f. 129v.
Madrid: Matrit. bibl. nac. 4631 (ol. N 110); a. 1474. f. 153.
Paris: Parisin. 2228; s. XIV—XI. f. 49.
Wien: Vindob. med.
27; s. XVI. f. 118v—121 (*Abschrift im Berol. fol. 39 [275]*).
29; s. XV. f. 464v—475 (Expl. τίθει δὲ ἐντὸς τῶν ὀφθαλμῶν περισσότερον. *Abschrift im Berol. fol. 39 [275]*).

Excerpta varia.

Lesbos: Βιβλ. τῆς τοῦ Λειμῶνος μονῆς 175; s. XVII.

Erasistratus.

Excerpta varia.

Paris: Parisin. 2324; s. XVI. f. 1 (Hipp., Gal., Magni et Erasistrati iatrosophium. Inc. Τὴν περὶ τῆς τῶν οὔρων).

[Diels II.37]

Erotianus.

Τῶν παρ' Ἱπποκράτει λέξεων συναγωγή.
Vocum Hippocraticarum conlectio.

Ed. Klein, Lips. 1865.

Inc. Τὴν Ἱπποκράτους πραγματείαν, ἀρχιατρὲ Ἀνδρόμαχε.
Expl. μάλιστα ἐν Θράκῃ καὶ Μακεδονίᾳ εὑρίσκειν.

Berlin: Berol. fol. 39 (275) —. (*Coll. vatikanischer Hdss.*).
Brüssel: Bruxell. 11345—48; s. XVI. f. 1.
Cambridge: Cantabr. 2049 (Kk V 7); s. XV—XVI.
Escurial: Scorial. y. I. 9; s. XVI. f. 158.
Florenz: Laurent. plut. 74, 1; s. XV.
München: Monac. 71; a. 1531.
Oxford:
Baroccian. 204; s. XV.
d'Orvill. X 1. 1. 3; s. XV ex. f. 166.
Paris: Parisin.
1868; s. XV.
2141; s. XV.
2142; s. XIII—XIV.
2143; s. XIV.
2144; s. XIV.
2145; s. XV.
2148; s. XV.
2151; s. XVI. f. 49 (A—O).
2177; s. XVI. f. 96.
2247; s. XVI.
2248; s. XV.
2254; s. XV.
2255; s. XV.
2614; s. XVI.
2615; a. 1533 *und* 1584. f. 1.
2651; s. XVI. f. 1.
Rom:
Urbin. 68; s. XIV.
Vallicell. 78 (F 9); s. XVI. f. 188—196v (Expl. παρὰ τὸ δόρυ (ει) παύειν· ὃ γὰρ ἡμεῖς. *Coll. Ilbergs, Vorrede u. p. 2—57, 14 Kl. in dessen Besitz*).

Vatic.
277; s. XIV. f. 2.
1133 (1134 Kl.); s. XVII (Apogr. codicis 277).
Venedig: Marcian. App. cl. V 15; s. XVI.
Wien: Vindob. med.
38ᶜ; s. — (*Coll. mit der Franzschen Ausgabe im Berol. fol. 39 [275]*).
43; s. XVI. f. 83—121ᵛ.

Dazu: Fonteblandensis Feuraei ap. Foesium. Mediceus Foesii. Imperialis Sambuci. Card. Sirleti.

Esdras Propheta.

Περὶ κρισίμων ἡμερῶν.
De diebus criticis.

Paris:
Parisin. 2149; s. XVI. f. 165ᵛ.
Suppl. 636; s. XVI. f. 134.
Wien: Vindob. med. 27; s. XVI. f. 121 (Περὶ τῶν δώδεκα μηνῶν τὰς ἐπιβαρεῖς ἡμέρας. Inc. Μηνὶ σεπτεβρίῳ γ'. Expl. Αὔγουστος δ' καὶ ιε').

Εἰς ὑδερικοὺς καὶ εἰς πάντα τὰ ψυχρὰ νοσήματα.
Pro hydropicis et omnibus morbis frigidis.

Inc. Μαμηρά, οὐγγιάνα.

München: Monac. 72; s. XVI.
Rom: Angelic. 4 (C. 4. 16); s. XVI in. f. 290.
Wien: Vindob. med. 31; s. —. *hinter* f. 127.

Ἡ ἀντίδοτος τοῦ Ἔσδρα. [Diels II.38]
Antidotus Esdrae.

Vgl. Paul. Aeg. VII 11.

Inc. Ἀμώμου γραμμάρια ιβ'.
Expl. καὶ ἔξωθεν ἐμπλάσας ἐπιτίθει.

Bologna: Bonon. 1808; s. XV. f. 124^v.
Oxford:
Baroccian. 150; s. XV in. f. 5b *und* 32^v.
Roe 14; s. XV. f. 280.

Euphemius Siculus.

[Περὶ συνθέσεως φαρμάκων.]
Medicamentorum compositiones ab Euph. S. et Philippo Nero Rheginensi collectae.

Paris: Parisin. 2194; s. XV. f. 454.

Eusebius.

Περὶ μέτρων καὶ σταθμῶν.
De mensuris et ponderibus.

Carpentras: nr. 1774 (P. V.); s. XVII. f. 162^v *und* 269.

Eustathius.

Excerpta.

Florenz: Laurent. App. 2; s. XV. f. 355 (Inc. Ἤκουσα καγώ Εὐστάθιος ὁ εὐτελὴς ἰατρός).
Rom: Vatic. 299; s. XV. f. 393^v (»Commemoratur ἐγὼ Εὐστάθιος ὁ εὐτελὴς ἰατρός«).

Eutecnius.

Παράφρασις εἰς Διονυσίου Ἰξιευτικά.
Paraphrasis in Dionysii Ixieutica. Libri II.

Inc. Ἐπειδή σοι τῆς γῆς ἁπάσης.
Expl. ἀπαρτίσαι τρίχας ἱππείους.

Athos: Βιβλ. Μον. Λαύρας; s. XII. f. 285 (Inscriptionis expers).
Escurial: Scorial. Σ. I. 17; s. XV. f. 259^v.

Wien: Vindob. med. 1; s. VI. f. 474—485^v (Inc. ...ψιεις, εἰ καὶ πόρρω που τελευτήσεις, τι τῶν ζώων. Expl. Ἀπόλλωνος δὲ μαλχεαι).

Παράφρασις ἐκ τῶν Νικάνδρου θηριακῶν. [Diels II.39]
Paraphrasis in Nicandri Theriaca.

Ed. Florentiae 1764 Nicandri p. 298 ss.

Athos: Athous Βιβλ. Μον. Λαύρας; s. XII. f. 242.
Cheltenham: Phillipps. 21975; s. IX. f. 360^v (*vgl.* f. 338 ss.).
Escurial: Scorial. Σ. I. 17; s. XV. f. 212.
Florenz: Florent. bibl. naz. II. III. 304; s. XVI (Inc. Τῶν ἑρπετῶν θηρίων ὁπόσα ἐστίν. Expl. οὗτός ποτε γένηται τοῦ πλῆξαι).
Rom: Urbin. 66; s. XV. f. 165^v.
Wien: Vindob. med. 1; s. VI. f. 393—437^v.

Παράφρασις ἐκ τῶν Νικάνδρου ἀλεξιφαρμάκων.
Paraphrasis in Nicandri Alexipharmaca.

Athos:
Βιβλ. Μον. Ιβήρων 4302. 181; s. XVI. f. 167.
Λαύρας; s. XII. f. 260.
Cheltenham: Phillipps. 21975; s. IX. f. 375.
Escurial: Scorial. Σ. I. 17; s. XV. f. 232^v.
Rom: Urbin. 66; s. XV. f. 183.
Wien: Vindob. med.
1; s. VI. f. 438^v.
5*; s. XVI—XVII. f. 9 (Inc. Νίκανδρος ὁ ποιητής. Expl. πρὸς σωτηρίαν τῶν ἀνθρώπων καὶ ὠφέλειαν ἐξεύρηται. *Aus* Vindob. med. 1).

Παράφρασις εἰς Ὀππιανοῦ Ἁλιευτικά.
Paraphrasis in Oppiani Halieutica.

Athos:
Βιβλ. μον. Ἰβήρων 4336. 216; s. XV (Inc. Αἱ ῥαφίδες τῷ λίνῳ πρὸς τὸν αἰγιαλόν).
Λαύρας; s. XII. f. 273 (Inc. *wie im* cod. Ἰβήρων. Expl. τοῖς ἰχθύσι οἱ θηραταί).
Escurial: Scorial. Σ. I. 17; s. XV. f. 246.

Rom: Urbin. 66; s. XV. f. 193ᵛ (Inc. Ταῖς ῥαφίσιν δὲ ὡς λεπταῖς διεξελθεῖν. Expl. ὥσπερ οὐδὲ τῶν παστάδων αἱ γυναῖκες).
Wien: Vindob. med. 1; s. VI. f. 460 (Inscriptionis expers).

Gregorius Nyssenus.

Περὶ κατασκευῆς ἀνθρώπου.
De hominis opificio.

Ed. Migne, Patrol. 44 p. 125—256.
Vgl. Nemesius *de natura hominis.*

Inc. Εἰ ταῖς διὰ τῶν χρημάτων τιμαῖς.
Expl. αἰῶνος τῶν αἰώνων. ἀμήν.

Athen: nr. 433 (132); s. XII. no. 2 (Κεφάλαια λ').
Athos:
Βιβλ. Μον. Διονυσίου
3748. 214; s. XV. no. 1 (Κεφ. λ').
3808. 274; s. XVI. f. 333 (Π. φύσεως ἀνθρώπου).
Ξενοφῶντος 739. 37; s. XVIII (Π. ἀνθρώπου κεφ. λ).
Berlin: Phillipps. 1432; s. XVI. f. 1.
Brüssel: Bruxell. 11354; s. —. f. 1 (De homine capp. 30. Inc. Θεωρία τις ἡ ἀκριβωτέρα [sic]. Expl. κεκριμένην μὲν ζῶσαν).
Cambridge: Cantabr. bibl. univ. L l IV 12; s. XV. f. 47.
Escurial: Scorial. Ψ. III. 7; s. XI. f. 202 (Des. in cap. 6 ἐδείχθη ἄρα λογικὴ ἡ ψυχή).
Jerusalem: Bibl. Mar-Saba 366; s. —. f. 101.
Genua: Bibl. della Missione urbana 17; s. IX ex.—x. f. 213.
Leyden: Gron. 12; s. XVI. f. 244 (Expl. cap. 23 καὶ εἴ τις ἐκ τῆς ἀνάγκης ταύτης ἀΐδ...).
Madrid:
Matrit. bibl. nac. 4861; s. XVI. no. VI (Π. εἰκόν. ἀνθρ.).
[Diels II.40] real bibl. 14 (ol. 13); s. XVI. f. 1 (*Wie im* cod. bibl. nac).
Mitylene: Bibl. gymnas. 1; a. 1598. no. 2.
Oxford: Miscell. 20; s. XIV. f. 321ᵛ.
Paris:
Coislin.
228; s. XI—XIV. f. 62.
229; s. X—XII. f. 83ᵛ.
235; s. X—XI. f. 121 (fine mutil.).

Parisin.
476; s. X. f. 64v.
479; s. XIII—XV. f. 79.
503; s. XIV. f. 144.
777 A; s. XVI. f. 246v.
940; s. XV. f. 140.
956; s. XIV. f. 82v.
968; s. XV. f. 109.
1007; s. XVI. f. 1.
1009; s. XVI. f. 1.
1010; s. XVI. f. 105.
1053; s. X—XI. f. 207.
1247; s. XIV—XV. f. 52.
1277; s. XIII. f. 55.
1542; s. X—XIII. f. 10.
Suppl. 341; a. 1533—1535. f. 10.
Saloniki: Bibl. gymnas. 17; s. XIV. f. 204.
Urbini et Pisauri: Bibl. Ducis —; s. — (De conditione hominis. *Verbleib unbekannt).*

Περὶ σφυγμῶν.
De pulsibus.

Escurial: Scorial. Φ. III. 11; s. XIV *und* XV. f. 49v (Περὶ σφυγμῶν καὶ ἑτέρων κινήσεως τοῦ σώματος).
London: Harleian. (Brit. Mus.) 6295; s. XV (XIV sec. catal.). f. 88v.
Paris: Parisin.
1884*; a. 1503. f. 78 (Fragmentum).
2316; s. XV. f. 194.

Λόγος πρὸς ἀστρονόμους.
Oratio adversus astronomos.

Berlin: Phillipps. 1527 (ol. Meerm. 217)*; s. XVI. f. 66v (Inc. Ὥσπερ οἱ ἰχθύες. Expl. ἕως ἑσπέρας).
Mailand: Ambros. Q 94 Sup.*; s. —. f. 366v (*Wie im* Phillipps.).
Paris: Parisin. 2155*; s. XIV. f. 305.

Excerpta varia.

Lesbos: Βιβλ. τῆς τοῦ Λειμῶνος μονῆς 175; s. XVII.

Gregorius Theologus.

Περὶ συνθέσεως καὶ διακρίσεως τοῦ ἀνθρωπείου σώματος.
De compositione et distinctione corporis humani.

Athos: Βιβλ. Μον. Διονυσίου 3748. 214; s. XVIII. no. 2 (Ποιήματα ... ιγ'. Περὶ φύσεως ἀνθρωπίνης).
Rom: Vatic. 300; s. XII—XIII. f. 293 (Inc. Δεύτερον ἐννοεῖ κόσμον. Expl. στοιχεῖα τοῦ ἀνθρώπου).

[Diels II.41] Ἀλάτιον.
Alatium.

Ed. Ideler, Phys. et Med. gr. I p. 297—298.

Inc. Ὀφθαλμίαν οὐ ποιεῖ ἕως γήρως.
Expl. χρῶ ἐν ἐδέσμασιν οἷς ἂν βούλῃ.

Athos: Βιβλ. Μον. Ιβήρων 4271. 151; s. XV. f. 70 B.
Bologna: Bonon.
1808; s. XV. f. 42.
3632; s. XV. f. 228.
Jerusalem: Bibl. patriarch. 148; s. XVI. f. 56.
London: Addit. (Brit. Mus.) 10, 058; s. XV. f. 47.
München: Monac.
105; s. XVI. f. 333.
288; s. XIV (Inc. Ὑσσώπου κρητικοῦ).
Oxford: Baroccian. 150; s. XV in. f. 32v.
Paris: Parisin. 2236; s. XV. f. 59v.
Turin: Taurin. 17 B VII 22 (B I 12); s. XVI *und* XVIII. f. 137 (*Verbrannt*).

Harpocration.

Περὶ φυσικῶν δυνάμεων ζῴων τε καὶ φυτῶν καὶ λίθων.
De facultatibus naturalibus animalium et herbarum et lapidum.

Inc. Ἄμπελος λευκή, ἥτις καὶ βρυωνία λέγεται.
Expl. μαινίδα ὀπτὴν δοὺς φαγεῖν θεραπεύσεις.

Madrid: Matrit. bibl. nac. 4631 (ol. N 110); a. 1474. f. 6ᵛ. 37. 53ᵛ. 67 (A—Y. »Consutum cum Hermetis Trismegisti Κυρανίδες.« Wellmann).
Moskau: Mosquens. 468; s. XVI. f. 114.
Paris: Coislin. 158*; s. XVI. f. 80 (De lapidibus, plantis A—Y).
[**Rom:** Vatic]
Toledo: Bibl. del cab. de la igl. cat. 101, 15*; s. XV. p. 280 (Περί ἀσπάλαγγος. Περὶ σαλαμάνδρας).
Venedig: Marcian. App. cl. V, 13; s. XIV—XV. f. 125 (*Specimen im Weigelschen Nachlaß Berol. fol. 39 [275]*).

[Ἐπιστολὴ πρὸς τὸν Καίσαρα.]
Epistula ad imperatorem.

Inc. Πολλῶν ἐπιχειρησάντων ἐν τῷ βίῳ, σεβαστὲ καῖσαρ.
Expl. σκευάζε καθ' ἑκάστην δύναμιν.

Madrid: Matrit. bibl. nac. 4631 (ol. N 110); a. 1474. f. 75.

Heliodorus.

Πρὸς Θεοδόσιον τὸν μέγαν βασιλέα.
Ad Theodosium regem.

Zweifelhaft, ob medizinisch.

Inc. Σκῆπτρα γῆς μέδοντες.

Rom: Vatic. 1174; s. XIV—XV. f. 68ᵛ.

[Diels II.42]

Περὶ μέτρων καὶ σταθμῶν.
De mensuris et ponderibus.

Inc. M^{v}. μνᾶ, < δραχμή, κΓο κοτίσχη (sic).
Expl. ὁ ξέστης τοῦ μέλιτος λίτρας δ'.

Escurial: Scorial. Υ. III. 14; s. XV. f. 236^{v}.
Florenz: Laurent. App. 2; s. XV. f. 240 (Expl. ὀβολοὺς ξε').
Leyden: Voss. fol. 25; s. XV.
Mailand: Ambros. S 3 Sup.; s. XV—XVI. f. 21.
Rom: Vatic. 299; s. XV. f. 451.

Excerpta varia.

Florenz: Laurent. plut. 74, 7; s. IX. p. 103 (Περὶ καταγμάτων. De fracturis. Inc. Ἐν πρώτοις. Cf. Orib. IV 154. Ed. A. Cocchius, Veterum medicorum chirurgica p. 90 sq.), p. 113 (Περὶ τερηδονισμοῦ κρανίου. De cranii carie. Inc. Τὴν τοῦ κρανίου. Cf. Orib. IV 187), p. 116 (Περὶ ὀστώδους ἐπιφύσεως. De osse excrescente. Inc. Ὀστώδης ἐπίφυσις. Cf. Orib. IV 204), p. 116b (Περὶ ἀλωπεκίας. De capillis fluentibus. Inc. Τῆς ἀλωπεκίας. Cf. Orib. IV 207), p. 128 (Περὶ ἀκρωτηριασμοῦ. De mutilatione. Cf. Orib. IV 247), p. 128b (Περὶ τῶν κατὰ τοὺς δακτύλους συμβαινόντων. De iis quae digitis accidunt. Inc. Ἐξαδακτύλοι γίνονται. Cf. Orib. IV 249), p. 136b (Περὶ ἐπιδέσμων. Cf. Orib. IV 281), p. 140b (Μεταγωγεύς. Adducens. Cf. Orib. IV 297), p. 141 (Κράτημα. Retinaculum. Cf. Orib. IV 299), p. 141b (Χειλοφύλαξ. Custos labiorum. Cf. Orib. IV 301), p. — (Περὶ διαφορᾶς καταρτισμῶν. Cf. Orib. IV 333) p. 154b (Νειλέως πλινθίον. Cf. Orib. IV 357).
Rom: Vatic. 1885; s. XIV. f. 2 (Περὶ τῶν ἐν κατακαλύψει ἀποστημάτων. Ex Orib. III 578).

[Diels II.43]

Heraclius.

Στίχοι πολιτικοί.
Versus politici.

Inc. Πέδον τίθηνον ἀκρίβου (?) πεφιλμένε.

Oxford: Baroccian. 220; s. XIII. f. 47^{v}.

Hermes Trismegistus.

Opera varia.

Sáros-Patak: Bibl. d. reform. Colleg. (Ἕρμους τρισμεγ. ἅπαντα. Mercurii ter maximi omnia quae exstant conquisita a. 1591.)

Ὄργανον.
Organum.

Edd. Berthelot-Ruelle, Alchim. gr. I p. 23.

Inc. Φιλοκαλίας χάριν ἐκκείσθω.
Expl. κ. κθ. λα. λδ.

Paris: Parisin. 2327; a. 1478. f. 293.

Κανόνιον.
Canon.

Rom: Vatic. 952; s. XIV. f. 184v.

Μέθοδος εἰς πᾶσαν καταρχὴν ἐπιτήδειος.
Methodus ad omne inceptum idonea.

Inc. Πρὸ πάντων.

Rom: Vatic. 1066; s. XVI f. 18.

Κυρανίδες.
Kyranides.

Ed. F. de Mély, Les lapidaires de l'antiquité II p. 3—124.
Vgl. Harpocration π. φυσικ. δυνάμ. κτέ.

Inc. Θεοῦ δῶρον μέγιστον ἀγγέλων
Expl. τὴν ἱστορίαν ποιήσομεν Θεοῦ ἡγήσει καὶ ἐνεργείᾳ.

Madrid: Matrit. bibl. nac. 4631 (ol. N 110); a. 1474. f. 6.
Moskau: Mosquens. —; s. XVI. XVIII.
Paris:
Coislin. 158; s. XVI. (L. I, A—Y).
Parisin.
2256; s. XV.
2419; s. XV.
2502; s. XVI. (Lib. III. II. IV).
2537; a. 1272.
Rom: Palat. 226; s. XV.
Venedig: Marcian. App. cl.
IV, 36 (olim Nanian. 258); s. XV—XVI.
V, 13 (olim Nanian. 247); a. 1377 (L. I. III. II. IV).
Wien: Vindob. med. 50; s. —.

[Diels II.44]

Ἰατρομαθηματικὰ πρὸς Ἄμμωνα Αἰγύπτιον.
Iatromathematica ad Ammonium Aegyptium.

Ed. Ideler, Phys. et Med. I p. 387—396).
Vgl. unten Π. κατακλίσεως νοσούντων.

Inc. Τὸν ἀνθρωπον, ὦ Ἄμμων, κόσμον φασίν.
Expl. τοῖς ἀνθρώποις οὐδὲν ἐπιγίνεται.

Cheltenham: Phillipps. 23007; s. XV. f. — (Inc. Τὸν ἄνθρωπον, ὦ Ἄμμων, φερέκοσμον. Expl. mutil. ἐὰν δὲ σελήνης οὔσης ἐν ταύρῳ κατακλιθῇ τις Κρόνου συνόντος αὐτῇ ἢ ἀναμετροῦντος = Ideler I p. 395, 20).
Erlangen: Bibl. Univ. 89; s. XV. no. 13.
München: Monac. 105; s. XVI. f. 213.
Paris:
Parisin.
1405; s. XVI. f. 42.
1991; s. XV. f. 25.
2139; s. XVII. f. 1.
2426*; s. XVI. f. 16v (Protagorae [Pythagorae] excerpta ex iatromathematicis Mercurii et Petosiridis etc. astrologica).
Suppl. 652; s. XV. f. 291.

Rom:
Angelic. 17 (C 5. 4); s. XIV. f. 339 (Inc. mutil. καὶ ῥωννύντα = Idel. I p. 388, 8).
Vatic.
1444; s. XV. f. 217.
1692 B; s. XV. f. 1.
Venedig: Marcian. 336; s. XV.

Περὶ κατακλίσεως νοσούντων.
Canon de decubitu infirmorum.

Ed. Ideler, Phys. et Med. I p. 430—440.
Vgl. oben Ἰατομαθηματικὰ πρὸς Ἄμμωνα.

Inc. Τὸν ἄνθρωπον, ὦ Ἄμμων, κόσμον φασὶν οἱ σοφοί.
Expl. τοῖς ἀνθρώποις οὐδὲν ἐπιγίνεται.

Paris: Parisin. 2139; s. XVII. f. 88.

Περὶ βοτανῶν χυλώσεως.
De succis plantarum.

Ed. W. Roether, Ioann. Laurent. Lydus de mensibus. Darmstadt 1827 p. 313—331.

Inc. prooem. Μακαρίας παρὰ θεῶν τιμῆς Ἑρμῆς τετυχηκώς.
cap. 1. Κριοῦ βοτάνης ἐστὶν ἐλελίσφακον.
Expl. ὥστε γενέσθαι μελίτος πάχος καὶ χρῶ.

Leyden: Vossian.
München: Augustan. 542; s. XV. f. 67.
Wien: Vindob. med. 23; s. XVI. f. 1—76 (Βίβλοι ἰατρικαὶ σύντομοι κατὰ μαθηματικῆς ἐπιστήμης ... ἐκδοθεῖσαι πρὸς μαθητὴν αὐτοῦ Ἀσκληπιόν, περὶ ἄστρων, βοτανῶν, τῶν ζώων, τῶν πηγῶν, τῶν τετραπόδων, τῶν ἐναλίων ἰχθύων τε καὶ ναυτῶν, τῶν ἄστρων τε καὶ λίθων δυνάμεως. Inc. f. 1 Κριοῦ ἐλελίσφακος. Expl. f. 76 ὡς ἔγωγε πεπείρακα).

Πρὸς τὸν Ἀσκληπιὸν λόγος καθολικός.

Athen: nr. 1180; s. XVIII no. 1.

[Diels II.45] [Περὶ ζῴων δυνάμεων καὶ τῶν ἐξ αὐτῶν φαρμάκων πρὸς Ἀσκληπίον.]
Ad Asclepium de animalium proprietatibus et remediis quae ex illis peti possunt, cum figuris.

Paris: Parisin. 2502; s. XVI. f. 30^{v}.

Περὶ δεκανῶν πρὸς Ἀσκληπιόν.
De decanis ad Asclepium.

Paris: Parisin.
2256; s. XV. f. 584^{v}.
2502; s. XVI. f. 19.
Wien: Vindob. med. 23; s. XVI. f. 18 (Inc. Τῶν ἐν τοῖς ζωδίοις τριακονταὲξ δεκανῶν. Expl. ἰδίαν γὰρ δύναμιν φυσικῶς ἔλαβεν βοτάνη).

Περὶ βοτανῶν τῶν ιβ' ζωδίων πρὸς Ἀσκληπιόν.
Ad Asclepium de plantis XII zodiaci signorum.

Bologna: Bonon. 3632; s. XV. f. 435^{v}.
Paris: Parisin.
2180*; s. XV. f. 85^{v}.
2256; s. XV. f. 588^{v}.
2419; s. XV. f. 265^{v}.
2502; s. XVI. f. 1.

Περὶ τῆς τῶν ιβ' τόπων ὀνομασίης καὶ δυνάμεως.
De XII locorum nomenclatura et facultate.

Erlangen: Bibl. Univ. 89; s. XV. no. 11.

Περὶ βοτανῶν τῶν ζ' ἀστέρων πρὸς Ἀσκληπιόν.
Ad Asclepium de plantis VII planetarum.

Bologna: Bonon. 3632; s. XV. f. —.
Paris: Parisin.
2180*; s. XV. f. 85^{v}.
2256; s. XV. f. 580.

Venedig: Marcian. App. cl. V 13, s. XIV—XV. f. 149 (Inc. Πρώτη βοτάνη ˝ὅ προσαγορευομένη κιχώ^ρ).

Περὶ σταθμῶν.
De ponderibus.

Wien: Vindob. med.
23; s. XVI. f. 76 (Περὶ τῶν δηλούντων τοὺς σταθμοὺς διὰ τῶν χαρακτήρων. Inc. Ὁ μακάριος τρισκαταιόφρων Ἑρμῆς. Expl. ἔτι δὲ καὶ οὕτως θ″ τὸ ἔνατον).
27; s. XVI. f. 104ᵛ (Περὶ σταθμῶν. Inc. Ὁ σταθμὸς βάρει μετρούμενος κρίνεται. Expl. μάλιστα συνήθων ἡμῖν ὁ λόγος).

Excerpta varia. [Diels II.47]

Escurial: Scorial. T. II 14; s. XVI. f. 178ᵛ (Ἀντίδοτος ἡ καλουμένη Ἑρμοῦ ἐκ τῶν ἀδύτων τοῦ Ἑρμοῦ εἰς μεμφίην παρεχώρησεν. »Ex Isaaci Iudaei libro τῶν ἐφοδίων videtur desumpta«).
Florenz: Laurent. App. 2; s. XV. f. 256ᵛ (Ἀντίδοτος αἰγυπτιακή. Inc. Πρὸς ποδαλγικούς. Expl. οὐκ ἀποτυγχάνει) *und* f. 361 (Ἀντίδοτος ἀρθρητική, ποδαλγικὴ καὶ νεφριτική. Inc. Ποδαλγικὴ ἀντίδοτος ἐκ τῶν Ἡφαίστου ἀδύτων ἐν Μεμφίδι).
Neapel: Bibl. Giovanni di Carbonara 15; s. XIV.
Orléans: Aurelian. 1032; s. XVII. p. 121 (Tabula smaragdina περὶ χημείας).
Oxford: Baroccian. 88; s. XVI. f. — (Inc. Πηγάνου φύλλων ξηρῶν, παιωνίας, ὀριγάνου, ὀποπάνακος, καρποβαλσάμου).
Paris: Parisin. 1991; s. XV. f. 29ᵛ (Exc. de rebus medico-astrologicis).
Wien: Vindob. med. 23; s. XVI. f. 77ᵛ (Περὶ τῶν μελῶν τοῦ ἀνθρώπου, ὅταν λαγγέβουν, γνώριζε οὕτως. Inc. Ὀφρὺς δεξιὸς ἐὰν ἅλυται [sic] ἐν ὀλίγῳ χρόνῳ. Expl. πολλῶν ἀγαθῶν ἐπιτυχίαν δηλοῖ) *und* f. 79ᵛ (Περὶ τῶν φριλτῶν [sic!], ὅπως τὸ ἕνα ὑπόκειται ὑπὸ τῆς δεκάδος καὶ ἡ δεκὰς ὑπὸ τῆς ἑκατοντάδος. Inc. [Kryptogr.] σεῆηνσωπεϛνωε. Expl. σλω· πθσ῾λ″ψ). [Diels II.48]

Herodotus.

Nach einer Vermutung von Wellmann gehört diesem der Anonymus Darembergii, den Fuchs publiziert hat.

Διάγνωσις περὶ τῶν ὀξέων καὶ χρονίων νοσημάτων.
Diagnostica de morbis acutis et chronicis.

Partim ed. R. Fuchs, Rhein. Mus. 49, 532 ff. 50, 576 ff. 58, 67 ff.
Festschrift f. Vahlen 145 ff.
Vgl. M. Wellmann, Hermes 40 p. 580 ff.

Inc. Φρενίτιδος αἰτία.

London: Medical Society We 29; s. XV ex. f. 366—403 (Expl. καὶ εἰ μὲν παρηγοροῖντο, ἐάσομεν· εἰ δὲ παροξύνοιντο = Parisin. Suppl. 636. f. 61ᵛ, 15. *Kalbfleischs Collation im Besitze der Berliner Akademie*).
Paris:
Parisin. 2324; s. XVI. f. 146ᵛ—209ᵛ (Inc. Τῶν σκοτωματικῶν τὴν αἰτίαν = Parisin. Suppl. 636. f. 46ᵛ. *Collation im Besitze der Akademie*).
Suppl. 636; s. XVII. f. 21—82 (Expl. καὶ ὑπὸ τῆς διαπύρου. *Vgl.* Costomiris, Rev. des ét. gr. III [1890] p. 146. *Abschrift im Besitze der Akademie*).
Wien: Vindob. med. 37; s. —. f. 13—38ᵛ (Inc. φάσκων = Parisin. Suppl. 636. f. 49, 8. Expl. καὶ τὸ διὰ τοῦ μυρο| ... = Paris. Suppl. 636. f. 82, 16. *Collation im Besitze der Akademie*).

Herophilus.

Περὶ πυρεσσόντων.
De febricantibus.

Wohl nur ein Excerpt.

Moskau: Mosquens. 466; s. XVI. f. 20ᵛ (Inc. Ὁ δὲ Ἡρ. πυρέσσειν ἀπεφήνατο).
Rom: Palat. 400; s. XV. f. 60ᵛ.

[Diels II.49] Σφυγμῶν ὅροι.
Definitiones pulsuum. Fragmentum.

Venedig: Bibl. Iosephi de Aromatariis (*Verbleib unbekannt*).

Hierophilus Sophista.

Περὶ τροφῶν δυνάμεων.
Κύκλος καθ' ἕκαστον μῆνα, ὁποίαι δεῖ χρᾶσθαι καὶ ὁποίοις ἀπέχεσθαι.
De alimentis, quae singulis mensibus sumenda aut vitanda sunt.

Ed. Boissonade, Not. et Extr. XI p. 192—273.
Ideler, Phys. et Med. I p. 409 sqq.

Inc. Μὴν Ἰανουάριος. Ἁρμόζει ἀπὸ κοίτης λαμβάνειν.
Expl. καὶ πληροῦται ὁ τῶν δώδεκα μηνῶν τοῦ ἐνιαυτοῦ χρόνος.

Berlin: Phillipps 1568 (ol. Meerm. 271); s. XVI. f. 22 (»Valde differt ab Ideleri editione«).
Oxford:
Baroccian. 150; s. XV in. f. 14v (»Valde differt ab Ideleri editione«).
Miscell. 278; a. 1780. p. 8. 22. 25—30. 39—54 (»The fragment on p. 8 is taken from codd. 396 and 985, the rest of the treatise from cod. 396 of the Paris library«).
Paris: Parisin.
396; s. XIII. f. 445.
985; s. XV. f. 315v.
2314; s. XIV—XV. f. 87.
Rom:
Palat. 400; s. XV. f. 75 (Inc. Ταύτης τῆς ἐπιτρέψεως).
Vatic. 285; s. XV. f. 301.
Venedig: Marcian. App. cl. V, 13; s. XIV—XVI. f. 1.
Wien: Vindob. med. 52; s. XV. f. 55—60.

Περὶ τροφῶν δυνάμεων.
De alimentorum facultatibus.

Inc. Τῶν διαιτημάτων τὰς τάξεις καὶ τὰς τούτων αἰτίας.

Oxford: Baroccian. 150; s. XV in. f. 18v (Expl. τὰ κητώδη πλὴν τῆς ὕσκας ... καὶ περιττωματικά. »Fragmentum, ed. ab Ideler p. 257—281 sub titulo Ἀνωνύμου περὶ χυμῶν, βρωμάτων καὶ πομάτων § 46 sqq., des. p. 281 in cap. Περὶ τῶν ἐκ τῶν ζῴων τροφῆς δυνάμεων. V. huius cod. § 12 et cod. Vindob. no. 28«. *Vgl.* Daremberg, Not. et Extr. I p. 21 sq.).

Rom: Palat. 400; s. XV. f. 83ᵛ.
Wien: Vindob.
28; s. —.
52; s. XV. f. 60—66ᵛ (Expl. mutil. φακῇ καὶ κράμβη διὰ τοῦτο καὶ τὴν ὄψιν ἀμβλύνουσι, πλὴν εἰ τύχοι ὑγρότερος ...).

[Diels II.50]

Hypatus.

Περὶ τῶν τοῦ σώματος μερῶν ἑρμηνεία.
Interpretatio partium corporis.

Inc. Βρέγμα, τὸ λεγόμενον ἁπαλόν.

Escurial: Scorial. Σ. I. 12; s. XVI. f. 51 (Sine auctoris nomine. Inc. Τὸ ἁπαλὸν βρέγμα. Expl. ταρσὸν καὶ πλατύπεδίον [sic]. *Vgl.* Rufus ed. Ruelle p. 599. *Collation in Wellmanns Besitz*).
Florenz: Laurent. plut. 74, 13; s. XV p. 301b.
Leyden: Vossian. 4° 54; s. XIII. f. 315—316.
Madrid: Matrit. 4636; s. XV. f. 209 (Sine auctoris nomine. Inscr. Περὶ τῶν μελῶν τοῦ ἀνθρωπίνου σώματος. Inc. *wie im* Scorial. *Wellmanns Collation in dessen Besitz*).

Iacobus Psychrestus.

Excerpta.

Florenz: Laurent. plut. 74, 2; s. XI. p. 282 (Emplastrum ἐντατικὸν λεγόμενον γαρέλαιον, ὃ ἐσκεύασεν ἡ λυσία, ἣ ἀρχηγός, ἢ τυφάς . Inc. Στέαρ καμήλου ἀνδριῶντος).
Paris: Parisin. 2210; a. 1537. f. 368.

Ioannes Zacharias Actuarius.

(*S. unter* ZACHARIAS.)

Ioannes Philoponus Alexandrinus.

Περὶ σφυγμῶν.
De pulsibus.

Inc. Σφυγμῶν ἐστιν αἴσθησις.
Expl. τέλος περὶ σφυγμῶν.

Rom: Vatic. 280; s. XV. f. 204.

Περὶ πυρετῶν.
De febribus.

Inc. Πρῶτον δεῖ εἰπεῖν, τί ποτε πυρετὸν καλοῦμεν.

Moskau: Mosquens. 466; s. XVI. f. 157 (Π. πυρετῶν θαυμάσιον).

Ioannes Alexandrinus (*nicht* Philoponus). [Diels II.51]

Σχόλια Ἱπποκράτους εἰς τὸ περὶ παιδίου φύσεως ἀπὸ φωνῆς Ἰωάννου.
Scholia in Hippocratis librum de natura pueri ab ore Ioannis.

Ed. Dietz, Scholia in Hipp. et Gal. II p. 205—235.
Von Dietz dem Ioannes Alexandr. zugeschrieben.

Inc. Ἦν ἡ γονὴ μείνῃ ἐπ' ἀμφοῖν ἐν τῇ μήτρᾳ.
Expl. Δύο τινὲς δόξαι γεγόνασι περὶ τοῦ ...

Florenz: Laurent. plut. 59, 14; s. XV. f. 227b (Fragmentum).

Ioannes Antiochenus Archiatrus.

[Συλλογὴ φαρμάκων.]
Collectio remediorum ex Dioscoride, Hippocrate et Galeno.

Paris: Parisin. 2315; s. XV. f. 117.

[Diels II.52]

Ioannes Archiatrus.

Παντοίων παθῶν θεραπεία.
Variorum morborum curatio.

Florenz: Laurent. plut. 75, 10; s. XV. f. 32 (Τοῦ σοφωτάτου Ἀριστοτέλους λόγοι καὶ προοίμια, κυρίου Ἰωάννου ἀρχιάτρου καὶ μαθητοῦ αὐτοῦ, περιέχων συνοπτικῶς πάντων τῶν παθῶν καὶ τῶν ἀδήλων τὰς θεραπείας. Inc. Πρὸς ὀξὺν πόνον κεφαλῆς. Ἔπαρον ἀγριαγκουρέας σπόρον. Expl. θέτ' ἐς τὸ μέτωπον).

München: Monac. 288; s. XIV. f. 7 (Ἑρμηνεία καὶ διδασκαλία καὶ ἐξήγησις τοῦ θαυμασιωτάτου καὶ λογιωτάτου ἀρχιητροῦ τοῦ Γαληνοῦ τοῦ σπεύσαντος εἰς τὸ [sic!] τῶν μορίων πάθη, ἀνίατα καὶ δυσίατα λέγω ἅμα καὶ εὔατα γενέσθαι ὠφέλειαν ἴασιν. Inc. Πρῶτον μὲν καὶ κοινῷ λόγῳ. »Esse commentarium in Galenum ab Ioanne Archiatro compositum ex fine concludi potest. In bibl. Paris, idem msc. habetur cuius titulus est: Ioannis Iatrosophistae λόγος καὶ ποίημα πάντων τῶν παθῶν καὶ τῶν ἀδήλων τὰς θεραπείας πρὸς ἓν ἕκαστον τὴν τάξιν. Capp. 252. Cod. 126 teste Fabricio vol. XII. p. 781«).

Paris: Parisin.
2224; s. XV. f. 80. (»Opus medicum«).
2236; s. XV. f. 1 (»Hoc opus ab Omont Actuario adscriptum Daremberg Not. et Extr. I 23 Ioanni Archiatro attribuit«).

Rom: Angelic. 17 (C. 5. 4); s. XIV. f. 1 (Λόγοι καὶ ποίημα ἰωάννου ἀρχιατροῦ περιέχων συνοπτικὸς παντοίων παθῶν ἀδήλων καὶ φανερῶν τὴν θεραπείαν. Inc. Πρὸς πόνων κεφαλῆς. Κισσὸν ξήρανον εἰς ἥλιον. »Cf. Hardt III 212«).

Ioannes Chrysostomus.

[Περὶ νόσων καὶ ἰατρῶν.]
De adversa valetudine et medicis.

Paris:
Coislin.
78; s. XI. f. 199.
79; s. XI—XII. f. 79.
Parisin. 912; s. XIV. f. 266.

Ioannes Chumnos.

Δίαιτα προφυλακτικὴ εἰς ποδάγραν.
Quali victus ratione podagra evitari possit.

Ed. Fr. Boissonade, Anecd. nova. Paris 1844. p. 220—222.

Inc. Βρώματα ταριχευτὰ πάντα.
Expl. διὰ τὴν μὴ φαινομένην μέλλουσαν τίσιν.

Paris: Parisin. 1000; s. XIV. f. 156 (?) (Sub nomine Nicephori Chumni?).

Ioannes Damascenus. [Diels II.53]

Excerpta.

Escurial: Scorial.
T. II. 14; s. XVI. f. — (Πόμα ἤτοι βοήθημα διὰ πειρας μεγάλης δόκιμον· ἄνθη τῆς βιόλας. »Ex Isaaci libro videntur desumpta. Cf. cod. Matrit. 166. f. 212.« Wellmann).
Υ. III. 14; s. XV. f. 89 (Ex Isaaci libro).

Ioannes Dioecetas Constantinopolitanus.

[Τέχνη ἰατρική?]
De medicina.

Paris: Parisin. Suppl. 638; s. XV. f. 1 (Libri VI—X).

Ioannes Esdra.

Περὶ οὔρων.
De urinis.

Inc. Ἐπειδὴ προεθέμεθα εἰπεῖν.

Rom: Reg. Suec. 182; s. XV. f. 4.

[Diels II.54]

Ioannes Iatrosophista.

[Περὶ νόσων καὶ θεραπείας.]
De morbis eorumque curationibus.

Paris: Parisin. 2316; s. XV. f. 51v.

Ioannes Pothus Pediasimus.

Vgl. Krumbacher, Sitz. Ber. d. Münch. Akad. d. Wiss. 1892 p. 350.

Rom: Vatic. 671; s. XIII—XIV. f. 237 (Τοῦ ὑπάτου τῶν φιλοσόφων κυρίου ἰωάννου πόθου τοῦ πεδιασίμου. Inc. Ἐζήτηται δι' ἣν αἰτίαν ἐννιάμηνος μὲν τόκος. Expl. ἀλλ' ἀρκοῦσι ταῦτα).

Ioannes Episcopus Prisdrianensis.

Παρεκβολαὶ ἐκ τῶν παλαιῶν ἰατρῶν συλλεγεῖσαι περὶ διαχωρημάτων.
Collectanea de excrementis.

Inc. Οἱ παλαιοὶ τῶν ἰατρῶν οἱ ἐξαίρετοι.
Expl. καὶ περὶ μὲν τῶν ἄνωθεν.

London: Addit. (Brit. Mus.) 17, 900; s. XVII. f. 271.
Paris: Parisin. 2286; s. XIV. f. 136.

[Diels II.55]

Συγγραφὴ περὶ οὔρων, συλλεγεῖσα ἀπὸ πολλῶν καὶ διαφόρων, παλαιῶν καὶ νέων ἰατρῶν.
Collectanea de urinis.

Inc. Ἐπειδὴ προεθέμεθα εἰπεῖν περὶ οὔρων.

Athen: Atheniens. 1481; s. XVI. no. 3.
Krakau: Cracov. bibl. univ. lagellon. 2526 FF VI 5; s. XV. f. 99 (Expl. ἢ ὑπὸ πλήθους τοῦ χυμοῦ).

Mailand: Ambros. D 13 Sup.; s. —. f. 300ᵛ (Inscr. man. rec. Ὀριβασίου π. οὔρων, in mg. Ἰωάννου ἐπισκόπου Πρισδριανῶν. Inc. Ἡ θεία φύσις ποιήσασα τὸν ἄνθρωπον. Expl. mutil.: ἐν τῷ οὔρῳ φαινόμενα τῆς κύστεως ...).

Palermo: Panormit. bibl. naz. XIII C 3; s. XVI. f. 85—94ᵛ (Expl. ἀπαρτίζομεν τὴν διδασκαλίαν).

Paris:

Parisin. 2286; s. XIV. f. 114.

Suppl. 637; s. XV. f. 50.

Rom: Vatic. 293; s. XVI. f. 22 (Συντάξεις θεοφόρου ἀνδρὸς καὶ ἐπισκόπου Ἰωάννου περὶ οὔρων καὶ ἄλλων πολλῶν).

Wien: Vindob. med. 8; s. —. f. 320.

[Συλλογὴ περὶ ἐντέρων, ἐκ Παλλαδίου, Ἀρχελάου, Στεφάνου κτέ]
Collectanea de intestinis, ex Palladio, Archelao, Stephano Alexandrino etc.

Paris: Parisin. 2286; s. XVI. f. 127ᵛ.

Ioannes Spensatus.

[Περὶ ἀνιάτων καὶ δυσιάτων νοσημάτων.]
Liber de incurabilibus et difficile curabilibus morbis.

Paris: Parisin. 2336; s. XVI.

Ioannes Staphidaces.

Σύνθεσις διαφόρων πράξεων.
De nonnullorum medicamentorum compositione.

Inc. Ἐπιθύμου ϛγδ μυροβαλάνου.
Expl. γῆς σαμίαν αἰγυπτί...

Rom: Vatic. 282; s. XVI. f. 433.

[Diels II.56]

Iustus.

Excerpta.

Bologna: Bonon. 3632; s. XV. f. 206 (Περὶ τῶν ἱερῶν καὶ πικρῶν ἀντιδότων, cap. ιθ' extr.: Ἱερὰ Ἰούστου κθ'. *Wohl aus* Aët. III 116).
London: Harleian. (Brit. Mus.) 5626; s. XV (XVI). f. 2* (Ἰατροσόφιον ποιηθὲν ὑπὸ διαφόρων φιλοσόφων τῶν πρὸς Ἱπποκράτους γιγνομένων αὐτοῦ μαθητῶν ... Ἰούστου ...).
Oxford: Baroccian. 150; s. XV (Ἀντίδοτος ἡ ἱερὰ Ἰούστου πρὸς κεφαλαγίαν).

Karastonus.

Περὶ μέτρων καὶ σταθμῶν.
Liber de mensuris et ponderibus, editus a Thebit filio Core.

Paris: Parisin. Suppl. 263; s. XVI. f. 183.

Kyranus.

(*Vgl.* Harpocration *und* Hermes Trismegistus.)

Περὶ φυσικῶν δυνάμεων.
Opus physico-magicum de naturalibus virtutibus.

Paris: Parisin. 2537; a. 1272.

Περὶ λίθων, βοτανῶν κτέ.
Lexicon de lapidibus, plantis etc.

Paris: Coislin. 158; s. XVI. f. 80 (Α—Υ).

[Diels II.57]

Lampudes.

Ἐκ τὸ χορτηνὸν (sic!) τοῦ Λαμπούδη.

Inc. Τί ἐστι συνοχή.

Paris: Parisin. 2244; s. XIV—XV. f. 95ᵛ.

Leo.

Σύνοψις ἰατρικῆς.
Synopsis artis medicae.

Ed. Ermerins, Anecd. med. gr. p. 79—221.

Inc. Οὐχ ἅπαξ οὐδὲ δίς, ἀλλὰ καὶ πολλάκις ᾔτησας.
Expl. ἐπείγονται πρὸς τὰ πράγματα, ἐν οἷς σὺν θεῷ τὸ τέλος.

Paris: Parisin. Suppl. 446; s. X. f. 147—168.

Σύνοψις εἰς τὴν φύσιν τῶν ἀνθρώπων.
Synopsis de hominis natura.

Inc. Τί ἐστι ψυχή; οὐσία ἀσώματος.
Expl. καὶ τῆς ψυχῆς ὡς ταύτης δώμημα (sic).

Escurial: Scorial. Φ. III. 7; s. XIV. f. 186v.

Περὶ ἰδιωμάτων ἀνθρώπων.
De hominum proprietatibus.

Inc. Ἄνθρωπος μετὰ μεγάλης κεφαλῆς.

Rom: Barberin. III 63 (= 245); s. XVI. f. 376.

Excerpta.

Oxford: Baroccian. 88; s. XVI. f. 18 (Περὶ μελαγχολίας et alia capita de Leone desumpta. *Vgl.* Ermerins, Anecd. med. gr. *a. a. O.*).

Libanius.

[Περὶ γενέσεως ἀνθρώπου.]
De hominis generatione.
Fragmentum.

Paris: Parisin. 2894; s. XIII. f. 336.

[Diels II.58]

Logadius.

Excerpta.

Athos: Βιβλ. μον. Ἰβήρων 4271. 151; s. XV. f. —. (Ἱερά. Inc. Κολοκυντίδι ἐτεριώνην ὀγκίας κ' σκίλλης ὀπτῆς).
London: Harleian. (Brit. Mus.) 5626; s. XV (XVI). f. 2* (Ἰατροσόφιον ποιηθὲν ὑπὸ διαφόρων φιλοσόφων τῶν πρὸς Ἱπποκράτους γιγνομένων αὐτοῦ μαθητῶν ... Λογαδίου ...).
Oxford: Baroccian. 150; s. XV in. f. 3b (*Wie im* Athous).
Rom: Angelic. 4 (C 4. 16); s. XVI in. f. 290 (Σκευασία τῆς ἱερᾶς. Inc. Εἰς ξανθο⟨χο⟩λικούς, μελαγχολικούς, φλεγματικούς).

Lucas.

(*Vgl.* Gregorius Theol[ogus])

Σκευασία ἀλατίου.
Compositio salsi intinctus.

Ed. Ideler, Phys. et Med. I p. 297.

Inc. Ἔχων ἐνεργείας τοσαύτας.
Expl. ἐν αὐτῷ τὰς τροφὰς πάσας.

Athos: Βιβλ. μον. Διονυσίου 3881. 347; s. XVI. f. 195.
Bologna: Bonon. 1808; s. XV. f. 42.
London: Addit. (Brit. Mus.) 10, 058; s. XV. f. 46ᵛ.
München: Monac. 72; s. XVI. f. 277.
Oxford: Baroccian.
150; s. XV in. f. 1 *und* 18.
224; s. XV in. f. 21b.

Paris: Parisin. [B. R. 349; s. —. f. 156].
Rom:
Angelic.
4 (C 4. 16); s. XVI in. f. 277ᵛ.
17 (C 5. 4); s. XIV. f. 326.
Vatic. 2250; s. XIV. f. 343ᵛ.
Turin: Taurin. 17 B VII 22 (B I 12); s. XVI. XVIII. f. 134 (*Verbrannt*).
Wien: Vindob. med.
28; s. XV. f. 156 (Inc. Ὀφθαλμῶν οὗ πιεῖ. Expl. ἀνὰ κοχλιαρίων δυοῖν ἢ καὶ τριῶν).
31; s. XV ex. *hinter* f. 127.

Excerpta varia.

Paris: Parisin. 2510; a. 1384. f. 125 (Remedia varia, inter quae S. Lucae etc.).

Lycus.

[Diels II.59]

[Περὶ μήτρας καὶ γυναικείου αἰδοίου.]
De vulva et muliebri pudendo.

Paris: Parisin. Suppl. 629; s. XIX. f. 94ᵛ (*Wohl aus* Oribas. III p. 382).

Excerpta varia.

London: Burneian. (Brit. Mus.) 94; s. XV—XVI. f. — (Ὅτι οὐκ ἐφικνεῖται τὸ σύμμετρον αἰδοῖον τοῦ ἄρρενος τοῦ στομίου τῆς ὑστέρας. Inc. Τοῦ κύτους τῆς μήτρας. Expl. βολῆς τινος προσδεῖν. *Aus* Oribas. III 382).
Turin: Taurin. 333b I 1; s. XVI. f. 170ᵛ (*Wie im* Burneian. *Durch Feuer stark beschädigt*).

Macarius Magnes.

Περὶ οὔρων.
De urinis.

Paris: Parisin. 1630; s. XIV. f. 205.

Macarius Maximus.

Περὶ ψυχῆς.
De anima.

Paris: Parisin. 2615; a. 1553. 1584. f. 9.

Magnus Emesenus.

Προγνωστικά.
Prognostica.

Rom: Vatic. 279; s. —. f. 280 (*Verbleib unbekannt*).

Περὶ οὔρων ἀπὸ φωνῆς Θεοφίλου.
De urinis ex ore Theophili.

Bologna: Bonon. 3632; s. XV. f. 57 (Inc. Τῶν οὔρων αἱ διαφοραὶ πολλαί. Expl. κατὰ τὰ εἰρημένα. »Concordat cum commentatione de urinis, quam Ideler Anonymo tribuit, ab initio usque ad II p. 315, 20«).
Escurial: Scorial. Υ. III. 14; s. XV. f. 55.
[Diels II.60] **Gallipoli:** Ἐκκλ. ἁγ. Νικολ. 38; s. XIV. f. 58 (Inc. *wie im* Bonon. *Vgl.* Daremberg Not. et Extr. I p. 55. 111. 161).
Paris:
Parisin. 2260; s. XVI. f. 9.
Suppl. 683; s. XV—XVIII. f. 58v (»De urinarum differentiis«).
Rom:
Palat. 279; s. XIV—XV. f. 292 (»f. 280v idem liber contractior«).
Vatic.
279; s. —. f. 280 (*Verbleib unbekannt*).
280; s. XV. f. 176v (*Vgl.* Ideler I p. 283).

Dazu: [Cod. Mich. Cantacuzeni].

Περὶ πυρετῶν.
De febribus.

Rom: Vatic. 279; s. —. f. 280 (*Verbleib unbekannt*).

Excerpta.

Oxford: Baroccian. 150; s. XV in. f. 77 (Pauca quaedam de simplicibus ex Dioscoride, Oribasio, Porphyrio, Paulo, Magno et Archigene).
Paris:
Parisin. 2324; s. XVI. f. 1 (Hippocratis, Galeni, Magni et Erasistrati iatrosophium. Inc. Τὴν περὶ τῆς τῶν οὔρων).
Suppl. 1202; s. XIII. f. 16 (Excerpta varia ex Dioscoride, Oribasio, Porphyrio, Paulo, Magno, Archigene etc.).

Mangens (?).

(= Macarius Magnes *oder* Magnus Emesenus?)

Σύνοψις περὶ οὔρων.
Synopsis de urinis.

Paris: Parisin. 2316; s. XV. f. 191 (Galeni et Mangentis synopsis de urinis).

Marcellinus.

Περὶ σφυγμῶν.
De pulsibus.

Bologna: Bonon. 3632; s. XV. f. 65.
Paris: Parisin. 2332*; s. XV. f. 149 (Inc. Τὴν δὲ περὶ σφυγμῶν. Expl. εἰς εὕρεσιν. *Hiervon oder von einem Vindob. Abschrift in Darembergs Nachlaß in Band 186*).
Wien: Vindob. med.
15; s. —. f. 101.
16; s. —. f. 319 (Μαρκέλλου περὶ σφυγμῶν. Inc. Σφυγμῶν θι..ειν καὶ σφυγμῶν ὅσα χρὴ μαθεῖν. Expl. παλαιας εἰς εὕρεσιν διδούς. *Abschrift im Berol. fol 39 [275]*).

Marcellus Sidetes. [Diels II.61]

Ἰατρικὰ περὶ ἰχθύων.
Medicina ex piscibus.

Ed. Ideler, Phys. et Med. I p. 134—137.
Duebner ap. Lehrs, Poet. bucol. et did. p. 169—171.

M. Schneider, Commentatt. in hon. Ribbeckii p. 124.

Inc. Εὖ δὲ καὶ εἰναλίων.
Expl. καλὸν χραισμήιον ἄφθαις.

Berlin: Berol. 4° 2 (301); s. XVII. f. 37v.
London: Burneian. (Brit. Mus.) 75; s. XV. f. 164v.
Paris:
Parisin.
2408; s. XIII. f. 216v.
2633; s. XIII. f. 743 (fine mutil.).
Suppl. 662; s. XIV. f. 257v.

Περὶ μέτρων καὶ σταθμῶν.
De mensuris et ponderibus.

Carpentras: nr. 1774 (P., V); s. XVII. f. 168 (*Vgl.* f. 315).

Marcianus.

Νευροχαλαστικόν.
Medicamentum ad nervos laxandos idoneum.

Florenz: Laurent. plut. 75, 3; s. XII. p. 263.

[Diels II.62]

Marianus.

Excerpta.

Rom: Barberin. II 58; s. XVI. f. 1 (Εὑρισκόμενα ἐν ταῖς οὐσίαις Μαριάνου θουκκίου ἰατροῦ).

Maximus (Planudes?).

Περὶ αἱμάτων.
De sanguinibus.

Inc. Μάθε καὶ τὰ αἵματα.
Expl. μακρονοσίαν δέ.

Rom: Barberin. I 127; s. XVI. f. 261ᵛ.

Melampus.

[Περὶ παλμῶν.]
De palpitationibus.

Paris: Parisin. 2154; s. XIV. f. 280.

Meletius Monachus.

Περὶ ψυχῆς.
De anima.

Escurial: Scorial.
Φ. I. 10*; s. XVI. f. 189ᵛ.
y. I. 15; s. XVI. f. 73ᵛ (»Περὶ ψυχῆς Meletii esse videtur«. Wellmann. Inc. Ὁ περὶ ψυχῆς ὅδε λόγος οὐ τὸ τί ἐστιν ἡ ψυχὴ κατ' οὐσίαν διδάσκει. Expl. οἱ γνῶσιν ἐν συνέσει κατωρθωκότες).
Paris: Parisin. 2299; s. XV. f. 89ᵛ.

Περὶ στοιχείων. [Diels II.63]
De quattuor elementis.

Paris: Parisin. 2299; s. XV. f. 99ᵛ.

Περὶ φύσεως ἀνθρώπου.
De natura hominis.

Ed. Gramer, Anecd. gr. Oxon. III p. 1—157.

Inc. Ἡ παροῦσα σύνοψις περὶ φύσεως ἀνθρώπου.
Expl. σώματι δὲ τὴν φράσιν. Δόξα Κυρίῳ κτέ. τῷ συνεργῷ τῶν καλῶν καὶ αἰτίῳ· ἀμήν.

Berlin: Berol. 4° 5 (304)*; s. XV—XVI. f. 53ᵛ (Διαθήκη τῶν τριῶν ἰατρῶν Γαλην. Ἱππ. καὶ Μελετίου ... περὶ τῆς τοῦ ἀνθρώπου κατασκευῆς καὶ πῶς δεῖ διεξιέναι τὸν καιρόν).
Brüssel: Bruxell. 5362—64; s. XVI. f. 105 (Expl. ἐν καρδίας διὰ τῆς ἀορτῆς ἀρ...).

Cheltenham: Phillipps. 3892 (ol. Meerm. 275); s. XV. no. 1.
Escurial: Scorial. y. I. 15*; s. XVI. f. 1 (Τὴν ἀρχὴν δὲ ἀπὸ τῶν τοῦ θαυμασίου πρεσβυτέρου ἡμῶν. Expl. Τὰ ἔργα σου, κύριε, πάντα ἐν σοφίᾳ ἐποίησας).
Florenz: Laurent plut. 75, 19; s. XIV. p. 8b.
Jerusalem:
Bibl. d. hl. Grabes
304; a. 1615. f. 103.
357; s. XVI. f. 304.
Bibl. patriarch.
203; s. XIX. f. 189.
470; s. XVIII. f. 1.
511; s. XVIII. XIX. no. 2.
Krakau: Bibl. Univ. Jagellon. misc. 2526 FF VI 5; s. XV. f. 1 (Inc. Τὰ περὶ τῆς τοῦ ἀνθρώπου κατασκευῆς. Expl. καὶ ἔξωθεν ἐμπλάσας ἐπιτίθει).
Leyden: Ruhnken 11; s. XVIII. (*Angefangene Ausgabe eines Freundes von Ruhnken.*)
München: Monac. 39; s. XVI. f. 1.
Neapel:
Bibl. dei Gerolamini XXII. I*; s. XV. f. 157ᵛ—160ᵛ (Μερικαί τινες παρεκβολαὶ ἐκ τοῦ περὶ φύσεως ἀνθρώπου πονήματος τοῦ ... Μελετίου. Inc. Οὗτός φησὶν ἄνθρωπός ἐστι ζῷον λογικόν. Expl. μετὰ τὴν γαστέρα κεῖται).
Oratorian. 152 (Pil. XXII. no. 1)*; s. XIV—XV. (Moschopuli Excerpta).
Oxford:
Baroccian. 131; s. XIV. f. 1 (Περὶ τῆς τοῦ ἀνθρώπου κατασκευῆς).
Roe
14 (Bodl. 260); s. XV. f. 210.
15 (Bodl. 261); s. XV. f. 1.
Paris:
Coislin. 384; s. XIV. f. 162.
Parisin.
2047 A; s. XIV. f. 113ᵛ.
2224; s. XV. f. 1 (Libri II).
2225; s. XIV. f. 1.
2226; s. XVI.
2227; s. XVI.
2257; s. XVI. f. 239.
2299; s. XV. f. 1.
2300; a. 1569.
Suppl.
49; s. XVI. f. 1.
84; s. XVI.
637; s. XV. f. 7.

Rom:
Ottobon. 145; a. 1363. f. 1.
Palat. 400; s. XV. f. 146v.
Vatic.
280; s. XV. f. 212.
1695; s. XV. f. 1.
Turin: Taurin.
6b IV 6; s. XVI. f. 110.
156b II 10; s. XVI. f. 1.
Upsala: Upsal. bibl. acad. 30; s. XIII—XIV.
Venedig: Marcian. 297; s. XIV.
Verona: Bibl. Capitolare CXXIX (118); s. XVI. no. 5.
Wien: Vindob. med.
8; s. XV. f. 1 (Τὰ περὶ τῆς τοῦ ἀνθρώπου κατασεκυῆς. Expl. καὶ αἰσχυνομένης ἐρυθρὸν σῶμα δείκνυται).
28*; s. XV. f. 164—183 (Ἐπιτομὴ π. τῆς κατασκευῆς τοῦ ἀνθρώπου κτλ. Inc. *wie im* Scorial. Expl. ἐν κόπρῳ ἐν οὔρῳ ἐν πτίσμασι ...).
45; s. XV. f. 1—27 (Inc. *wie im* Scorial.).

Ἐξήγησις εἰς τοὺς Ἱπποκράτους ἀφορισμούς.
Commentarius in Hippocratis aphorismos.

Vgl. Dietz, Scholia in Hipp. et Gal. II p. XI sq., p. 236—544.
Vgl. Stephanus Atheniensis *und* Theophilus.

Paris: Parisin.
2222; s. XV. f. 104.
2223; s. XVI. f. 158.

Excerpta varia. [Diels II.64]

Athen: nr. 1506; s. XIX (Μελετίου ἰατροσόφιον).
Athos:
Βιβλ. μον. Ἰβήρων 4655. 535; s. XVI (Ἰατροσόφη ἐκλελεγμένον ὑπὸ ... Γαλ. Ἱππ. καὶ Μελ. καὶ ἄλλων δοκίμων ἰατρῶν. Cap. I. Ὅτι ὁ κόσμος ὑπὸ τεσσάρων στοιχείων).
Παντελεήμονος
5768. 261; s. XVIII (Τοῦ πανιερωτάτου καὶ λογιωτάτου μητροπολίτου Ναυπάκτου καὶ Ἄρτης κυρίου, κυρίου Μελετίου, Εἰσαγωγὴ διαφόρων ἀκουσμάτων καὶ ἰατρικῶν).

5769. 262; s. XVIII. f. 15 (Ἰατροσόφιον ἐκλελεγμένον ὑπὸ ... Γαλ. Ἱππ. Μελ. Μοναχοῦ καὶ Παύλ. τοῦ Αἰγ., συγγραφὲν δὲ παρὰ Κοσμᾶ ἱερομονάχου τοῦ Μακεδόνος).

6372. 865; s. XIX. f. 205 B (Ἀποσημειώσεις τινὲς ψυχωφελεῖς. *Darunter* Τοῦ ἁγίου Μελετίου τοῦ ὁμολογητοῦ Περὶ διαίτης ὁλικῶς).

Berlin: Berol. 4° 46 (348); s. XVI. ρνθ' (Στίχοι πάνυ ὠφέλιμοι Μελετίου) *und* ρξ' (Περὶ τοῦ παραγενομένου εἰς ἰατρίαν ἀδελφοῦ).

Jerusalem: Bibl. Mar-Saba 432; a. 1662. f. 1 (Ἰατροσόφιον ... Γαλ. Ἱππ. καὶ Μελετίου).

Lesbos: Βιβλ. τῆς τοῦ Λειμῶνος μονῆς 175; s. XVII.

Paris:

Coislin. 335; s. XV. f. 75 (Gal. Hipp. et Meletii iatrosophium, capita 604).

Parisin.

2240; s. XVI. f. 151ᵛ (Versus politici de urinis illarumque differentiis).

2315; s. XV. f. 11ᵛ (*Wie im* Parisin. 2240).

Rom:

Angelic. 17 (C 5. 4); s. XIV. f. 141 (Ἕτερα περὶ τροφῶν δυνάμεων ἐκβληθέντα ἐκ τῆς βίβλου τοῦ μοναχοῦ κυρίου Μελετίου· ἐκ τὸν μικρὸν [sic!] κόσμων) *und* f. 141—236 (Περὶ ἄρτου κατὰ ἀλφαβήτου. Inc. Τῶν ἄρτων ὅσοί ῥυπαροί. Expl. πρὸς ἀνθρωπίνου σώματος ὁμοιότητα).

Barberin. III 63 (245); s. XVI. f. 394—414ᵛ (Ἰατροσόφιον ἐκλελεγμένον Γαλ. Ἱππ. καὶ Μελετίου περὶ γυναικός. Expl. εἰς τὰ νευροχαλαστικά).

Turin: Taurin. 17 B VII 22 (B I 12); s. XVI. XVIII. f. 30ᵛ (Γαλ. Ἱππ. Μελ. περὶ φλεβοτομίας) *und* f. 154 (Ἰατροσόφιον περὶ ἐντέρων. *Verbrannt*).

Wien: Vindob. med. 53; s. XVI. f. 129—189 (Ἰατροσόφιον. Capita 112. Inc. Περὶ ἐντέρων ὅταν ἐξέβουν. Expl. διὰ τί ἔνε καλὸς καιρός).

Menander Iatrosophista.

Περὶ γυναικῶν.
De mulieribus.

Paris: Parisin. 1630; s. XIV. f. 212ᵛ.

Mercurius Monachus.

Περὶ σφυγμῶν.
De pulsibus.

Ed. Ideler, Phys. et Med. II p. 254—256.

Inc. Πιάσον τὸν σφυγμὸν ἅμα τοῖς τέσσαρσι δακτύλοις.
Expl. εἰς τὰς πύλας τοῦ θανάτου ἐστίν.

Berlin: Phillipps. 1531 (ol. Meerm. 223); s. XVI. f. 230 (»Mercurius?« Inc. Ἅψαι τοῦ σφυγμοῦ μετὰ τῶν τεσσάρων δακτύλων. Expl. καὶ τὰ τούτοις περιεχόμενα. *Vgl.* Daremberg, Not. et Extr. I p. 143 sq.).
Dresden: Dresd. Da 5; a. 1519 f. 247 (Sine auctoris nomine. Inc. *wie im* Phillipps.).
Florenz: Laurent. App. 2; s. XV. f. 83ᵛ (»Περὶ σφυγμῶν. Sunt nr. 25—28 tractatus Mercurio tributi, Ideler II p. 256, sed post n. 25 inseruntur Κράτησον τὸν σφυγμὸν, [Diels II.65] καὶ εἰ μὲν ῥίπτει ὅλον ἔξω ἀραιά, ἕως ἡμέρας τρεῖς ἐστιν ἡ ζωὴ αὐτοῦ«).
London: Harleian. (Brit. Mus.) 6295; s. XV (XIV sec. catal.). f. 111ᵛ.
Mailand: Ambros. R 20 Sup.; s. —. f. 533.
Neapel: Neapolit. 307 III D 23; s. XV. f. 137.
Paris: Parisin.
2307; s. XVI. f. 599.
2315; s. XV. f. 1.
Rom: Vatic.
299; s. XV. f. 101.
7152; s. —. f. —. (*Vgl.* Daremberg *a. a. O.*).

Methodius Causocalybitus.

Περὶ διαίτης ἀνθρώπου.
De diaeta hominis.

Paris: Parisin. Suppl. 654; s. XIX. f. 224ᵛ.

Methodius Patriarchus.

Excerpta varia.

Venedig: Marcian. App. cl. V 13; s. XIV—XVI. f. 6 (Inc. Ὁ στόμαχος ἢ κατὰ ποιότητα τρέπει τοὺς σφυγμούς, ἥτις θεωρεῖται. Expl. ὁ ἀνίσως πλήττων τὴν ἀφήν).

Metrodora.

Περὶ τῶν γυναικείων παθῶν τῆς μήτρας.
De mulierurn morbis uteri.

Vgl. Costomiris, Rev. des ét. gr. III [1890] p. 147.

Inc. Τῶν γυναικείων παθῶν πολλῶν τε.
Expl. οὗ ἐπίχριε τὸν στόμαχον.

Florenz: Laurent. plut. 75, 3; s. XII. f. 4—33 (*Vgl.* Daremb. Orib. I p. XXV. *Abschrift besitzt Mr. E. O. Winstedt, Oxford*).

Mnesitheus Cyzicenus.

Excerpta varia.

Paris: Parisin. 2240; s. XVI. f. 156 (Fragmentum de brassica. Inc. Κράμβην χρὴ κατακόψαι (*Aus* Oribas. I 278 sq.).

[Diels II.66]

Moschion.

Ὑποθῆκαι.
Praecepta vitae.

Inc. Παραφύλαττε σεαυτὸν ἐν παντὶ τῷ βίῳ.
Expl. ἐν τῷ τρόπῳ κιβδηλείας.

Oxford: Baroccian. 173; s. XII. XIII. f. 349.

Muscio.

Περὶ γυναικείων παθῶν.
De morbis mulierum.

Leyden: B. P. 62 A; s. XV.
München: Monac. 511; s. XVI.

Paris: Parisin. 2152; a. 1539. f. 1.
Wien: Vindob. med. 39; a. 1561. f. 5v—52v (Inc. Ὁπηνίκα συνεχῶς ἡμῖν ἐν ταῖς γυναιξὶν ἡ μαῖα ἐγεγόνει. Expl. ἢ φόβου ἢ ὀργιλότητος. *Collation mit der Ausgabe von Dewezius 1793 im Berol. fol. 39 [275]*).

Nemesius Emesenus.

(*Vgl.* Gregorius Nyssenus.)

Περὶ φύσεως ἀνθρώπου.
De natura hominis.

Ed. Chr. Fr. Matthaei, Halae 1802.
Migne Patrol, gr. 40 p. 503—818.
Vgl. Burkhard, Wiener Stud. X 93—135. XI 143—152. 243—267.

Inc. Τὸν ἄνθρωπον ἐκ ψυχῆς νοερᾶς καὶ σώματος κατεσκευασμένον.
Expl. διὰ τὸ συμφέρειν ἐκείνοις ἀφείλοντο.

Athen: nr.
375; s. XIII. no. 11.
447 (146); s. XVI. no. 16.
Athos: Βιβλ. μον. Διονυσίου 3799. 265; s. XV. no. 2.
Berlin: Phillipps. 1557; s. XVI. f. 1 (Inc. mutil. [τοί]νυν ὡς ἐν εἰκόνι = Migne Patrol. 40 p. 529, 16).
Bologna: Bonon. A I 13; s. XVI. f. 1. [Diels II.67]
Breslau: Vratisl. Rhedig. bibl. urb. 34; s. XV. f. 1—54v.
Brüssel: Bruxell. 11351—52; s. XVI (Inc. cap. 2 διαφωνεῖται σχεδόν).
Dresden: Dresd.
Da 57; s. XII. f. 1.
Da 58*; s. XV. f. 1 (capp. 35—38).
Escurial: Scorial.
Σ. III. 17*; s. XVI. f. 141 (Inc. Μέχρι τοῦ βάθους διϊκνεῖσθαι πέφυκεν ἡ ὄψις. Expl. ἐπειδὴ δὲ τῶν αἰσθητικῶν ἡδονῶν οἱ μὲν ἄλλαις ...).
X. I. 11; s. XVI. f. 1.
X. II. 9; a. 1564. f. 1 (fine mutil.).
Florenz: Laur. plut.
7, 2; s. XV (*aus Dresd. Da 57 abgeschr.*).
7, 35; s. XIV. f. 196.
56, 21; s. XV (*aus Monac. 419 abgeschr.*).
86, 6; s. XII. f. 1 (Ἀδαμαντίωνος τοῦ καὶ Νεμεσίου).

Jerusalem:
Bibl. d. hl. Grabes
273; s. X. f. 182b.
405; a. 1717. f. 124.
Bibl. patriarch. 15; s. XI. *hinter* f. 137.
Karlsruhe: Caroliruh. 451; s. XVI. f. 1—128 (*aus Monac. 419 abgeschr.*).
London: Harleian. (Brit. Mus.) 5685; s. XII—XI (s. XIII *nach M. Thompson*). f. 1.
Lyon: Lugdun. Bibl. des Dép. 52*; s. XVI—XVII. f. 134 (Theodoreti, Cyri episcopi, Nemesii etc. excerpta et interrogationes de rebus theologicis).
Madrid: Matrit. bibl. nac. 4759 (ol. N 138); s. XVI. f. 167.
Mailand: Ambros.
B 39 Sup.*; s. XIV—XV. f. 26.
D 338 Inf.; s. XV. f. 1.
F 88 Sup. s. XV. f. 163^{v} (Expl. δόγμασι παραλειπτέον = 144, 10 Matth.).
Modena: Mutin.
18 (III A 4); s. XV.
240 (III F 17); s. XV—XVI. f. 111 (Expl. καὶ τῆς ἐνεργείας λαμβάνοντες, δέον = Migne 40 p. 601, 5).
München: Monac.
29; s. XVI. f. 108—159. 170^{v}—175^{v}. (Expl. ἐπιδέουσιν ἀπαράβατον = 301, 4 Matth.).
100; a. 1551. f. 152—170^{v} (*Ergänzung der vorhergehenden Hds.*).
419; s. XIV. f. 1 (Expl. τὰ αὐτὰ παρὰ πᾶσιν = 331, 2 Matth.).
536; s. XV. f. 1 (Inscr. Ἀδαμαντίωνος λόγος κεφαλαιώδης).
562; s. XVI. XI. f. 1.
Oxford:
Baroccian.
82; s. XV. f. 156 (Expl. mutil. καὶ μηδένα edit. Oxon. 1671 p. 305, 13).
94*; s. XV. f. 43 (Liber Nemesii . . in epitomam redactus, forsan ab Andrea Dono).
Canonic. 56; s. XVI. f. 55.
Miscell.
69; s. XI (?). f. 23b (In capita 58 distributus. De hominis opificio).
162; s. XV.
d'Orvillian.
X 1. 4. 3; *nach* 1500 (Expl. τὸ δὲ ἀντικείμενον ἀδύνατον).
X 2. 6. 2 (= 432); s. — (»*A copy of the 1671 Oxford edition, with a collation of a ms. by J. P. d'Orville*«).
Paris:
Coisl.
115*; s. XII. f. 131^{v}. 170^{v}.

120*; s. X. f. 99. 116v.
259*; a. 1056. f. 128.
294*; s. XII. f. 18.

Parisin.
825; s. XVI. f. 1.
826; s. XVI.
827; s. XVI.
827 A*; s. XVI. (Nemesii? Inc. Τὴν κακίαν Πλωτῖνος μέν).
1044; s. XIV. f. 1 (*beginnt c. 2 p. 102, 1 Matth., schließt* 368, 10; *abgeschr. aus Dresd. Da 57*).
1045; a. 1501. f. 1.
1046; s. XVI.
1268; s. XII. f. 53.
1603; s. XVI. f. 224.
1739; s. XV. f. 340.
2077; s. XV. f. 66.
2225; s. XV. f. 50.
2295; s. XIV. f. 50.
2299; s. XV. f. 104.
2428; s. XVI. f. 116 (Sub nomine Adamantionis).

Suppl.
86; s. XVII.
148; s. XVI.
194; s. XVI. f. 2 (Sub nomine Adamantii).
640; s. XVI.
641; s. XVIII.
702; s. XV—XVI. f. 43v.

Bibl. de Paris 42*; s. XVI. f. 131v (Excerpta varia, ed. Oxon. 1671 capp. 39—41. 29—34. 42. 44. 35. 38).

Rom:

Barber.
V 18*; s. XI. f. 136v.
VI 5*; s. XIV/XV. f. 71.

Ottobon.
275*; s. XVII. f. 76.
464; s. XVI. f. 1.

Palat.
370; s. XV. f. 1v.
385; s. XV—XVI. f. 121.

Vatic.
423; s. XIII. f. 227v (Inc. Τὸν ἄνθρωπον ἴσμεν. Expl. τῆς αὐτοῦ βασιλείας. Frgm.?).

489; s. XV—XVI. f. 3.
Patmos: Patmiac. —; s. X.
Venedig: Marc. 266; s. XV. f. 99ᵛ.
Wien: Vind.
phil.
34 s. XVI (*aus Dresd. Da 57*).
181*; s. XVII. f. 171 (ἀδαμαντίνου νεμεσίνου [!]; *capp. 9—11. 16 Schl. 18—44 fehlen*).
theol.
68; s. XVI (*aus Monac. 419 abgeschr.).*
199*; s. XVI. f. 1.

[Diels II.68]

Neophytus Prodromenus.

Συλλογὴ κατὰ στοιχεῖον περὶ βοτανῶν.
Remediorum collectio alphabetica.

Inc. Ἀμάρακον καὶ λευκάνθεμον.

Berlin: Phillipps. 1570; s. XVI. f. 55.
Mailand: Arch. del Capitolo Metrop. 2; s. XV. f. 129—132ᵛ (Expl. ὤκυμον τὸ βασιλικόν).
Oxford: Miscell. 278; a. 1780. p. 135.
Paris: Parisin.
2256; s. XV. f. 540.
2286; s. XIV. f. 105. 108ᵛ.
Rom: Palat. 77; s. XIV. f. 3.
Venedig: Marcian. App. cl. V, 13; s. XIV—XVI. f. 8—25 (Expl. mutil. τῶν ὀλεθρίων ὑφισταμένων τὰ μέν ἐστι κριμνώδη ...).

Περὶ τῶν τοῖς ὀδοῦσι παθῶν.
De dentium doloribus.

Athen: nr. 1481; s. XVI. no. 1.

Nepualius.

Περὶ τῶν κατὰ συμπάθειαν καὶ ἀντιπάθειαν.
De sympathicis et antipathicis.

Ed. Fabricius, Bibl. gr. IV p. 295—301 [edit. I].
Gemoll, Progr. Striegau 1884 p. 1—3.
Vgl. E. Rohde, Kl. Schriften I p. 383 sq.

Inc. Ἐπιστάμενός σου τὸ φιλομαθὲς καὶ εἰς πάντα φιλότιμον.
Expl. ὅπου ἂν γάρον ἀφ' ἑσπέρας ῥάνῃς.

Mailand: Ambros.
R 111b; s. —.
S 3 Sup.; s. XV ex.—XVI in. f. 117—120b.
Rom:
Vallicell. — (Allatianus); s. —.
Vatic. 299; s. XV. f. 495b.

Nicolaus Myrepsus.

[Diels II.69]

Δυναμερόν.
De compositione medicamentorum, alphabetice.

Berlin: Phillipps. 1583 (ol. Meerm. 300); s. XV. f. 1 (Sine auctoris nomine).
Escurial: Scorial. Σ. II. 3; s. XVI. f. 12.
Oxford: Baroccian. 171; s. XV. f. 8 (Inc. Ἀντίδοτος Ἀλεξανδρεία).
Paris: Parisin.
2149; s. XVI. f. 102 (»Desunt B—Z«).
2237; s. XIV. f. 7.
2238; s. XV. f. 1.
2243; a. 1339. f. 11v.

Περὶ ἐμπλάστρων.
De emplastris.

Paris: Parisin. 2315; s. XV. f. 276.

Excerpta.

Oxford: Baroccian. 150; s. XV in. f. — (Medicamentum. *Vgl.* Medicae artis principes ed. Stephanus, col. 408).

Nicomedes Iatrosophista.

Lexicon medicum.

Athos: Βιβλ. μον. Ἰβήρων 4271. 151; s. XV. f. 11 (Inc. Ἀκτὶς ἡ κουφοξυλέα. Expl. Ὤνια τὰ ἐν ταῖς δρύαις [?] ζῷα. ὑποσταθμὴ ἐλαίου τρυγαῖα).
Paris: Parisin. 2224; s. XV. f. 71.

Nicomedes.

Εἰς Ἱπποκράτην.
Versus in Hippocratem.

Inc. Ἱπποκράτης φάος ἦν μερόπων.
Expl. ἦν σπάνις εἰς ἀίδη.

Wien: Vindob. med. 31; s. XV ex. f. 166ᵛ.

[Diels II.70]

Ocianus.

Περὶ συνθέσεως φαρμάκων λόγος πέμπτος.
De compositione medicamentorum liber V.

Inc. Ἐπὶ τοῖς προεκτεθεῖσι βιβλίοις.
Expl. μέλιτος τὸ ἀρκοῦν.

Athos: Βιβλ. μον. Ἰβήρων 4271. 151; s. XV. f. 184.

Olymnius Alexandrinus.

Περὶ κατακλίσεως.
De decubitu.

Inc. Κατεκλίθη τοίνυν ὁ νοσῶν ἐν ἀρχῇ.
Expl. ἐπὶ τοῦ προγνωστικοῦ ἡμᾶς ἐδίδαξεν.

Cheltenham: Phillipps. 6763; s. XV (XIV Cat. *und* Schenkl). f. 29ᵛ.

Excerpta.

Cheltenham: Phillipps. 6763; s. XV (XIV Catal. *und* Schenkl). f. 29 (Inc. Τῶν κρισίμων ἡμερῶν αἱ μὲν κατὰ σύλληψίν εἰσιν. Expl. καὶ ἐν ἐνιαυτῷ καὶ ἐν ἑπτὰ ἔτεσι).
Paris: Parisin. 2286; s. XIV. f. 55 (Excerpta de criticis diebus etc.).

Oribasius.

Opera varia.

Padua:
Bibl. Ioannis Rhodii (*Verbleib unbekannt*).
Bibl. S. Ioannis in Viridario, ad dextr. plut. XVI (*Verbleib unbekannt*).
Salamanca: Bibl. Univ. (Epistt. septem).

Ἰατρικαὶ συναγωγαὶ πρὸς Ἰουλιανόν.
Medicae collectiones ad Iulianum.
Libri I—X. XIV—XV. XXI—XXII. XXIV—XXV. XLIV—LI.

Edd. Daremberg-Bussemaker tom. I—IV.

Inc. (prooem.) Τὰς προσταχθείσας ἐπιτομὰς παρὰ τῆς σῆς θειότητος, αὐτόκρατορ Ἰουλιανέ.
Expl. (lib. 51) καὶ τὰ νέα καὶ ἁπαλὰ σφαιρία σὺν ἀλφίτοις.

Berlin:
Phillipps.
1532 (ol. Meerm. 225); s. XVI. f. 1ᵛ (L. XXIV. XXV).
1533 (ol. Meerm. 226); s. XVI. f. 1 (L. XLVI—XLVIII fine mutil.).
fol. 35 (271)*; s. IX (? Fragmentum. Inc. προσήσθαιτο· πολλοῖς γοῦν καὶ μόνον ἐξήρκεσεν = L. VII 26, 167; Dbg.-Buss. II p. 134, 7. Expl. πρῶτον μὲν τὸ δύσεργον καὶ τοῦτο = ibid. 26, 179; Dbg.-Buss. p. 138, 5. 6).
Budapest: Mus. nat. Hungar. 9 fol.; s. XVI. f. 23ᵛ—35ᵛ (L. III *z. T. in veränderter Fassung*).
Cambridge: Coll. St. Johann. A 6; s. XV—XVI (L. I—XV).
[Diels II.71] **Escurial:** Scorial. Φ. I. 2; s. XVI. f. 16ᵛ. 43ᵛ (L. XXIV. XXV).
Florenz: Laurent. plut.
74, 7; s. IX. p. 89b (L. XLVI—XLIX).
74, 17; s. XII. f. 1 (Inc. Ἡ ὠμαία κατ' ἀγκῶνα).
Heidelberg: Bibl. Univ. 375; s. XIV. no. 3 (Liber XXIV, init. et fine mutil.).
Leipzig: Lipsiens. 59; s. XIX. no. 1 (L. XLIII).
Leyden: Vossian. 9.
London:
Burneian. (Brit. Mus.) 94; s. XV (XVI). f. 170 (L. XXIV. XXV. Expl. ἀλλὰ καὶ βολῆς τινος προσδεῖν).
Medical Society Wf 6; s. — (L. I—X. XIV).
Moskau: Mosquens.? (*Abschrift von Buch 4. 6. 9. 14 des cod. Mosquensis im Berol. fol. 39 [275]*).
München: Monac. 29*; s. XVI. f. 81 (L. VII 2 *und* 13).
Neapel:
Neapolit. 304 D III 20; s. XIV (L. I—XV).
Bibl. S. Giovanni di Carbonara 42; s. XV (L. I—XV).
Oxford: Baroccian. 224*; s. XV in. f. 1 (*Wie im* Monac. 29).
Paris:
Parisin.
1883; s. XIV (L. III 65 [bis]. VII 26 [*vgl.* Oribas. II praef. p. 5 *und* p. 90 sq.]. cap. 26—40 libror. incert.).
2151; s. XVI. f. 12 (L. XXIV. XXV).
2189; s. XVI (Libri XV).
2190; s. XV (L. I—X).
2237; s. XIV (L. IX 52—55. X 13. 14. 19—36. XXI. XXII. LIV. XXIV 30—36. c. 21 librorum incert. XXI 7 bis).
2247; s. XVI (L. XLVI—XLIX).
2248; s. XVI (*Wie im* Parisin. 2247).
2261; s. XVI. f. 37 (L. XXIV. XV).
2262; s. XVI. f. 31 (*Wie im* Parisin. 2261).

2263; s. XVI. f. 28v (*Wie im* Parisin. 2261).
2321; s. XVI. f. 11v (*Wie im* Parisin. 2261).
2510; s. XIV. (L. I 5. 15—65. II 1—53. III. 21 26—28. 31—34 abbrev.).
Suppl. 446*; s. X (L. XLIV 5—8. 23. XLV 26 *und* Ἐκλογαὶ βοηθημάτων).
Bibl. de Paris 57; s. XVII. f. 18 (L. XLVIII).

Rom:
Ottobon. 235; s. —. f. 17 (L. XXIV—XXV 58).
Palat. 375; s. XII. f. 230 (L. XXIV. XXV).
Vatic.
288; s. XV. f. 1 (L. I—XV).
1835; s. —. f. — (L. XLIV—LI).
1885*; s. XIV. f. 1 (Inc. Τῶν τοιούτων .... αὐτῷ μέν. *Vgl.* A. Mai, Auctor. class. IV p. 276—278).

Turin: Taurin.? (L. XXIV. XXV).
Vicenza: Bertolian. 44 (1. 6. 15); s. XVI. no. 2—4 (Libri XXIV. XXV).
Wien: Vindob. med. 16 (ol. 35); s. — (Capp. 43 extr. 44 librorum incert. = Oribas. III p. 230 sq. Dbg.-Buss.).

Σύνοψις πρὸς Εὐστάθιον τὸν υἱὸν αὐτοῦ.
Conspectus ad Eustathium filium. Libri IX.

Dbg.-Buss. V 1—556.

Inc. (lib. 1) Κελεύσαντος τοῦ Ἰουλιανοῦ ποτε τοῦ θειοτάτου αὐτοκράτορος.
Expl. (lib. 9) ἡ δὲ λοιπὴ χρῆσις ἡ αὐτή.

Athos: Βιβλ. μον. Ἰβήρων 4436. 316*; s. XVII. f. 102 (Inc. Ὅσα θερμαίνει μετρίως).
Berlin: Phillipps. 1581 (ol. Meerm. 297)*; s. XVI. f. 289v (Π. ὑδάτων = Dbg.-Buss. V p. 192—193, 6).
Budapest: Mus. nat. Hungar. 9 fol.*; s. XVI. f. 1—10v.
Escurial: Scorial. y. I. 9; s. XVI. f. 1.
Florenz: Laurent. plut.
74, 15; s. XIV. p. 1.
74, 17. s. XII. p. 1.

Mailand: Ambros. D 13 Sup.; s. —. f. 1.
Moskau: Mosquens. 498; s. XVI. f. 2.
Oxford: d'Orvill. X 1. 1. 3; s. XV ex. f. 1.
Paris:
Facult. med. 145 (ol. Bibl. de Paris 59); a. 1841—42 (*Apographon des* Parisin. 2188).

Parisin.
2188; s. XV. f. 1.
3099*; s. —. f. 13 (Fragmentum).
Rom:
Barberin. I 118; s. XIV. f. 1.
Ottobon. 129; s. XVII. f. 1.
Vatic.
287; s. XV. f. 1.
1427*; s. XVI. f. 1.
Salamanca: Bibl. Univ. 1. 1. 11; a. 1524. f. 1.
Venedig: Marcian. 294; s. XIV.
Wien: Vindob. med. 42; s. XVI—XVII. f. 1—333 (Expl. βέβαιον λάβωμεν περὶ τοῦ μένειν κατεσταλμένον. »Die letzten Capitel des I. Buches, von Buch IV das Cap. de aquis u. die Bücher V—XI [*IX?*] Abschrift« *im* Berol. fol. 39 [275]).

[Diels II.72]

Πρὸς Εὐνάπιον περὶ εὐπορίστων.
Ad Eunapium de parabilibus medicamentis. Libri IV.

Dbg.-Buss. V 557—797.

Inc. (lib. 1) Ἐξ ὧν ἡμῖν διελέχθης, Εὐνάπιε κράτιστε.
Expl. (lib. 4) ἑψήσας μόνον ἐν τῇ προγεγραμμένῃ συμμετρίᾳ.

Athos: Βιβλ. μον. Ἰβήρων 4436. 316*; s. XVII. f. 102.
Berlin: Phillipps. 1568 (ol. Meerm. 271)*; s. XVI. f. 1 (L. I 14—17).
Budapest: Mus. nat. Hungar. 9 fol.; s. XVI. f. 11—23. 66—158v (Expl. τοσοῦτον ἐμβάλῃς ὄξους ὅσον μέλιτος).
Moskau: Mosquens. 499; s. XVI. f. 3.
München: Monac. 72; s. XVI. f. 1.
Paris: Parisin.
2177; s. XVI. f. 10.
2335; s. XVI.
Rom:
Ottobon. 129; s. XVII. f. 38.
Vatic. 1427; s. XVI. f. 70 (Expl. in cap. Ἐφημέρων πυρετῶν ἰάσεις).
Venedig: Marcian. 294; s. XIV. f. 9.

Excerpta varia. [Diels II.73]

Athos:

Βιβλ. μον Ἰβήρων 4302. 181; s. XVI. f. 29 B—145 (Ἰατροσόφιον κατ' ἀλφάβητον).

Κουτλουμουσίου 3321. 248; s. XVII.

Berlin: Berol. 39 (275); s. — (»Collationen kleinerer Stücke«).

Bologna: Bonon.

1808; s. XV. f. 30^{v} (φουλ$^{\overline{\iota\gamma}}$ σκευασία) *und* f. 267 (Πρὸς πάρεσιν τοῦ αἰδοίου μάλιστα γερόντων).

3632; s. XV. f. 204 (Περὶ τῶν ἀντιδότων cap. ρλθ', extremum ἀληθυριακὸν Ὀρ.).

Budapest: Mus. nat. Hungar. 9 fol.; s. XVI. f. 35^{v}. 36 (Inc. Συκάμινα βάτινα. Expl. ἐπεμβάλλειν αὐτῷ) *und* f. 36—65^{v} (Περὶ τῆς δυνάμεως τῶν ἁπλῶν κατὰ στοιχεῖον. Inc. Ὅσα μὲν εἰδέναι τέ σε καὶ ποιεῖν. Expl. καὶ ἀδήκτως ξηραίνει).

Carpentras: nr. 1774; s. XVII. f. 140^{v} (De ponderibus et mensuris manifestum experimentum medicum).

Dresden: Dresd. Da 5; a. 1519. f. 249 (Περὶ οὔρων).

Florenz: Laurent.

— (Ἐκ τῶν Ὀρ. ὑγιεινῶν παραγγελμάτων).

plut. 74, 7; s. IX. p. 89b (Ἐκ τῶν Γαλ. περὶ καταγμάτων. Inc. Ἐπειδὴ λέλυται), p. 117 (Ἐκ τῶν Γαλ. περὶ ἐξαρθρημάτων. Inc. Τῶν ἐξαρθρημάτων), p. 129 (Ἐκ τοῦ Ἡρακλᾶ πῶς πλέκεται βρόχος ὁ ἐρτός), p. 129b (Ἐκ τῶν Γαλ. περὶ ἐπιδέσμων), p. 148b (Ἐκ τῶν Ἡλιοδώρου περὶ διαφορᾶς καταρτισμῶν).

Mailand: Ambros. D 13 Sup.; s. —. f. 300^{v} (Περὶ οὔρων. Inc. Ἡ θεία φύσις ποιήσασα τὸν ἄνθρωπον. Expl. mutil. ἐν τῷ οὔρῳ φαινόμενα, τῆς κύστεως ... Inscr. man. rec. [Diels II.74] Ὀριβασίου περὶ οὔρων, in mg. ┌ᴾ Ἰωάννου ἐπισκόπου Πρισδριανῶν).

Messina: Messan. bibl. univ. 84; s. — (*Vgl.* Rühl, Philol N. S. I p. 577—588).

Moskau: Mosquens. 260; a. 1630. f. 254^{v} (Inc. Εὐεξίας τράπεζαν, εἰ θέλεις, μάθε).

Oxford: Baroccian. 150; s. XV in. f. 20^{v} (Περὶ ἁπλῶν φαρμάκων κράσεων καὶ μίξεων ὑγιεινῶν κτηνῶν ὁμοῦ καὶ πτηνῶν τῆς ἄγρας κτέ. Inc. Ἐν ἀγρῷ εἰς ἕνα τόπον. Expl. χυλὸς σὺν οἴνῳ ἐγχυματιζόμενος) *und* f. 77 (Pauca de simplicibus ex ... Oribasio).

Paris:

Facult. med.

—; s. — (De fracturis fragmenta).

14 (ol. Bibl. de Paris 57); s. XVII. f. 18 (De ligamentis et machinamentis chirurgicis, ex Heraclide Ephesio [lib. 48]).

Parisin.

1883; s. XIV (*Vgl.* D.-Buss. I p. XXXVI).

2149; s. XVI. f. 159 (De mensuris et ponderibus ex Orib. et Gal.) *und* f. 201 (Orib. et Gal. capita varia de re medica).

2208; s. XI—XV. f. 285^{v} (Opuscula) *und* f. 385 (Orib. et Adamantii fragmenta de ponderibus et mensuris).

2237; s. XIV. f. 165[v] (Collectionis medicinalis ex Galeno Orib. Aetio libri IV—X).

2240; s. XVI. f. 45 (De antidotis, emplastris, oleis) *und* f. 92[v] (De plantis et metallis).

2243; a. 1339. f. 640 (De mensuris et ponderibus).

2337; s. XV—XVI. f. 1 (Anon. collectio medicorum, ex Oribasio etc.).

2408; s. XIII. f. 224[v] (S. Artemii martyris, Iuliani imp. et Oribasii medici dialogus de Apolline Delphico).

2510; a. 1384. f. 125 (Remedia varia, inter quae ... Oribasii).

3076; a. 1616. f. 56 (De nephritide).

Suppl.

446; s. X. f. 35[v]—38[v] (Ὀφθαλμικά; *vgl.* Costomiris Revue des ét. gr. III 148) *und* f. 168 (Eclogae ex Orib. *Vgl.* Dbg.-Buss. I p. XXXVI. Littré, Revue de philologie II [1846—47]).

683; s. XVIII. f. 1[v].

1202; s. XIII. f. 16 (Exc. ex Diosc. Orib. aliis).

Rom:

Angelic. 17 (C 5. 4); s. XIV. f. 91 (Βίβλος περιέχουσα περὶ ἁπλῶν φαρμάκων, κράσεων καὶ μίξεων ὑγιεινῶν νοσούντων καὶ κτηνῶν ὁμοῦ καὶ τῶν πτηνῶν τῆς ἄγρας κτλ. Inc. Ἀπείρου σκευασία ξυροῦ. *Vgl.* Baroccian. 150. f. 20[v]).

Vatic. 876; s. XV. f. 3 (*Wie im* Laurent. —. *Vgl.* Dbg.-Buss. I p. XXXV.).

Turin: Taurinens. 333b I 1; s. XVI. f. 66 (Γαληνοῦ περὶ ἀνατομῆς sive potius Oribasii anatomica ex libris Galeni desumpta. Libri IV. *Durch Feuer stark beschädigt*).

Venedig: Marcian. 293; s. XV. f. 291 (»Quaedam instar prologi generalis in medicinam quae Oribasio tribuantur«. Inc. *wie im* Ambros. D 13 Sup. Expl. mutil. καὶ ἐὰν διὰ τέλους ...).

Wien: Vindob. med. 27; s. XVI. f. 122 (Περὶ τὸ πῶς χρὴ γιγνώσκειν τὸ αἷμα. Inc. Δεῖ σε γινώσκειν τοῦτο ὅτι τὸ αἷμα ὃ προφαίνεται. Expl. ἵνα μὴ διαβοῦν καὶ τὰ ἔγκατα αὐτῆς).

[Diels II.75]

Orpheus.

Περὶ λίθων.
De lapidibus.

Ed. E. Abel, Orphei Lithica. Berol. 1881. p. 138—153.
F. de Mély, Les lapidaires de l'antiquité II p. 160—173.

Inc. Λίθος κρύσταλλος ὁ πᾶσι γνώριμος.
Expl. φανεροῦσαν τὰ μέλλοντα τῷ φοροῦντι.

Oxford: Baroccian. 131; s. XIV in. f. 175ᵛ.
Paris: Parisin.
2228; s. XIV—XI. f. 50.
2419; ca. a. 1460. f. —.
Rom: Vatic. 578; s. XV.
Wien: Vindob. med. 30; s. XV. f. 477 (Expl. mutil. καὶ εὐόμιλον καὶ εὐπειθῆ καὶ δυνατόν. *Abschrift im Berol. fol. 39 [275]*).

Palladius.

Περὶ πυρετῶν σύντομος σύνοψις.
Stephani philosophi vel Palladii synopsis de febribus.

Ed. I. St. Bernard, Lugd. Bat. 1745.
Ideler, Phys. et Med. I p. 107—120.
Vgl. Stephanus *und* Theophilus.

Inc. Σκοπὸν ἔχομεν ἐν τῷ παρόντι.
Expl. αἱ διαφοραὶ τῶν πυρετῶν.

Bologna: Bonon. 3632*; s. XV. f. 132 (Initium tantum [Ideler p. 107, 1—17] comparari potest cum libro Palladii).
Escurial: Scorial. T. II. 14*; s. XVI. f. 177 (Inc. Ὁπηνίκα γὰρ πλεονάσει. Expl. πρὸς τὴν διαφορὰν τῆς ὕλης. *Vgl.* Ideler p. 109, 35 sq).
Florenz: Laurent. plut. 74, 11; s. XIII. f. 211ᵛ (Scholia in Galeni de febrium differentiis. *Vgl.* Palat. 297).
Oxford: Baroccian. 88; s. XV—XVI. f. 51ᵛ—54ᵛ (Expl. διαφοραὶ τῶν πυρετῶν. ἁλμυρώδεας δὲ λέγει τοὺς συμβαίνοντας τοῖς ὑπερκοπωθεῖσιν, ὡς γινομένου ξηροτέρου τοῦ δέρματος οἷον ἐπὶ τῶν ταριχευομένων σωμάτων. Verba ἁλμυρώδεας κτλ. apud Idelerum desunt).
Paris: Parisin.
2218; s. XVI. f. 1.
2269; s. XV. f. 84.
Rom:
Palat. 297; s. XV—XVI (Ex Galeno de febrium substantia et differentiis praevio indice. *Vgl.* Laurent. 74, 11. Inc. prol. Σκοπὸν οὖν ἔχομεν).
Vatic. 283; s. XIV. f. 16ᵛ.

Περὶ βρώσεως καὶ πόσεως.
De cibo et potione.

Ed. Dietz, Schol. in Hipp. II praef. p. VII.

Inc. Δεῖ εἰδέναι ὅτι τὸ στόμα.
Expl. δέχεται τὴν κόπρον.

Florenz: Laurent. plut. 74, 2; s. XI. p. 282b.
Rom: Reg. Suec. 176; s. XIV. f. 302.

[Diels II.76] Σχόλια εἰς τὸ περὶ ἀγμῶν Ἱπποκράτους.
Scholia in Hippocratis de fracturis.

Ed. Foesius, Hippocr. Opera [Genevae 1657] I p. 917—933.
Vgl. Stephanus Alexandr.

Inc. Τὰ εἰωθότα προλέγεσθαι ὀκτὼ κεφάλαια.
Expl. κατὰ τὸ κείμενον παραδιδούς. ἐν οἷς σὺν θεῷ ἡ θεωρία.

Florenz: Laurent. plut. 74, 7; s. IX. p. 299b.

Σχόλια τῆς ἕκτης ἐπιδημίας ἀπὸ φωνῆς Παλλαδίου σοφιστοῦ.
Scholia in Hippocratis de popularibus morbis librum sextum, sectiones VIII.

Ed. Dietz, Scholia in Hipp. II p. 1—204.

Inc. Ἄρτι ταῖς μεθόδοις τὰ ὀξέα.
Expl. οὐ βραδέως γενομένη ἐπίληπτος.

Berlin: Phillipps. 1525 (ol. Meerm. 215); s. XVI. f. 1.
Escurial: Scorial. y. I. 8; s. XVI. f. 82.
Florenz: Laurent. plut.
75, 21*; s. XIII. p. 251 (»Sextae et septimae sectionis fragmentum« = Dietz II p. 161, 21—171, 34. 177, 18—198, 19).
75, 22; s. XV. p. 1.
Mailand: Ambros. B 113 Sup.; s. XIV in. f. 85.
Paris: Parisin. 2295; s. XVI.
Rom: Urbin. 64; s. XIII. f. 94 (Sub Galeni nomine).

Εἰς Γαληνοῦ περὶ αἱρέσεων σχόλια.
In Galeni librum de sectis scholia.

Florenz: Laurent. plut. 74, 11; s. XIII. p. 200—242ᵛ (Expl. mutil. *Abschrift besitzt Dr. E. Bianchi, Florenz*).

Excerpta varia.

Paris: Parisin. 2210; a. 1357. f. 368.

Pamphilus.

Excerpta.

Bologna: Bonon. 1808; s. XV. f. 33 (Θυμίαμα ῥοδάτον τοῦ ἐπισκόπου Π.).

Pancharius.

Περὶ κατακλίσεως νοσούντων ἐπιτομή.
Compendium de decubitu infirmorum.

Paris: Parisin. 2139; s. XVII. f. 70ᵛ.
Rom:
Barberin. I 127; s. XVI. f. 197ᵛ.
Vatic. 1444; s. XV. f. 235ᵛ.

Excerpta. [Diels II.77]

Paris: Parisin. 1991; s. XV. f. 29ᵛ (Excerpta de rebus medico-astrologicis).

Paulus Aegineta.

Ἐπιτομῆς ἰατρικῆς βιβλία ἑπτά.
Epitomae medicae libri septem.

Ed. Basileae 1538.
Liber VI ed. René Briau, Paris 1855.

Inc. Οὐχ ὡς τῶν παλαιοτέρων ἐν τοῖς κατὰ τὴν τέχνην.
Expl. διὰ σκίγκου ταχθεῖσαν εὑρήσεις.

Athos: Βιβλ. μον. Ἰβήρων 4436. 316; s. XVII. f. 134 B (Lib. I Διόρθωσις τῶν θερμῶν δυσκρασιῶν) *und* f. 136 A (Ἴασις τῶν ξηρῶν δυσκρασιῶν κτλ.).
Basel: Bibl. univ. F VI 46; s. XVI. f. 9 (L. VI 15. 16).
Bologna: Bonon. 3636*; s. XIV—XV. f. 140ᵛ (L. III 26. 25. 52. 54. 81. L. VI 85. 86. 87. L. III 58. L. I 43—46. 51. 203. L. III 27. L. II 12).
Escurial: Scorial.
R. I. 12; s. XV. f. 91ᵛ (Liber VI).
Y. III. 14; s. XV. f. 188 (Liber VII init. mutil.).
Φ. I. 2; s. XVI. f. 73ᵛ (L. VI 8 ἀνωτέρω τῶν κατὰ φύσιν τριχῶν. Expl. τὸν ἁρμόζοντα δεῖ ποιεῖσθαι χειρισμόν).
Φ. III. 12; s. XV. f. 421 (Liber II).
Ω. I. 8*; s. XIV. f. 1. 26. 31ᵛ. 42 etc.
Florenz: Laurent. plut.
74, 2; s. XI. p. 1.
74, 7*; s. IX. p. 239b (Libri VII. capp. 89—112) *und* p. 252b (Libri VI. cap. 42).
74, 17*; s. XII. p. 106b (Libri I. capp. 1—30).
74, 21*; s. XV. p. 1 (Libri VI. capp. 89—122), p. 36b (L. V 1. part. 2. 28. 29. 7. 11. L. VII 1. part. 17. 3), p. 46 (»X capp. forte eiusdem Pauli Aeg.«).
74, 23*; s. XIV. p. 204 (L. VII 26 extr. Inc. Ὁ σταθμὸς βάρει).
74, 24; s. XV. p. 1 (Liber VI).
74, 26; s. XIV. p. 1 (L. V—VII. »L. VI saec. xv scriptus est«),
74, 27; s. XIV. p. 1.
74, 29; s. XI. p. 1 (L. I—IV. L. V 22. 23. 26. 3).
74, 31; s. XIV. p. 1 (L. I—VII 25).
Jerusalem: Bibl. patriarch. 273; s. XVIII. f. 107 (L. III 15).
Leipzig: Lipsiens. 62; s. XIX (»Paul. Aeg. ex editione Aldina descriptus cum coniecturis Salmasii«).
Leyden: Voss. fol. 22; s. XV (Libri V).

London: Medical Society A Ac 2 = Wf 15; s. XV in. (L. I—VII. Expl. ψὼς ὅ ἐστι κόρος, $μο^{δι}$ λ̄).
Madrid: Matrit. bibl. nac.
4581 (ol. N 45); s. XII. f. 1 (L. IV inde a cap. 56) *und* f. 3ᵛ. 28ᵛ. 124 (L. V. VI. VII).
4616 (ol. N 84)*; s. XV. f. 132 (Liber VII c. 1—3).
4631 (ol. N 110); a. 1474. f. 86 (Liber VII c. 1—3 »alienis additis«. Wellmann).
Mailand: Ambros. B 126 Sup.; s. XIV. f. 1 (L. I—VII 2) *und* f. 143 (L. III 21).
Neapel: Neapolit. 306 III D 22; s. XIII (L. I—III lacunos.).
Oxford: Baroccian.
88; s. XVI (L. II 1—5).
224; s. XV in. f. 21ᵛ (L. V 1—47).
Padua: Bibl. S. Ioannis in Viridario ad dextr. plut. XVII (*Verbleib unbekannt*).
Paris:
Coislin.
8*; s. X. f. 1—283 (»Frgmta. l. III, sine auctor. nom. trad.«).
168; a. 1355. f. 1.
Parisin.
2047; s. XV. f. 30.
2149; s. XVI. f. 177 (Lib. de fracturis).
2191; s. XIV. f. 435 (L. VI usque ad c. 120 χειρισμόν).
2192; s. XV. f. 317ᵛ (L. VI 8—122).
2204; s. XVI. f. 43 (Liber VI).
2205; s. XI (Libri VII, fine mutili).
2206; s. XI (Libri VII, fine mutil.).
2207; a. 1299 (1294). f. 1.
2208; s. XIV. f. 1.
2209; s. XV. f. 1 (Libri VII, fine mutil.).
2210; a. 1357. f. 1.
2211; s. XVI.
2212; s. XV (Libri VII, fine mutil.).
2213; s. XVI.
2214; s. XVI.
2215; s. XVI (Libri VII, fine mutil.).
2216; s. XVI—XI (L. I—III, fine mutil.).
2217; s. XI—XV. f. 1 (L. III 28—VII). [Diels II.78]
2292; s. XIV.
2293; s. XIV (L. I—III, initio et fine mutili, graece et arabice).
2294*; s. XV. f. 1 (L. VII 3).
Suppl.
338; s. XIV. f. 1.
446; s. X. f. 114 (L. VI 1—63 omissis capp. 15—21).

494; s. XV. f. 5.
1156*; s. IX—XI. f. 23 (L. V—VI).
Patmos: Bibl. monast. St. Johannis 111; s. — (»paraît fort ancien«).
Rom:
Angelic. 17 (C 5. 4)*; s. XIV. f. 236 (L. III 49).
Reg. Suec. 176; s. XIV. f. 2.
Vatic.
295; s. XV. f. 1.
296; s. XV. f. 1.
299; s. XV. f. 153ᵛ (L. VII 26).
Salamanca: Bibl. univ. 1. 1. 14; s. XIV. f. 1.
Upsala: Bibl. acad. 8 (Sparfwenf. 49)*; s. XV. f. 104 (L. I 73 sq.).
Venedig:
Marcian.
292; a. 1306. f. 5.
293; s. XV. f. 1 (*Abschrift von* 292).
App. cl. V, 1; s. XV.
Wien: Vindob. med.
8; s. XV. f. 64 (L. I—VI χειρισμόν; *vgl.* Parisin. 2191).
48; s. XIV—XV. f. 197—236ᵛ (L. I—III in. Expl. διὰ τῆς ἱερᾶς ἀντιδότου καθαίρωμεν φλέγματός τε ...).
Wolfenbüttel: Guelferbyt. 2 (Gud. 47); s. —.

Dazu: Cod. Michael. Cantacuzeni *bei* Foerster de antiquit. et libris Constantinop. Progr. Rostock 1877.

De venenis
(= Epit. lib. V?).

Paris: Parisin. gr. 2293; s. XIV. (L. I—III, initio et fine mutili, graece et arabice).

Περὶ ἀντεμβαλλομένων ἐκ τῶν Γαληνοῦ.
De succedaneis, ex Galeno.

= Ἐπιτομ. ἰατρικ. L. VII c. 25.

Inc. Ἐν Ἀλεξανδρείᾳ.
Expl. ἀντὶ ὠκυμοειδοῦς ἡδύοσμον ἄγριον.

Athos: Βιβλ. μον. Ἰβήρων 4271. 151; s. XV. f. 8v. 125.
Berlin: Phillipps.
1570; s. XVI. f. 70.
1583; s. XV. f. 65v.
Dresden: Dresd. Da 5; a. 1519. f. 176v.
Escurial: Scorial.
R. I. 12; s. XV. *hinter* 'Επιτ. lib. VI.
Υ. III. 14; s. XV. f. 1v. 77v.
Φ. III. 12; s. XV. f. 467.
Florenz: Laurent.
plut.
74, 23; s. XIV. f. 200v.
75, 4; s. XV. p. 235.
75, 9; s. XV. p. 460. [Diels II.79]
75, 11; s. XV. p. 286.
75, 16; s. XV. p. 383b.
App. 2; s. XV. f. 245.
Magliabecch. 44; s. XII. f. 2.
Riccard. 71 (K II. 16); a. 1428. f. 108.
Jerusalem: Bibl. patriarch. 339; s. XVI. f. 64v.
London:
Brit. Mus.
Addit. (Brit. Mus.) 10, 058; s. XV. f. 151 (Expl. ὤκιμον τὸ βασιλικόν).
Harleian. (Brit. Mus.) 6305; s. XVI. f. 151 (?).
Medical Society H Hi 17 = We 30; s. XV in. f. 50 (Expl. ἀντὶ ὠοῦ τὸ λευκὸν γάλα γυναικίῳ).
Madrid: Matrit. bibl. nac. 4631 (ol. N 110); a. 1474. f. 147v.
Mailand:
Ambros. R 20 Sup.; s. —. f. 536.
Arch. del Capitolo Metrop. 2; s. XV. f. 135v—137.
Modena: Mutinens. 61 (III B 9); s. XV. f. 14.
München: Monac. 69; s. XV. f. 298.
Oxford: Miscell. 241; s. XV. f. 182.
Paris:
Coislin. 335; s. XV. f. 69.
Parisin.
2153; s. XV. f. 424v.
2240; s. XVI. f. 40.
2315; s. XV. f. 64v.
2318; s. XV. f. 72.
Suppl. 1193; s. XVI. f. 17.

Rom: Angelic. 68 (C 2. 7); s. XV.
Venedig: Marcian. 92; s. XIII. f. 39.
Wien: Vindob. med.
8; s. XV. f. 240.
21; s. —. f. 303—306.
26; s. XV. f. 303—305ᵛ (Expl. ἀντὶ ὠκίμου σισύμβριον).
29; s. XV. f. 459ᵛ.
40; s. XV. f. 65—71 (Expl. *wie im* Vindob. 26).

Περὶ οὔρων.
De urinis. Libri VII.

Paris: Parisin. 2153; s. XVI. f. 458.

Περὶ μέτρων καὶ σταθμῶν.
De mensuris et ponderibus.

Aldin. I. VII c. 26. f. 138.

Inc. Ὁ σταθμὸς βάρει μετρούμενος.
Expl. ὡς ἀληθῶς ἄριστοι.

Escurial: Scorial. R. I. 12; s. XV. *hinter* περὶ ἀντεμβαλλομένων.
Florenz: Laurent. plut. 74, 23; s. XIV. f. 204.
London: Harleian. (Brit. Mus.) 6305; s. XVI (?). f. 159 (Expl. διαφορά = Ald. f. 138ᵛ, 18).
Paris: Parisin. Suppl. 1297; s. XI. f. 119ᵛ.
Venedig: Marcian. 295; s. XIV. f. 176ᵛ (*Apographon des* Parisin.).
Wien: Vindob.
med.
8; s. XV. f. 281ᵛ (Expl. *wie im* Harleian.).
23*; s. XVI. f. 76 (Inscr. Ἑρμοῦ τοῦ τρισμεγίστου. Inc. Ὁ μακάριος τρισκραταιόφρων Ἑρμῆς. Expl. καὶ οὕτως θ'' τὸ ἔννατον).
25*; s. XV. f. 10 (Περὶ τῶν δηλούντων τοὺς σταθμοὺς καὶ τὰ μέτρα χαρακτήρων. Inc. Ἀλλ' ἐπειδή τινες. Expl. *wie im* Harleian.).
27*; s. XVI. f. 104ᵛ (Inc. Ἀλλὰ διὰ τῶν χαρακτήρων ταῦτα. Expl. *wie im* Vindob. med. 23).
32*; s. XVI. f. 31 (Inc. Τὸ ἡμίεκτον. Expl. ἑρμηνία τῶν σταθμῶν καὶ μέτρων καὶ ⟨π⟩ερὶ ἐλαίου καὶ οἴνου ... ἐτελειώθησαν).
phil. 178; s. XV. f. 24ᵛ—25ᵛ (Inc. Ὁ σταθμός. Expl. μικρὸν μύστρον <θ).

Excerpta varia.

Athen: nr. 1479; s. XIX (Ἰατροσόφιον ἀπηνθισμένον ἀπὸ Γαλ. Παύλου τοῦ Αἰγ. etc.).
Athos: Βιβλ. μον. Παντελεήμονος 5769. 262; s. XVIII. f. 15 A (Ἰατροσόφιον ἐκλελεγμένον ὑπὸ πολλῶν ἰατρικῶν βιβλ. Γαλ. Ἱππ. Μελ. καὶ Παύλ. τοῦ Αἰγ. συγγραφὲν δὲ παρὰ Κοσμᾶ ἱερομονάχου τοῦ Μακεδόνος).
Berlin:
Phillipps. 1571 (ol. Meerm. 279); s. XVI. f. 4v (Π. φλεβοτομίας. Inc. Φλεβοτομία λέγεται φλεβὸς ὀρθῶν τμῆμα. Expl. μακρονοσίαν σημαίνει, οὐ θάνατον).
fol. 39 (275); s. XVIII—XIX. (»Probecollation von P. Aeg. περὶ διαφορᾶς καὶ αἰτίας νοσημάτων nach d. Hds. des Beatus Rhenanus, verglichen mit der Baseler Ausgabe durch Schneider«). [Diels II.80]
Bologna: Bonon.
3632; s. XV. f. 16v (Imaginum quae P. Aeg. chirurgiam illustrant index), f. 114v Capita nonnulla P. Aeg. tributa), f. 209v (Ἀρχὴ π. τροχῆσκον [*l.* τροχίσκων] capp. 77; cap. 2—41 concordant cum lib. VII 12 P. Aeg.), f. 259 (Χρήσματος ἀπὸ τοῦ κόδητος [sic!] τοῦ Π.), f. 379. 382. 383v (Ad titulum περὶ δεσμῶν imagines), f. 419—434v (Ad tit. de repositionibus, lib. VI c. 114. 102. 118. 117 imagines; *vgl. Apollon. Citiensis*).
3636; s. XIV—XV. f. 61v (Κατὰ στοιχεῖον ἁπλαῖ θεραπεῖαι. Inc. Ἄβροτα διατηρεῖ σκωλύκων. Expl. καὶ γάλακτι γυναικείῳ ἐγγλυόμενον).
Florenz: Laurent. App. 2; s. XV. f. 273v (Commemoratur Paul.), f. 327v (πρὸς ἑλμίνθας), f. 328 (Ἐκ τοῦ Παύλου), f. 339 (εἰς κοιλιοστόμαχον), f. 339v (π. λυγμοῦ), f. 340 (πρὸς τὸ ποιῆσαι ὄρεξιν), f. 349v (π. ἥπατος), f. 356 (Παύλ. καὶ Δημοκρίτου π. πόνων ἰσχίου), f. 358 (ἐπὶ ἰσχιδιακῶν), f. 359 (π. κιονίδος).
London:
Addit. (Brit. Mus.) 10, 058; s. XV. f. 102 (Exc. apud Anonymum π. δυνάμεως ζουλαπίων καὶ ἑτέρων πομάτων).
Medical Society H Hi 17 = We 30; s. XV in. no. 21 Dbg. (Remedia).
Madrid: Matrit. bibl. nac.
4616 (ol. N 84); s. XV. f. 132.
4631 (ol. N 110); a. 1474. f. 86.
Mailand: Ambros. Q 87 Sup.; s. —. f. 271—278v (Inc. mutil. ...|ραγία γένηται, μοθοῖς. Expl. γυμνωθῆναι· εἰ μὲν αἱμορ|...).
Mitylene: Bibl. gymnas. 33; a. 1774. no. 2. 3. 4 (2: Δίαιτα διὰ τὴν γεροντικὴν ἡλικίαν. 3: ἐπιστολὴ πρὸς Διοκλέα ... προφυλακτική. Inc. Ἐπειδή σοι συμβαίνει. 4: περὶ τῶν κενωτικῶν τῆς κεφαλῆς ἀποφλεγματισμῶν τε καὶ ἐρρίνων καὶ διαχιστῶν. μς'. Inc. Τοὺς ἐν τῇ κεφαλῇ χυμούς).

Oxford: Baroccian.

150; s. XV in. f. 77 (Pauca de simplicibus).

224; s. XV in. f. 2ᵛ (*Wie im* Bonon. 3636. f. 61ᵛ) *und* f. 21ᵛ (Ἄλειμμα πρὸς ῥαγάδας χειρῶν καὶ ποδῶν, πρὸς δὲ τὰς γινομένας ἐν αὐτοῖς ἐγκαύσεις ἀπὸ δὲ τοῦ προσομιλῆσαι χιόνι ἢ ἀνέμῳ χειμερίῳ. Expl. τὸ ζάμβακα καὶ τὸ νάρδον).

Paris:

Parisin.

36; s. XIV—XV. f. 96 (Pauli Aeg. excerpta ex Hipp. et Gal. de venae sectione).

1865; s. XV. f. 133.

2153; s. XV. f. 435 (De spiritu animali, ad Josephum rhacendytam), f. 447 (De diaeta, ad Josephum rhacendytam).

2178; s. XV. f. 9 (De praenotionibus), f. 11ᵛ (De febrium differentiis), f. 42 (De morbis hominum et remediis).

2294; s. XV. f. 73ᵛ (Collectio remediorum), f. 124 (Exc. medica).

2313; s. XIV. f. 1 (Remedia varia).

2316; s. XV. f. 229ᵛ.

2320; s. XVI. f. 12ᵛ (Π. φλεβοτομίας).

2337; s. XV—XVI. f. 11 (De fracturis etc.).

2510; a. 1384. f. 108 (Praecepta medica et remedia varia).

Suppl.

924; s. XV—XVI. f. 1 (De differentia et causa aegritudinum).

1202; s. XIII. f. 16.

Rom:

Angelic. 17 (C 5. 4); s. XIV. f. 238—238ᵛ.

Barberin. I 127; s. XVI. f. 206ᵛ (Περὶ τῶν ἀπὸ τῶν γευστῶν ποιοτήτων δηλουμένων κράσεων. Inc. Οὔτε ἐξ ὀσμῆς. Expl. καὶ στυπτηρία), f. 252 (Ὀδόντων προφυλακτικά. Inc. Οἱ ὀδόντες οὐκ. Expl. γλώττης φλέβας), f. 276 (Πρὸς τεθλασμένους ὄνυχας, πρὸς ὑφαίμους ὄνυχας etc.), f. 311 (Π. ἰχθύων Inc. Ὅτι μὲν πᾶς ἰχθύς. Expl. ὕδωρ ὁμοίως), f. 323 (Π. ἑρμαφροδίτων. Inc. Τὸ ἑρμαφρόδιτον πάθος. Expl. θεραπευομένων), f. 334ᵛ (Ἡδυχρόου τοῦ ἐν τῇ θηριακῇ σκευασία).

Palat.

279; s. XIV—XV. f. 212ᵛ (De phlebotomia, exc. ex Galeno et Paulo Aeg. Inc. Οἱ πρῶτοι καὶ κυριώτατοι σκοποὶ τῆς φλεβοτομίας) *und* f. 214ᵛ (Π. φλεβοτομίας. Inc. Ὁ τῆς φλεβοτομίας τρόπος).

400; s. XV. f. 383 (Simplicium et compositorum pharmacorum experimenta).

Urbin. 158; s. XIII. f. 269 (Σύντομοι καὶ εὐσύνοπτοι ἰατρεῖαι διαφόρων νοσημάτων).

Vatic.

279; s. —. f. 214 (Π. φλεβοτομίας. »Hic codex deest«; *Verwechslung mit dem* Palat. 279?).

294; s. —. f. 296 (Π. ἀντιβαλλομένων).

Venedig: Marcian. App. cl.
V, 13; s. XIV—XVI. f. 119ᵛ.
V, 16; s. XVI. f. 160ᵛ (*Wie im* Bonon. 3636. f. 61ᵛ. Expl. θαυμάσεις πάνυ).
Wien: Vindob. med.
28; s. XV. f. 186ᵛ. 187ᵛ (Π. φλεβοτομίας. Inc. *wie im* Palat. 279. f. 212ᵛ. Expl. καὶ τῶν ἀλλοτρίων ἀποκριτικήν).
29; s. XV. f. 12—22ᵛ (Inc. *wie im* Palat. 279. f. 212ᵛ. Expl. τὸν καθαρισμὸν τοῦ ἐγκεφάλου ἐξάγον).

Paulus Italus.

[Diels II.81]

Excerpta.

Oxford: Baroccian. 88; s. XV (XVI). f. 47 (Ἱπποκρ. διδασκάλου καὶ Γαλ. σοφοῦ καὶ Παύλου Ἰτάλου καὶ Ἀθηναίου ῥήτορος καὶ Ἰωάννου Τζέτζου διάγνωσις περὶ ἰαλίων [l. ὑαλίων] ἀρρώστων καὶ τελευτῆς ἀνθρώπων. Inc. Τὸ α'. ἄσπρον . Expl. σημαίνει καὶ θάνατον).

Paulus Nicaeensis.

[Περὶ διαγνώσεως καὶ θεραπείας διαφόρων νοσημάτων.]
De cognitione et curatione variorum morborum.

Inc. Πολλῶν τε καὶ ποικίλων.
Expl. πανταχόθεν ἀπὸ τοῦ ὄνυχος.

[**München:** Monac. Hardt I p. 448 (*Wahrscheinlich Irrtum*)].
Rom: Angelic. 4 (C 4. 16); s. XVI in. f. 165 (*Abschrift im Berol. fol. 39 [275]*).
Wien: Vindob. med.
31; s. XV ex. f. 1—126ᵛ (*Collation im Berol. fol. 39 [275]*).
41; s. XIV. XV. f. 1 (Inc. mutil. cap. ιη' med. διακρατήσω οὖν καὶ μαλακῶς τρίψας. *Collation im Berol. fol. 39 [275]*).

Perzoe.

Βιβλίον φυσιολογικὸν μετακομισθὲν ἐκ τῆς Ἰνδίας
καὶ δοθὲν τῷ βασιλεῖ Χοσρόῃ ἐν Περσίδι παρά τινος Περζῶε σοφοῦ κτέ.
Liber physiologicus ex India translatus et Chosroe regi Persarum traditus a Perzoe etc.

Inc. Περὶ τῆς εὑρέσεως τοῦ παρόντος βιβλίου.
Expl. ὅπερ λέγεται στεφανίτης καὶ ἰχνηλάτης.

Rom: Barberin. I 72 (440); s. XVI. f. 1.

[Diels II.82]

Petosiris.

Vgl. E. Rieß, Nechepsonis et Petosiridis fragmenta magica. Philol. Suppl.VI p. 325—394.

Ἐπιστολὴ πρὸς Νεχεψὼ βασιλέα.
Epistula ad regem Nechepso.

Florenz: Laurent. plut.
28, 14; s. XIV. cap. σμα' (Ἑτέρα μέθοδος Πετ. scil. περὶ νόσου ζωῆς καὶ θανάτου).
28, 34; s. XI. f. 21 (Inc. Ἡ δὲ ὑπὸ Πετ. προσαχθεῖσα μεθόδος. Expl. ὁ κίνδυνος ἢ οὔ) *und* f. 61 (Περὶ μηνὸς ἀγαθοῦ καὶ φαύλου. Inc. Οὐδὲ τοῦτο ἄτοπόν σε γνῶναι. Expl. τῶν λοιπῶν ἀστέρων δυνόντων).
86, 14; s. XV. f. 96 (Inc. Περὶ ἑνὸς ἑκάστου. Expl. *wie im* plut. 28, 34. Ed. Rieß *a. a. O.* p. 385).
Krakau: Cracov. bibl. univ. 2526; s. XV. f. 98 (Inc. Ἐπειδὴ βεβάρηταί σου. Expl. ἐν τῷ ὑπογείῳ ἀποθνήσκει. *Vgl.* Rieß *a. a. O.* p. 384).
Madrid: Matrit. bibl. nac. 4616 (ol. N 48); s. XV. f. 89. 90.
Modena: Mutinens. 174 (II F 9); s. XV. f. 262 (Inc. Περὶ τῶν κατακλινομένων ἐν ἀρρωστίαις εὑρήσονται [l. εἰ ῥύσονται]. Expl. ὄργανον ὑπέργειον ἀστρονομικόν. Ed. *im* Catal. cod. astr. IV p. 120 sq.).
Neapel: Neapolit. II C 33 (ol. 34); a. 1495. f. 307ᵛ (Inc. Περὶ ἑνὸς ἑκάστου τῶν ὑπ' ἐμοῦ; *vgl. den* Laurent. 86, 14. Expl. ταχέως τελευτήσει).
Paris:
Parisin. 2139; s. XVII. f. 115.
Suppl. 446; s. X. f. 43 (Inc. Ψῆφος σεληνιακός).

Venedig: Marcian.
335; s. XV (»In indice adnotatur, in codice deest«).
336; s. XV—XVI. f. 259 (Μέθοδος περὶ νόσων. Inc. *wie im* Laurent. 28, 34).
Wien: Vindob.
med. 8; s. XV. f. 294 (*Wie im* Cracov.).
phil. 37; s. XV—XVI. cap. ρκη'.

Περὶ κατακλίσεως νοσούντων.
De decubitu infirmorum.

Modena: Mutinens. 174 (II F 9); s. XV. f. 263 (Inc. Ἐὰν ἐν κυριακῇ ἢ τετράδι κατακλιθῇ τις. Expl. ἡ πέμπτη ♃". »Post Petosiridis epistulam neque vero sub eius nomine traditur«).
Paris: Parisin. 2139; s. XVII. f. 90.

Περὶ ζωῆς καὶ θανάτου.
Organum de vita et morte.

Modena: Mutinens. 174 (II F 9); s. XV. f. 263 (Inc. Μάθε πότε κατεκλίθη ὁ ἄρρωστος. Expl. ζωὴ σκότος ὑπὲρ γῆν. »Post Petosiridis epistulam neque vero sub eius nomine traditur«).
Paris: Parisin. 2426; s. XVI. f. 6^v^.
Wien: Vindob. phil. 108; s. XVI. f. 162 (Περὶ Πετ. ὄργανον πρὸς Νεχεψὼ τῷ βασιλεῖ. *Vgl. oben die* Ἐπιστολὴ πρὸς Νεχ.).

Excerpta.

Florenz: Laurent. plut. 86, 14; s. XV. f. 95^v^ (Κύκλος Πετοσίρι⟨δος⟩).
Paris: Parisin.
1991; s. XV. f. 29^v^ (Excerpta de rebus medico-astrologicis).
2426; s. XVI. f. 16^v^ (Protagorae [Pythagorae] excerpta ex iatromathematicis Mercurii et Petosiridis etc. astrologica).
Turin: Taurin. C VI 21 (b VI 18); s. XVI. f. 66 (Ἐκ τῶν ἰατρομαθηματικῶν Ἑρμοῦ καὶ Πετοσίρεως καὶ τῶν συναγωγῶν Πρωταγόρου).
Wien: Vindob. phil. 108; s. XVI. f. 232 (Περὶ συμφώνων τῶν τετραγώνων θαυμάσιον. Inc. Ὑπολαμβάνουσι πάντες. Expl. τὸ πράσσειν ἔχοντες ἐστηριγμένοι. Ed. *im* Catal. cod. astrol. gr. VI p. 62).

[Diels II.83]

Philagrius.

Excerpta varia.

Berlin: Phillipps. 1532 (ol. Meerm. 225); s. XVI (In Anonymi opere περὶ οὔρων commemorantur Σχόλια περὶ οὔρων Philagrii).

Bologna: Bonon. 1808; s. XV. f. 102 (Διαφορητικὸν βρογκοκήλων καὶ σκληριῶν, θαυμάσιον φάρμακον) *und* f. 267ᵛ (Περὶ ὀνειράξεων [l. ὀνειρώξεων]. »Ex Aetio?« Wellmann).

Paris: Parisin.

2228; s. XIV—XI. f. 63 (Opusculum de urinis, ex Galeno, Philagrio etc.).

2276; s. XVI. f. 217 (Archigenis et Philagrii opusculum de renum calculis, ex Aëtio).

Philaretus.

Περὶ πραγματείας σφυγμῶν.
De pulsuum scientia.

Ed. lat. *in* Articella, Venedig 1493. f. 3ᵛ—4ʳ.
Basel 1538.
Vgl. Theophilus de pulsibus.

Inc. Τριχῇ τῶν σφυγμῶν.
Expl. τὰ πρὸς τὰ ἐσόμενα.

Florenz: Laurent. plut. 59, 14; s. XV. p. 162.

[Diels II.85]

Philo.

Excerpta varia.

Madrid: Matrit. N 116 (ol. Tolet. 97, 15); s. XV. f. 214ᵛ (Ἀντίδοτος ἡ τοῦ Φίλωνος).

Oxford: Baroccian. 150; s. XV in. (Ἀντίδοτος ἡ Φίλωνος, ληφθεῖσα περὶ [l. παρὰ ?] τοῦ φιλοσόφου).

Rom: Angelic. 17 (C 5. 4); s. XIV. f. 318 (Ἀντίδοτος ἡ τοῦ Φίλωνος. Τοῖς ὑσακολητικοῖς, πλευριτικοῖς καὶ πρὸς πᾶσαν ὀδύνην τὴν ἐντὸς κτλ. Expl. διάκλυζε καὶ στύονται· σκευάζεται δὲ ...)

Philo, Herennius.

Γνῶσις τῶν ἡλικιῶν.
De aetatibus hominis.

Ed. Studemund, Anecd. var. I p. 245 adn.
Vgl. A. Fresenius, De λέξεων Aristophanearum et Suetonian. excerptis Byzantinis. Aquis Mattiacis 1875 p. 82—89.

Inc. Βρέφος μὲν τὸ γεννηθὲν εὐθύς.
Expl. εἶτα πρεσβύτης, εἶτα ἐσχατόγηρως.

Berlin: Phillipps. 1527 (ol. Meerm. 217); s. XVI. f. 68ᵛ.
Mailand: Ambros. C 222 Inf.; s. XIII. f. 41ᵛ.

Philumenus.

Vgl. Puschmann, Berliner Studien V, 2. p. 8 sq.

Excerpta varia.

Rom: Vatic. 284; s. XI—XII (?). f. 264ᵛ (Περὶ ἰοβόλων ζῴων καὶ τῶν ἐν αὐτοῖς βοηθημάτων).

Photius Monachus.

Carmina.

Paris: Parisin. 2224; s. XV. f. 76 (Carmina de terra, oceano, nubibus et sanguine).

Excerpta. [Diels II.86]

Bologna: Bonon. 3632; s. XV. f. 217 (Ζουλάπιον).
Venedig: Marcian. App. cl. V, 13; s. XIV—XVI. f. 5. 12 (Στιχηρὰ ... δοθέντα τῷ εὐσεβεστάτῳ βασιλεῖ κυρίῳ Ἰωάννῃ περὶ μεθόδου ὑαλίων Photii Philosophi. Expl. τῇ δὲ ἕκτῃ ἀπελθέτω εἰς λουτρόν).

Porphyrius.

Excerpta varia.

Oxford: Baroccian. 150; s. XV in. f. 77 (Pauca quaedam de simplicibus ex Diosc., Orib., Porphyrio, Paulo, Magno, Archig. etc.).

Paris:

Parisin. 2183; s. XV. f. 7.

Suppl. 1202; s. XIII. f. 16 (Exc. varia ex Diosc., Oribas., Porphyrio, Paulo, Magno, Archigene etc.).

Posidonius.

Excerpta varia.

Venedig: Marcian. 279; s. XV (De atra bile, ex libris Galeni, Rufi, Posidonii, Aëtii. »Ex Aetio.« Wellmann).

[Diels II.87]

Proclus.

Excerpta.

Rom: Barberin. I 127; s. XVI (Ἡ Πρόκλου ποδαγρικὴ καὶ πρὸς ἰσχιάδας).

Protagoras.

Protagorae [Pythagorae] excerpta ex iatromathematicis Mercurii et Petosiridis etc. astrologica.

(*S. oben* PETOSIRIS Excerpta.)

Paris: Parisin. 2426; s. XVI. f. 16v.

Turin: Taur. C VI 21 (b VI 18); s. XVI. f. 66.

Ptolemaeus.

Excerpta varia.

Bologna: Bonon. 3632; s. XV. f. 317ᵛ (Ἐκ τῆς γενεθλιακῆς βίβλου τῆς ἀποτελεσματικῆς μερικὰ περί τε ἀρρένων καὶ θηλέων τέκνων) *und* f. 320ᵛ (Περὶ τῶν ιβ' ζωδίων).
Wien: Vindob. med. 49; s. XVI. f. 22—30ᵛ (Καρπός. Προεκθέμενοι, ὦ Σύρε. Expl. ἐγχώριος ἔσται ὁ ἐχθρός).

Pythagoras.

Ψῆφοι.
Supputationes prognosticae.

Madrid: Matrit. bibl. nac.
4616 (ol. N 84); s. XV. f. 66. 74ᵛ. 80ᵛ. 82ᵛ. 83ᵛ. 84ᵛ. 86ᵛ. 87. 87ᵛ.
4631 (ol. N 110); a. 1474. f. 158. 159ᵛ.
München: Monac. 287; s. XV. f. 135 (Ψῆφος περὶ ζωῆς καὶ θανάτου).

Protagorae [Pythagorae] excerpta ex iatromathematicis Mercurii et Petosiridis etc. astrologica. [Diels II.88]
(*S.* PETOSIRIS Excerpta.)

Paris: Parisin. 2426; s. XVI. f. 16ᵛ.

Romanus.

Περὶ τῶν ὀξέων καὶ μακρῶν νοσημάτων.
De morbis acutis et chronicis.

Rom: Vatic. 280; s. XV. f. 162ᵛ (Ῥωμανοῦ καὶ κουβουκλησίου τῆς τοῦ Θεοῦ ἐκκλησίας ἁγίας καὶ πτορομηνιτου [sic] τοῦ βασιλικοῦ ξενῶνος τοῦ μυρελαίου καὶ τῆς περιδόξου. Inc. Οὐ παραιτητέον. Expl. αἷς ὑγιεινόν ἐστιν).
Wien: Vindob. med. 48; s. XIV—XV. f. 1—46 (Inscr. Ῥωμανοῦ κουβουκλισίου κτλ. Expl. κἂν συνάγῃ στύφοντα κἂν σκληρύνῃ μαλάγματα).

Rufus.

Περὶ τῶν ἐν νεφροῖς καὶ κύστει παθῶν.
De vesicae renumque affectibus.

Daremberg-Ruelle 1—63.

Inc. (προοίμ.) Ὅσα περὶ τοὺς νεφροὺς καὶ τὴν κύστιν.
Expl. τὸ δὲ ψυχρὸν [ἀκ]ρατέστατον τῇ κύστει

Berlin: Phillipps. 1536 (ol. Meerm. 231); s. XVI. f. 9v.
Jerusalem: Bibl. d. hl. Grabes 38; s. XVII. no. 2.
Leyden: Bibl. Univ.
(Catal. p. 395); s. XV.
Voss. 4° 9; s. XIV (*Vgl.* Bodleian. Catal. mss. Angl. et Hib. I 1 no. 2182).
München: Monacens. 469; s. XV. f. 148—160.
Oxford: Laudian. C 58 (nunc 59, Bodleian. 708); s. XV. f. 375.
Paris:
Parisin.
2288; s. XVI. f. 161.
2331; s. XVII. f. 11v.
Suppl. 629; s. XIX. f. 65.
Petersburg: Petropol. 164; s. XVIII. f. 1.
Rom:
Barberin. 382 (= I 91); s. XV. f. 27v.
Vatic. 291; s. XV—XVI. f. 1 (*Vgl.* Mai, Classici auct. IV. p. 198).

Περὶ σατυριασμοῦ καὶ γονορροίας.
De satyriasi et gonorrhoea.

Dbg.-R. p. 64—84.

Inc. Ἄνθρωπός τις ἦν ᾧ τὸ αἰδοῖον ἐπάλλετο.
Expl. [εἰς τὸ παν]τελῶς ὑγιαίνειν.

München: Monac. 469; s. XV. f. 161—165 (»Fragmentum huius opusculi esse censet Daremberg p. XVI sq.«).

Περὶ ὀνομασίας τῶν τοῦ ἀνθρώπου μορίων. [Diels II.89]
De corporis humani appellationibus.

Dbg.-R. p. 133—167.

Inc. Τί πρῶτον ἔμαθες ἐν κιθαριστικῇ.
Expl. Τὰ πολλὰ ἀτιμάσαι διά τινα ὀλίγα παροφθέντ .

Berlin: Phillipps. 1536 (ol. Meerm. 231); s. XVI. f. 22.
Bern: Bernens. 459; s. XV. f. 1.
Escurial: Scorial.
  Σ. I. 12*; s. XVI. f. 51 (Sine inscriptione).
  Φ. I. 2; s. XVI. f. 1.
Florenz: Laurent. plut. 74, 7; s. IX. p. 275 (*H. Schoenes Collation im Besitz der Berl. Akademie*).
London:
  Burneian. (Brit. Mus.) 94; s. XV (XVI). f. 154 (*Vollständig*) *und* f. 197^{v} (*Excerpte.* Inc. Ἀναγκαιότατόν ἐστι προδιδαχθῆναι. Expl. ἀνάλογον τοῖς ἐν χερσίν· οὕτω δὲ καὶ ὅσα).
  Medical Society H Hi 23 = We 32^{a}; s. XVI in. no. 2 Dbg., Not. et Extr. (Expl. ἐνδεχόμενον, καὶ ἡ τῶν ὀστέων φύσις).
Madrid: Matrit. bibl. nac. 4636 (ol. N 115)*; s. XV. f. 209.
Mailand: Ambros.
  duo (*Vgl.* Montfaucon I p. 504).
  T 141; s. XVI (*Vgl.* Darembg. Ruf. p. XXIII).
Montpellier: Montepess. bibl. episcopatus (*Vgl.* Montfaucon II p. 1199).
Paris:
  Facult. med. 14 (ol. Bibl. de Paris 57); s. XVII. f. 58.
  Parisin.
    2151; s. XVI. f. 1.
    2220; s. XVI. f. 44.
    2247; s. XVI (*Apographon des* Laurent.).
    2248; s. XVI (*Apographon des* Laurent.).
    2264; s. XVI (Fine mutil.).
    2321; s. XVI. f. 1 (Sine auctoris nomine. Inc. Περὶ ὀφθαλμοῦ. Τῶν δὲ τοῦ ὀφθαλμοῦ).
  Suppl. 629; s. XIX. f. 72.
Rom:
  Fonds Colonna 12; s. —.
  Ottobon. 235; s. —. f. 1.
  Palat. 302; s. XVI. f. 40.

Vatic. 2304 (ol. 2217)*; s. XV. f. 6[v] (Inc. *wie im* Burneian. 94. f. 197[v]. Expl. τῆς χειρὸς ὀνομάζονται).
Turin: Taurin. 333b I 1; s. XVI. f. 1 (*Durch Feuer stark beschädigt*).
Vicenza: Bertolian. 44 (1. 6. 15); s. XVI. no. 1.
Wien: Vindob. phil. 303; s. XVI. f. 1—16[v].

Dazu: Président de Mesmes (*Vgl.* Montf. II 1327. Dbg. p. XXIII).

Ὀνομασίαι τῶν κατὰ ἄνθρωπον.
Nomenclatura rerum ad hominem pertinentium. Libri III.

Inc. Εἴ τις τὴν κιθαριστικὴν μέλλοι διδαχθήσεσθαι.
Expl. καὶ ἡ τῶν ὀστέων θέσις.

Berlin: Phillipps. 1536 (ol. Meerm. 231); s. XVI. f. 30[v] med.
Bern: Bernens. 459; s. XV. f. 23.
Escurial: Scorial. Φ. I. 2; s. XVI. f. 8[v].
London:
Burneian. (Brit. Mus.) 94; s. XV (XVI). f. 161[v].
Medical Society H Hi 23 = We 32[a]; s. XVI in. no. 2 Dbg., Not. et Extr.
Paris: Parisin.
2151; s. XVI. f. 6—12.
2261; s. XVI. f. 1.
2262; s. XVI. f. 1.
2263; s. XVI. f. 1.
Petersburg: Petropol. 164; s. XVIII. f. 138.
Rom: Vatic.
12*; s. XIV. f. 236[v] (*Vgl.* Dbg. p. 236).
291; s. XV—XVI. f. 20 (*Vgl.* Dbg.-R. praef. p. XXV).
Zaragoza: Bibl. d. cat. d. Pil. 1106 (ol. 562); s. XV. f. 2.

Περὶ ἀνατομῆς τῶν τοῦ ἀνθρώπου μορίων.
De dissectione partium corporis humani.

Dbg.-R. p. 168—185.

Inc. Παραδόντες τὴν τῶν ἔξωθεν θεωρουμένων ὀνομασίαν.
Expl. διαπαντὸς ὑπὸ ὀστῶν περιεχόμενος.

Rom: Vatic. 12; s. XIV. f. 236v (Fragmenta. *Vgl.* Daremberg p. 236).
Zaragoza: Bibl. d. cat. d. Pil. 1106 (ol. 562); s. XV. f. 6v.

Περὶ ὀστῶν. [Diels II.90]
De ossibus.

Dbg.-R. p. 186—194.

Inc. Ἐπειδὴ τὴν τῶν ἐντοσθίων θεωρίαν.
Expl. καὶ ἡ τῶν ὀστῶν θέσις.

Florenz: Laurent. plut. 74, 7; s. IX. p. 283b (*H. Schoenes Collation im Besitz der Berl. Akademie*).
Zaragoza: Bibl. d. cat. d. Pil. 1106 (ol. 562); s. XV. f. 16.

Ἰατρικὰ ἐρωτήματα.
Quaestiones medicinales.

Dbg.-R. p. 195—218.

Inc. Ἐρωτήματα χρὴ τὸν νοσοῦντα ἐρωτᾶν.
Expl. τὸν μέλλοντα ὀρθῶς ὑπὲρ ἁπάντων γνώσεσθαι.

Paris: Parisin. Suppl. 637; s. XV. f. 65v.
Wien: Vindob. med. 8; s. XV. f. 283.

Σύνοψις περὶ σφυγμῶν.
Conspectus de pulsibus.

Dbg.-R. p. 219—232.

Inc. Τὴν περὶ σφυγμῶν πραγματείαν δεόντως.
Expl. τὸ παρὰ τὸν ῥυθμόν.

Florenz: Laurent. plut. 75, 7; s. XIV. p. 214 (*Vorangeht:* Ἐγὼ προσέθηκα τοῦτο τὸ π. σφυγμῶν μονόβιβλον· τὸ γὰρ σύνταγμα οὐκ εἶχε· νομίζω δὲ αὐτὸ μὴ εἶναι Γαληνοῦ, ἀλλὰ Ῥούφου τοῦ Ἐφεσίου).
Paris: Parisin. 2193; s. XIV. f. —.

Περὶ τῶν φαρμάκων καθαρτικῶν.
De medicamentis purgantibus.

= Orib. Coll. med. VII 26, ed. Daremberg Orib. II p. 90—145.

Berlin: Phillipps. 1536 (ol. Meerm. 231); s. XV. f. 1.
Florenz: Laurent. plut. 75, 7; s. XIV. p. 219 (Inc. Οὔτε πάντας τοὺς ὅπως).
Leyden:
Bibl. Univ. (Catal. p. 395).
Voss. 4° 9; s. XVII.
München: Monac. 469; s. XV. f. 137—147.
Paris: Parisin. 2331; s. XVII. f. 1.
Petersburg: Petropol. 164; s. XVIII. f. 40.
Rom: Barberin. I 91 (382); s. XV. f. 1 (Μονόβιβλον τίνας δεῖ καιθαίρειν καὶ ποίοις καθαρτηρίοις καί πότε. Inc. Οὔτε πάντας. Expl. στήθους καὶ πνεύματος).

[Diels II.91]

Excerpta varia.

Berlin: Berol. fol. 39 (275) — (*Coll. kleinerer Stücke*).
Bologna: Bonon.
1808; s. XV. f. 267 (Χρῖσμα ἐπεργὸν ἐντεῖνον τὸ αἰδοῖον).
3632; s. XV. f. 265 (Περὶ αἵματος).
Florenz: Laurent. plut. 74, 7; s. IX. p. 173 (Ἐκ τῶν Ῥούφου τὸ Ἱπποκράτους βάθρον. Inc. Ὁ θαυμασιώτατος Ἱπποκράτης. *Aus* Oribas. IV p. 432).
Jerusalem: Bibl. patriarch. 273; s. XVIII. f. 108 (Ἡ Ῥούφου ἱερά).
London: Harleian. (Brit. Mus.) 5626; s. XV—XVI. f. 2 (Ἰατροσόφιον ... Ἱπποκράτους ... Ῥούφου).
Moskau: Mosquens. 436; s. XIII *und* XIV. f. 115 (Περὶ τῆς τοῦ πηγάνου χρήσεως. Inc. Πηγάνου οὐδὲν εἰς τὴν ἰατρικὴν χρησιμώτερον).
München: Monac. 469; s. XV. f. 161—165 (»Frgm. fortasse ex libello περὶ ἀφροδισίων.« *Vgl.* Daremberg p. XI).
Paris:
Coislin. 335; s. XV. f. 8 (De aquis. »*Aus* Orib.« Wellmann).
Parisin.
2152; a. 1539. f. 6 (Frgm. de rebus venereis. »*Aus* Orib.« Wellmann).
2240; s. XVI. f. 146v (Gal. et Rufi excerpta de venereis. »*Aus* Orib.« Wellmann).
Rom: Vatic.
12; s. XIV. f. 236v *(Vgl.* Daremb. p. 236).

1885; s. XIV. f. 154v (Ἐκ τῶν Ῥούφου τοῦ Ἱππ. βάθρον ἀπὸ τῶν προοιμίων τοῦ μονοβίβλου τοῦ ἐπὶ γῆρας ἄνθρωπος, τινὲς δὲ αὐτὸ περὶ ἐξαρθημάτων ἐπιγράφουσιν. »*Stammt aus* Orib. IV 432 *mit* Scholion.« Wellmann. *Vgl.* den Laurent. 74, 7).

2256; s. XIV. f. 26 (Ἱερὰ υγ τῶν μελαγχολικῶν).

Venedig:

Marcian. 279; s. XV (De atra bile ex libris Gal., Rufi, Posidonii et Aëtii).

App. cl. II 171; s. XV (Περὶ ἐμέτων).

Salomo.

[Παραγγελίαι.]
Praecepta.

Athos:

Βιβλ. μον. Ἰβήρων 4302. 182; s. XVI. f. 7 (»Praecepta quorum nonnulla secundum Salomonicum«).

Παντελεήμονος 6351. 844; s. XVIII. f. 42 (Σολομωνικὴ μετὰ προγνωστικῶν).

Severianus.

Ὁρισμοί.
Definitiones.

Florenz: Laurent. plut. 74,11; s. XIII. p. 150 (Inc. Τί Θεὸς ὄνομα κυρίως. Expl. Τί φρὴν κτέ.).

Περὶ τῆς προσηγορίας τοῦ ἀνθρώπου.
De hominis nomine.

Inc. Τοῦ ἀνθρώπου προσηγορία τῇ ἑβραΐδι διαλέκτῳ.
Expl. τοῦ Ἀδὰμ ἀρραβὼν ἦν τῆς οἰκουμένης.

Wien: Vindob. med. 27; s. XVI. f. 113v—114.

[Diels II.92]

Severus.

Περὶ ἐνετήρων ἤτοι κλυστήρων πρὸς Τιμόθεον.
De instrumentis infusoriis seu clysteribus ad Timotheum.

Ed. Dietz, Regiomonti 1836 p. 1—43.

Inc. Ἐν τῇ τῆς (vel τῶν) κατὰ τὴν τέχνην.
Expl. πονοῦσιν ἐξεθέμεθα.

Berlin: Phillipps. 1532 (ol. Meerm. 225); s. XVI. f. 177 (*Vgl.* Daremberg Not. et Extr. I p. 148).
Bologna: Bonon. 3636; s. XIV—XV. f. 134v.
Florenz: Laurent. plut. 75, 7; s. XIV. p. 225b.
Paris: Parisin. 2228; s. XIV—XI. f. 57v (De intestinis).

Socrates.

Excerpta.

Paris: Parisin. Suppl. 1202; s. XIII. f. 16 (Excerpta varia ex Dioscoride, Oribasio, Porphyrio, Paulo ... Socrate).

Soranus.

Περὶ γυναικείων παθῶν.
De muliebribus affectionibus.

Ed.Val. Rose, Lips. 1882 p. 171—379. *Vgl.* Muscio.

Inc. Ἐπεὶ πρὸς τὸ τῶν ἀποδοθησομένων.
Expl. τῆς διακρίσεως ἴσης ἀποτελεσθῆναι.

Leyden: Voss. 8° 18; s. XVI (Apogr. *des* Parisin.).
Paris: Parisin. 2153; s. XV. f. 220. (*Vgl.* Buss.-Dbg. Oribasius I p. XXV.)
Rom: Barberin. I 49 (= 359); s. XVI. f. 1—165 (Apogr. *des* Parisin.).

Περὶ ἐπιδέσμων.
De fasciis.

Ed. Charterius *in* Hipp. et Gal. Opp. XII p. 505—517.

Florenz: Laurent. plut. 74, 7; s. IX. p. 227.

Περὶ σημείων καταγμάτων.
De signis fracturarum.

Ed. Cocchi, Graecor. chirurgici libri, Florent. 1754 p. 44—51.
Ideler Phys. et Med. I p. 248—252.

Inc. Κάταγμά ἐστι διαίρεσις.
Expl. δέχεται τὴν ἐπίδοσιν. Καὶ περὶ καταγμάτων ἀπόχρη τοσαῦτα.

Berlin: Phillipps. 1533 (ol. Meerm. 226); s. XVII. f. 115.
Florenz: Laurent. plut. 74, 7; s. IX. p. 224b.

Ἱπποκράτους γένος καὶ βίος κατὰ Σωρανόν. [Diels II.93]
Hippocratis genus et vita secundum Soranum.

Hippocr. edit. Venet. 1588 I p. 1.
Ideler Phys. et Med. I p. 252—255.
Westermann, Biographi p. 449—452.

Inc. Ἱπποκράτης γένει μὲν ἦν Κῷος.
Expl. παῖδας, λέγεται καταλιπών.

Cambridge: Caius Coll. 50; s. XV—XVI. f. 1.
Florenz: Laurent. plut.
  74, 1; s. XV. p. 8b.
  74, 13; s. XV. p. 3.
Kopenhagen: Hauniens. ant. fund. reg. 224; s. XVI.
Leyden: Voss. fol. 10; s. XVI (*Vgl.* Hipp. ed. Ermerins prf. p. IX).
München: Monacens. 71; a. 1531. f. 9.
Oxford: Baroccian. 204; s. XV. f. 8.

Paris:

Parisin.

2140; s. XII—XIII. f. 8ᵛ.

2141; s. XV. f. 8.

2142; s. XIII—XIV. f. 12.

2143; s. XIV. f. 10.

2144; s. XIV. f. 12.

2145; s. XV.

2255; s. XV. f. 53ᵛ.

2596; s. XIV. f. 184.

Suppl. 688; s. XVI. f. 39.

Rom:

Urbin. 68; s. XIV. f. 4.

Vatic.

277; s. XIV. f. 24ᵛ (*Coll. Ilbergs in dessen Besitz*).

278; a. 1512. f. 25ᵛ.

1879; s. XV. f. 159.

Venedig: Marcian. 269; s. XI.

Wien: Vindob. med. 43; s. XVI. f. 122 (Inc. Πρῶτον τὴν ἐπωνυμίαν. Expl. ἐν περιόδοισιν ὅτι ἑβδομήκοντα κινέεται. »Wahrscheinlich nicht hierhergehörig.« Schoene).

Περὶ μήτρας καὶ αἰδοίου γυναικείου.
De matrice et muliebri pudendo.

Ed. Ideler Phys. et Med. I p. 255—260.
Aus Orib. III p. 369 sq.; *vgl.* Soran. ed. Rose p. 175.

Inc. Μήτρα καὶ ὑστέρα λέγεται καὶ δελφύς.
Expl. αὕτη δὲ μικροτέρα καὶ εὐθυτράχηλος.

Leyden: Voss. 8° 18; s. XVI (*Vgl.* Soranus ed. Ermerins praef. p. CX).
Paris: Parisin. Suppl. 629; s. XIX. f. 91.
Turin: Taurin. 333b I 1; s. XVI (*Durch Feuer stark beschädigt*).

Περὶ μέτρων καὶ σταθμῶν.
De ponderibus et mensuris.

Inc. Τῶν τοίνυν μέτρων.

Berlin: Phillipps. 1547; s. XVI. f. 120 (Inc. Τῶν τοίνυν μέτρων καὶ σταθμῶν).

London: Addit. (Brit. Mus.) 10, 058; s. XV. f. 46 (Inc. Τῶν μέτρων καὶ σταθμῶν οὐ μόνον. Expl. ὁ ξέστης ⫵' ἅς":).
Paris: Parisin. Suppl. 1297; s. XI. f. 127ᵛ.
Rom: Vatic. 1347; s. XV—XVI. f. 1.

Excerpta varia. [Diels II.94]

Rom: Ottobon. 192; s. XVI—XVII. f. 285 (Σωρανὸς ὁ Ζωγράγος).

Splenius Philosophus.

Περὶ γενέσεως ἀνθρώπου.
De generatione hominis.

Ed. Rohde, Acta soc. philol. Lips. I p. 28 not.
Krumbacher, Münchener Sitz.-Ber. 1892, II p. 345—347.
Vgl Rohde, Acta V p. 303—306.

Inc. Τὸ σπέρμα ἐν τῇ μήτρᾳ καταβαλλόμενον.
Expl. ἐπιτελειοῦται τοῖς τεθνεῶσιν.

Florenz: Laurent.
plut.
4, 10; s. XI. p. 299b (Sine auct. nomine).
58, 24; s. XIV. f. 126 (Sine auctoris nomine).
Conv. soppr. 627 (Abb. 2728); s. XIII. f. 92ᵛ (Sine auctoris nomine).
München: Monac.
308; s. XII. f. 223 (Sine auctor. nomine).
498; s. XIII. f. 227 (Sub nomine Ioannis Damasceni).
Neapel: Neapolit. II C 33; a. 1495. f. 7ᵛ (Inscr. Σπλίνου φίλοσ. π. γεν. ἀνθρ. καὶ διαλύσεως).
Paris: Parisin.
1310; s. XV. f. 443ᵛ (Sine auct. nomine).
1346; s. XI—XII. f. 274 (Sine auct. nomine).
1766; s. XVII. f. 437 (Sine auct. nomine).
1788; a. 1440. f. 238ᵛ (Σπλ. φίλοσ. π. γενέσ. καὶ ὅθεν τρίτα καὶ ἔννατα καὶ τεσσαρακοστά).
2894; s. XV—XVI. f. 336 (Sub nomine Libanii).
3023; s. XV—XVI. f. 46ᵛ (Sine auctor. nomine).

Rom:
Palat.
[Diels II.95] 13; a. 1167. f. 347^v (Sine auct. nomine).
328; s. XV. f. 154^v (Π. γενέσ. ἀνθρ. Σπλ. φιλοσ.).
Vatic.
12; s. XIV. f. 206^v (Inscr. Π. γεν. ἀνθρ. ὅθεν τά τε τρίτα καὶ ἔννατα καὶ τὰ τεσσαρακοστά).
854; s. XI. f. 265^v (Sine auct. nomine).
855; s. XVI. f. 312^v (Sine auctor. nomine. Expl. mutil. τῆς ἐπιρροῆς καὶ θηλύ⟨νεται⟩).
1277; s. XV—XVI. f. 55 (Sine auct. nomine).
Tübingen: Tubing. 2; s. XIII. f. 291 (Σπληνίου φιλοσόφου περὶ γεννήσεως ἀνθρώπου καὶ ὅθεν τρίτα καὶ ἔννατα καὶ τεσσαρακοστὰ τοῖς τεθνεῶσιν ἐπιτελοῦσιν, παρελθόντος τοῦ ἀνθρώπου).
Venedig: Marcian. 173; s. XIII—XIV (?). f. — (Sine auct. nomine. Inscr. Π. γεν. ἀνθρ. καὶ ὅθεν τρίτα καὶ θ̄ καὶ μ̄).
Wien: Vindob. theol. 207; s. —. f. 61^v (Sub nomine Splenii).

Stephanus Alexandrinus.

(*Vgl.* Usener, De Steph. Alexandr. Index lect. Bonnens. 1879.)

Πρᾶξις περὶ τοῦ ἐνόλου κόσμου.
De mundo. Libri IX.

Ed. Ideler, Phys. et Med. II p. 199—253.

Inc. Θεὸν τὸν πάντων ἀγαθῶν αἴτιον.
Expl. φάρμακον τρέχον εἰς πᾶν σῶμα ἀκωλύτως.

Escurial: Scorial. y. III. 18; s. XV *und* XVI. f. 86.
Rom: Vatic. 2259; s. —. f. 16.

Περὶ τῆς ἱερᾶς καὶ θείας τέχνης τῆς τοῦ χρυσοῦ ποιήσεως.
De sacra divinaque arte auri faciendi.

Ed. Ideler, Phys. et Med. II 199—202.

Inc. Θεὸν τὸν πάντων ἀγαθῶν αἴτιον.
Expl. τὴν ὑπεράγαθον τοῦ θεοῦ ἀγαθότητα.

Berlin: Phillipps. 1540; s. XVI. f. 29.
Escurial: Scorial.
Φ. I. 11; s. XVI. f. 36ᵛ.
Ψ. I. 13; s. XVI. f. 1.
Leipzig: Lipsiens. 66; s. XVII. f. 1 (Περὶ χρυσοποιΐας).
Venedig: Marcian. 299; s. XI.

Ἐπιστολὴ πρὸς Θεόδωρον.
Epistula ad Theodorum.

Ed. Ideler, Phys. et Med. II p. 208.

Inc. Περὶ τοῦ ἀγροῦ γνῶθι ὡς πολλοὺς γεωργούς.
Expl. καὶ μυστικῶν λόγων μάθῃ.

Rom: Vatic.
1174; s. XIV—XV. f. 70ᵛ.
2259; s. —. f. 25.

Περὶ τῆς ἱερᾶς καὶ μεγάλης ἐπιστήμης τῆς ἡλίου πορείας [Diels II.96]
πρὸς Ἡράκλειον τὸν μέγαν βασιλέα.
De magna sacraque scientia solis itineris ad regem Heraclium.

Ed. Ideler, Phys. et Med. II p. 243—253.

Inc. Ὁ ἄναρχος καὶ ὑπεράρχιος θεός.
Expl. τρέχον εἰς πᾶν σῶμα ἀκωλύτως.

Rom: Vatic. 1174; s. XIV—XV. f. 54.

Σχόλια εἰς τὸ προγνωστικὸν Ἱπποκράτους.
Scholia in Hippocratis praenotiones. Sectiones III.

Ed. Dietz, Scholia in Hipp. et Gal. I p. 51—232.

Inc. Τὰ εἰωθότα ἐπὶ ἑκάστου συγγράμματος προλέγεσθαι.
Expl. καὶ τὰ σχόλια τοῦ προγνωστικοῦ· δόξα τῷ θεῷ. ἀμήν.

Florenz: Laurent. plut. 59, 14; s. XV. p. 12.
Gallipoli: Ἐκκλησ. ἁγ. Νικολάου 38; s. XIV. in fine codicis.
Mailand: Ambros.
A 27 Inf.; s. XVI. f. 2 (»Operi sine auctoris nomine tradito praemittitur poëma«).
L 30 Sup.; a. 1524. f. 127.
Paris: Parisin. 2296; s. XVI. f. 131ᵛ—277ᵛ (*Vgl.* Costomiris, Rev. des ét. gr. II [1889] p. 356).
Venedig: Venet. bibl. Josephi de Aromatariis (*Verbleib unbekannt*).

Προλεγόμενα εἰς τὸ περὶ ἀγμῶν Ἱπποκράτους.
Prooemium in Hippocratis de fracturis.

Vgl. Palladius.

Inc. Τὰ εἰωθότα προλέγεσθαι.

Moskau: Mosquens. 466; s. XVI. f. 89.

Εἰς τὸ Μάγνου σοφιστοῦ περὶ οὔρων.
In Magni sophistae librum de urinis.

Ed. Bussemaker, Rev. de philologie I [1845] p. 423—438. 543—560.
Vgl. Bussemaker, Ianus 1847 p. 273 sqq.
Daremberg, Not et Extr. p. 119 sq.
Vgl. Magnus Emesenus.

Inc. Περὶ οὔρων προθέμενος γράψαι, δέον ἔδοξέ μοι.
Expl. καὶ τοῖς βουλομένοις ἀναγινώσκειν ἐπαφήκαμεν.

Cheltenham: Phillipps. 6763; s. XV (XIV sec. catal. et Schenkl). f. 1 (Μάγνου σοφ. ἐξήγησις εἰς τὸ περὶ οὔρων καὶ ἄλλων πολλῶν παλαιῶν σοφῶν τε καὶ διδασκάλων, συντεθεῖσα παρὰ τοῦ φιλοσόφου Στεφ. τοῦ Ἀλεξ.).
Paris: Parisin.
2220; s. XVI (Στεφάνου σχόλαια μάγνου εἰς τὸ περὶ οὔρων).
2229; s. XIII (Σχόλια Στεφάνου μάγνου εἰς τὸ περὶ οὔρων).
2260; s. XVI. f. 178ᵛ. (Inscr. *wie im* Phillipps. 6763).
Venedig: Marcian. App. cl. V 16; s. XVI. f. 148.

Stephanus Atheniensis.

[Diels II.97]

Σχόλια σὺν θεῷ τῶν ἀφορισμῶν Ἱπποκράτους ἐξήγησις.
In aphorismos Hippocratis commentarius.

Ed. Dietz, Scholia in Hipp. et Gal. II p. 236—344.

Inc. Σκοπός ἐστι τῷ συγγραφεῖ.
Expl. οὗτος γοῦν ἐκείνῳ κατὰ πάντα ὅμοιός ἐστιν.

Escurial: Scorial. Σ. II. 10; s. X. f. 1 (Inc. ⟨Αἱ⟩ μεταβολαὶ τῶν ὡρέων. Expl. φύσει ἀνώμαλον εἶναι τὸ φθινόπωρον).
Mailand: Ambros. S 19 Sup.; s. — (Stephani et Theophili in aphor. Hipp. comm.).
Paris: Parisin.
2222; s. XV (Sub nomine Meletii).
2223; s. XVI (Apogr. *von* nr. 2222).
Wien: Vindob. med.
16; s. XV—XVI. f. 185 (Sine auctoris nomine. Σχόλια εἰς τοὺς Ἱππ. ἀφορ. κατὰ σύνοψιν. Inc. Ὅρος ἀφορισμοῦ. Ἀφορισμός ἐστι λόγος σύντομος. Expl. δηλοῖ γὰρ ἐπίτασιν ξηρότητος).
44; s. XV—XVI. f. 1 (Inc. ἐν τῇσι = Dietz p. 283, 3).

Ἐξήγησις εἰς τὴν πρὸς Γλαύκωνα Γαληνοῦ θεραπευτικήν.
Enarratio Galeni de methodo medendi ad Glauconem librorum.

Ed. Dietz, Schol, in Hipp. et Gal. I p. 233—344.

Inc. Ὅτι μὲν οὖν τὴν κοινήν.
Expl. χυμὸν ἀπελάσαι συναγωνίζεται.

Kopenhagen: Hauniens. bibl. univ. e donatione variorum fol. 29; s. XV—XVI.
Leyden: B. P. 2 A; s. XVI.
Mailand: Ambros. L 110 Sup.; s. XV—XVI. f. 131 (Inc. Τὸ προοίμιον δύο ταῦτα ...).
Padua: Bibl. Ioannis Rhodii (*Verbleib unbekannt*).

Βίβλος Διοσκορίδου καὶ Στεφάνου Ἀθηναίου τοῦ φιλοσόφου
περιέχουσα φαρμάκων ἐμπειρίας κατὰ ἀλφάβητον.
Dioscoridis et Stephani Atheniensis de pharmacis ordine litterarum.

Ed. lat. Casp. Wolf. Basel 1581.

Jerusalem: Bibl. patriarch. 148*; s. XVI. f. 56^{v}.
Padua: Bibl. Ioannis Rhodii (*Verbleib unbekannt*).
Paris: Parisin.
2151; s. XVI. f. 65.
2181; s. XVI. f. 1.
Wien: Vindob. med. 18; s. — (»Proben« *im* Berol. fol. 39 [275]).
Zürich: Turicens. C 50; s. XVI. f. 1.

Περὶ διαφορᾶς πυρετῶν ἀπὸ φωνῆς Θεοφίλου.
De febrium differentiis ex ore Theophili.

Ed. Ideler, Phys. et Med. I p. 107.
Dem. Sicuri, Florenz 1862.

Inc. Σκοπὸν ἔχομεν.
Expl. ἐν οἷς αἱ διαφοραὶ πυρετῶν.

Berlin: Phillipps. 1532 (ol. Meerm. 225); s. XVI. f. 173 (Inc. Ἡ μὲν παράδοσις ἡ περὶ τῶν πυρετῶν σύντομός ἐστι. Expl. οἷα τῶν ταριχευομένων σωμάτων. »Congruunt fere cum Palladii comm. de febribus«).
[Diels II.98] **Escurial:** Scorial. T. II. 14; s. XVI. f. 177 (Inc. Ὁπηνίκα γὰρ = Ideler I p. 109, 35. Expl. πρὸς τὴν διαφορὰν τῆς ὕλης).
Florenz: Laurent. plut. 86, 20; s. XV. f. 64 (*Collation besitzt Dr. E. Bianchi, Florenz*).
London: Medical Society H Hi 17 = We 30; s. XV in. no. 24 Dbg. (Expl. *wie im* Berol. Phillipps. »Est opus traditum sub nomine Palladii«).
Mailand: Ambros. Q 94 Sup.; s. —. f. 24^{v}.
Paris:
Parisin.
985; s. XV. f. 71.
2218; s. XVI. f. 1 (Stephani [vel Palladii] synopsis de febribus).
2228; s. XIV—XI. f. 55 (Stephani synopsis de variis febrium generibus).
2267; s. XIV. f. 55^{v}.
2276; s. XVI. f. 191.
Suppl. 446; s. X. f. 107.

Rom:
Ottobon. 311; s. XV—XVI. f. 79.
Vatic. 285; s. XV. f. 196.
Wien: Vindob. med.
16; s. XV—XVI. f. — (Sine auctoris nomine. Περιτομὴ τοῦ περὶ διαφορᾶς πυρετῶν).
44; s. XV—XVI. f. 127—135ᵛ (Expl. τοῦ ἐπὶ ζέσει τοῦ αἵματος γινομένου πυρετοῦ).

Excerpta varia.

Oxford: Baroccian. 111; s. XV. f. 122 (Γυναῖκα ὁμολογῆσαι, ὑπὸ πόσων ἀνδρῶν ἐμιδύθη κτλ.).

Stephanus Ἀρχιατρὸς τῶν Μαγγάνων.

Ἐπιστολή.
Epistula.

Florenz: Laurent. App. 2; s. XV. f. 343 (Ἐπιστολὴ ἀπὸ Θεσσαλονίκης παρὰ Στεφάνου ἀρχιατροῦ τῶν Μεγγάνων [sic] etc.).

Excerpta varia.

Berlin: Phillipps.
1529; s. XVI. f. 191ᵛ (Κολλύριον ὀφθαλμικὸν παρὰ Στεφάνου ἰατροῦ τοῦ μαγίστρου. Ed. Studemund, Ind. lect. Vratisl. 1888/89 p. 12—14).
1540; s. XVI. f. 5 (Περὶ ἀσβέστου. Inc. λαβὲ ἐκ τῶν τεσσάρων στοιχείων ἀρσενικοῦ).
Palermo: Panorm. bibl. naz. XIII C 3; s. XVI. f. 914ᵛ—915ᵛ (Ἀποφλεγματισμὸς ἐαρινὸς κατασπῶν τὰ ἐν τῷ κρανίῳ φλέγματα καὶ χυμούς. Inc. Ὑσσώπου ὄγγ. δ'. Expl. καὶ ὅταν γένηται χλιαρὸν χρῶ. *Vgl.* Daremberg, Not. et Extr. I 33).
Paris: Parisin. 2147; s. XVI. f. 30.

Stephanus Magnes. [Diels II.99]

Ἐμπειρικά.
Empirica.

Paris: Parisin. 2298; s. XVI.

Σχόλια εἰς τὸ περὶ οὔρων (Θεοφίλου?).
Scholia in (Theophili?) tractatum de urinis.

Vgl. Bussemaker, Rev. de philologie I [1845] p. 423 ff.

Paris:
Parisin.
2220; s. XVI. f. 24v.
2229; s. XIII. f. 42.
2260; s. XVI. f. 98—120.
Suppl. 629; s. XIX. f. 43.

Symeon S[anctus] Mamas.

[Περὶ ἀέρων, στοιχείων, τροφῶν δυνάμεων].
De mutationibus quae corpori et animae accidunt ex aëre, elementis et cibis.

Paris: Parisin. 1010; s. XVI. f. 175.

Syncellus.

Excerpta.

Oxford: Baroccian. 150; s. XV in. f. 5b (Ἀντίδοτος ἡ βασιλική) *und* f. 32b (Ἀντίδοτος).

Synesius.

Περὶ ἐνυπνίων προθεωρία.
De insomniis.

Holkham: nr. 293; s. XV. f. 1 (c. comm.).
Oxford: Miscell. 130; s. XVII. p. 330.

Πρὸς Διόσκορον εἰς τὴν βίβλον Δημοκρίτου ὡς ἐν σχολίοις. [Diels II.100]
Ad Dioscorum, scholia in librum Democriti.

Edd. Berthelot-Ruelle, Alchim. gr. I p. 56—69.

Inc. Διοσκόρῳ ἱερεῖ τοῦ μεγάλου Σαράπιδος κτέ. Τῆς πεμφθείσης μοι ἐπιστολῆς.
Expl. ἀποχωρίζονται. Θεοῦ δὲ βοηθοῦντος ἄρξομαι ὑπομνηματίζειν.

Berlin: Phillipps. 1540 (ol. Meerm. 236); s. XVI. f. 24.
Florenz: Laurent. plut. 86, 16; a. 1492.
Mailand: Ambros. (*bei* Berthelot-Ruelle p. 56).
Paris:
Parisin.
2275; a. 1465. f. 14 (§§ 1—5).
2325; s. XIII. f. 20.
2327; a. 1478. f. 72v.
Suppl. 1022; s. XVII.
Rom: Vatic. 1174; s. XIV—XV. f. 79.
Wien: Vindob. (*bei* Berth.-Ruelle *a. a. O.*).

Ἐπιστολὴ ὑπὲρ τοῦ σιλφίου τῷ ἀδελφῷ.
Epistula de silphio ad fratrem.

Inc. Ἠρόμην τὸ μειράκιον ὑπὲρ τοῦ σιλφίου.
Expl. ὅσα φέρουσιν ὧραι.

Mailand: Arch. del Capitolo Metropolit. 2; s. XV. f. 2.

Taronitus (?).

Excerpta.

Bologna: Bonon. 3632; s. XV. f. 138 (Ἐπίθεμα καταρκοικον [sic!]) *und* f. 189v (Ἀντίδοτος).
Rom: Vatic. 429; s. XV—XVI. f. 341v (Κατάστοιχον εἰς δυσουρίαν. Inc. Ἀλθαίας σπέρματα. Expl. μέλιτος τὸ ἀρκοῦν).
Venedig: Marcian. App. cl. V, 8; s. XIV. f. 102v (Ἀντίδοτος. λίθος θριπτική).

Theodoretus.

Ἀντίδοτα.
Antidota.

Vgl. Medicae artis principes ed. Stephanus, col. 415.

Berlin: Phillipps. 1571 (ol. Meerm. 279); s. XVI. f. 13ᵛ (Ἡ λεγομένη ἀνακάρδιος).
Oxford: Baroccian. 150; s. XV in.

Theodorus.

Excerpta.

Florenz: Laurent. App. 2; s. XV. f. 342ᵛ (Εἰς ἔμφραξιν στομάχου δοθὲν παρὰ Θεοδώρου τῶν Μαγγάνων) *und* 343 (Πρόσταξις στομαχικὴ τοῦ ξενῶνος τῶν Μαγγάνων).
Rom: Ottobon. 311; s. XV—XVI. f. 117ᵛ (Θεραπεία εἰς ἐπιληπτικοὺς καταπίποντας, ἐκ τοῦ δευτέρου Θεοδώρου).

[Diels II.101]

Theophilus.

Περὶ τῆς τοῦ ἀνθρώπου κατασκευῆς λόγοι Ε'.
De hominis fabrica libri V.

Ed. Greenhill, Oxford 1842.

Inc. Ὅτι μὲν πάντα τὰ ζῷα τετράποδα καὶ ἑρπετά.
Expl. τὸ δὲ θῆλυ γίνοιτο. Καὶ περὶ μὲν τούτων ὧδε ἔχει ...

Berlin: Phillipps. 1527 (ol. Meerm. 217); s. XV. f. 3 (lacunos. Expl. τὸ δὲ σχῆμα).
Mailand: Ambros. L 110 Sup.; s. XVI. f. 173 (Expl. mutil. τὸν ἀδένα ἔχοντες, τὸ δὲ σχῆμα. *Vgl. den* Phillipps.).
Paris: Parisin.
825; s. XVI. f. 108.
2155; s. XIV. f. 1ᵛ *und* 265.
2297; s. XVI.
Venedig: Marcian. App. cl. V, 12 (ol. Nanian. 246); s. X—XIII. XV. f. 39.

Ἐπισυναγωγὴ περὶ κοσμικῶν καταρχῶν.
De principiis mundi collectanea.

Rom: Vatic. 1444; s. XV. f. 243v.

Θεραπευτικὴ Θεοφίλου συλλέξαντος ταύτην ἐκ διαφόρων ξενωνικῶν βίβλων.
Therapeutica Theophili, quam ipse ex variis libris valetudinariis collegit.

Inc. Ὅτι μὲν ἀσήπτου.

Florenz: Laurent. plut. 75, 19; s. XIV. p. 82b.

Περὶ σφυγμῶν.
De pulsibus.

Ed. Ermerins, Anecd. med. gr. 1840 p. 1—77.

Inc. Ὅτι μὲν δύο κοιλίαι τῆς καρδίας.
Expl. καὶ ὀλίγον πυκνοὶ καὶ ταχεῖς. Καὶ περὶ μὲν τῶν σφυγμῶν διδασκαλίας ἱκανὰ τὰ εἰρημένα, Χριστοῦ συμπράξαντος ἡμῖν.

Florenz: Laurent. plut. 74, 31; s. XIV. p. 34.
Leyden: Voss. fol.
31*; s. xv (Inc. Ἐπὶ τῶν πυρεκτικῶν σωμάτων).
59; s. XIV.
London: Medical Society H Hi 17 = We 30; s. XV in. no. 39 Dbg. (Expl. τὰ δὲ ἄλλα φυλάττουσι κατὰ φύσιν).
Paris:
Parisin.
2184; s. XVI. f. 221v.
2219; s. XV. f. 1.
2220; s. XVI. f. 28.
2229; s. XIII. f. 46v.
2257; s. XVI. f. 363v.
Suppl. 629; s. XIX. f. 45.
Rom: Vatic. 2304 (ol. 2217); s. XV. f. 1v.
Venedig:
Bibl. losephi de Aromatariis (*Verbleib unbekannt*).
Marcian. App. cl. V, 12; s. X—XIII. XV. f. 126.

[Diels II.102]

Περὶ διαχωρημάτων.
De alvi excrementis.

Ed. Ideler, Phys. et Med. I 397—408.

Inc. Ἐπειδὴ τὰς διαθέσεις τοῦ σώματος.
Expl. ἀφανεῖς τύπους, ἐπικαλούμενον Χριστὸν τὸν ἀληθινὸν θεὸν ἡμῶν εἰς τοὺς αἰῶνας. ἀμήν.

Athen: nr. 1494; s. XVIII. no. 2.
Berlin: Phillipps.
1532 (ol. Meerm. 225); s. XVI. f. 180ᵛ.
1566; s. XVI. f. 23ᵛ.
Bologna: Bonon. 3636; s. XIV—XV. f. 133ᵛ (Expl. ἀπολείπεται τὸ διαχώρημα = Idel. I 399, 31).
Escurial: Scorial. Υ. III. 14; s. XV. f. 22.
Florenz: Laurent. plut. 74, 31; s. XIV. p. 34.
London:
Addit. (Brit. Mus.) 17, 900; s. XVII. f. 101ᵛ.
Medical Society H Hi 21. 22 = We 28. 29; s. XV ex. f. 354ᵛ.
Oxford: Roe 15 (Bodl. 261); s. XV ex. f. 97ᵛ.
Paris:
Parisin.
1630; s. XIV. f. 22.
2306; s. XV. f. 338.
2307; s. XVI. f. 523ᵛ.
Suppl.
629; s. XIX. f. 9ᵛ.
637; s. XV. f. 40.
Rom:
Barberin. I 127; s. XVI. f. 271 (Expl. τῷ συνετῷ δυνάμενον).
Vatic. 280; s. XV. f. 197ᵛ (Fine mutil.; expl. 408,1 Idel.).
Venedig: Marcian. App. cl.
V, 8; s. XIV. f. 131 (Expl. καὶ τῶν διὰ μελαγχολικόν).
V, 12; s. X—XIII. XV. f. 114.
Wien: Vindob. med.
8; s. XV. f. 57ᵛ.
37; s. XV. f. 75ᵛ (»Ein Blatt«).

Περὶ οὔρων.
De urinis.

Ed. Ideler, Phys. et Med. I 261—284.

Inc. Τὴν περὶ τῶν οὔρων πραγματείαν.
Expl. ἐκ πάσης προαιρέσεως μανθάνειν.

Berlin: Phillipps.
1524 (ol. Meerm. 214); s. XV. f. 36 (Inc. Κατὰ πόσας αἰτίας γίνεται ἡ ἀπεψία. Expl. καὶ τοῦτο εἰπὼν παρέλιπε).
1531; s. XVI. f. 91.
Bologna: Bonon. 3632; s. XV. f. 51v.
Escurial: Scorial.
Υ. III. 14; s. XV. f. 31.
Φ. III. 11; s. XIV—XV. f. 1.
Florenz: Laurent. plut.
74, 10; s. XIV. p. 15 (De urinarum coloribus) *und* p. 18b (Inc. Τὴν π. τῶν οὔρων).
11; s. XIII. p. 131b (Inc. Οὖρόν ἐστι τὸ περιήθημα).
Gallipoli: Ἐκκλ. ἁγ. Νικολ. 38; s. XIV. f. 64v.
Krakau: Bibl. Univ. Iagell. misc. 2526 FF VI 5; s. XV. f. 86v.
London:
Addit. (Brit. Mus.) 17, 900; s. XVII. f. 95.
Medical Society H Hi 17 = We 30; s. XV in. no. 28 Dbg.
Mailand: Ambros.
A 95 Sup.; s. XV. f. 52 (= Idel. I 261—264, 20).
L 110 Sup.; s. XVI. f. 117 (»Falso Philotheus pro Theophilo scriptum est«).
Modena: Mutin.
61 (III B 9); s. XV. f. 2.
115 (II D 16)*; s. XV. f. 9.
Oxford: Roe 15 (Bodl. 261); s. XV ex. f. 90v.
Palermo: Panormit. bibl. naz. XIII C 3; s. XVI. f. 96—119v (Inscr. Σχόλια εἰς τὰ π. οὔρων).
Paris:
Parisin.
1630; s. XIV.
2204; s. XVI. f. 23.
2220; s. XVI. f. 1.
2229; s. XIII. f. 35v.
2257; s. XVI. f. 345.
2306; s. XV. f. 329.

2307; s. XVI. f. 508v.
2308; s. XV. f. 27.
2316; s. XV. f. 170.
Suppl.
629; s. XIX. f. 1.
637; s. XV. f. 44.

Rom:
Angelic. 17 (C 5. 4); s. XIV. f. 247 (lacunos. et fine mutil.).
Barberin. I 127*; s. XVI. f. 265 (Inc. λευκὸν ὡς ὕδωρ. Expl. τὰ ἐλαιώδη καὶ δυσώδη).

Venedig: Marcian. App. cl. V 12; s. X—XIII. XV. f. 98.

Wien: Vindob. med.
8; s. XV. f. 320v.
29*; s. XV. f. 1—8v (Inc. Ἐρώτησις πῶς γίνεται. Expl. ἐγκυμονούσης ἐστίν).

[Diels II.104]

Σχόλια εἰς τοὺς Ἱπποκράτους ἀροφισμούς.
Commentarius in Hippocratis Aphorismos.

Ed. Dietz, Schol. in Hipp. II 245—544.

Inc. Ἀφορισμός ἐστιν λόγος σύντομος.
Expl. κατὰ πάντα ὅμοιός ἐστιν.

Berlin: Phillipps. 1524 (ol. Meerm. 214); s. XV. f. 1 (Inc. κείμενον· ὁ βίος βραχύς. Expl. ὅθεν ἡ ἔκλυσις γίνεται. »Codex verbis ab editione discrepat nec totum commentarium continet«).

Erlangen: nr. 90; s. XVI (Inde ab aphor. XXIV).

Escurial: Scorial. y. l. 8; s. XVI. f. 1.

Florenz: Laurent. plut. 74, 11; s. XIII. p. 1 (Initio mutilus).

Göttingen: Hist. nat. 5; s. XVII.

Mailand: Ambros.
A 95 Sup.; s. XV. f. 165 (= »Dietz II 245 sub finem, 247, 7—300,15 passim«).
B 113 Sup.; s. XIV in. f. 4 (= Dietz II 245—543).
L 30 Sup.; a. 1524. f. 1 (= Dietz II 245—543, 4. »Falso Philotheus pro Theophilo scriptum est«).
L 110 Sup.; s. XVI. f. 1 (»In prooemio non semper verba eadem atque apud Dietz II 245«).
S 19 Sup.; s. — (»Stephani et Theoph. in aphor. Hipp. comm.«).

Oxford:
Baroccian. 204; s. XV in. f. 1 (Initium solum).
Roe 14 (Bodl. 260); s. XV. f. 87v (= Dtz. II 245—543 ἴαμα).

Paris:

Parisin.

1883; s. XIV. f. 74v—156 (Sine auctor. nomine. Inc. mutil. τεχνικῆς φάμεν. *Vgl.* Costomiris, Rev. des ét. gr. II p. 357).

2149; s. XVI. f. 1—94v.

2222; s. XV (Sub nomine Meletii).

2223; s. xvi (*Apograph. von* 2222).

2228; s. XIV—XI. f. 95—149v.

2296; s. XVI. f. 1—131v.

Suppl. 64; s. XV—XVII. f. 207—230v (Sine auctor. nomine. Expl. λειποθυμία καὶ συγκοπὴ ἕπεται. *Vgl.* Costomiris l. l. p. 357).

Rom: Vatic.

1062; s. XVI. f. 1.

2254; s. X—XI. f. 25 (Sine auctor. nomine. Expl. καὶ οἷον ὑποχόνδρια μετέωρα = Dtz. II 500, 2. *Collation Reitzensteins von Hipp. IV 458—466, 7 L. in Ilbergs Besitz*).

Upsala: Upsal. 34; s. XV—XVI. f. 2 (Expl. νομίζειν ἀνίατα).

Wien: Vindob.

med.

16; s. XV—XVI (Expl. δηλοῖ γὰρ ἐπίτασιν ξηρότητος. *Abschrift im Berol. fol. 39 [275]*).

44; s. XV—XVI. f. 1—126v (*Vgl.* Stephanus).

phil. 74; s. XVI. f. 52—107v (Expl. πάντως ἂν εἴη ἴαμα. *Vgl.* Oxford Roe 14).

[Diels II.105]

Ἐκ τῶν Ἱπποκράτους καὶ Γαληνοῦ περὶ ἰατρικῆς ἐπιστήμης σύντομος παράδοσις.
De arte medica, ex Hippocrate et Galeno.

Inc. Ἐπειδὴ πᾶν τὸ ἀναγκαιότερον τῆς ἰατρικῆς τέχνης.
Expl. καὶ μεγάλης γινομένης ἐπὶ ταύτης τῆς διαιρέσεως.

Escurial: Scorial. Σ. III. 17; s. XVI. f. 126v.

Περιτομὴ τοῦ περὶ διαφορᾶς πυρετῶν (Γαληνοῦ).
Epitome librorum Galeni de febrium differentiis.

Ed. Dem. Sicuri, Florenz 1862.
Vgl. Palladius *bei* Ideler Phys. et Med. I 107 ss. *und* Stephanus Atheniens.

Inc. Σκοπὸν ἔχομεν ἐν τῷ παρόντι συγγράματι.
Expl. ἐν οἷς αἱ διαφοραὶ τῶν πυρετῶν. τέλος Γαληνοῦ τοῦ περὶ διαφορᾶς πυρετῶν.

Florenz: Laurent. plut. 86, 20; s. XV ex. f. 64 (*Collation besitzt Dr. E. Bianchi, Florenz*).
Wien: Vindob. med.
16; s. XV—XVI. f. 325ᵛ—328ᵛ.
28; s. XV. f. 18 (Πόσαι διαφοραὶ πυρετῶν. Inc. Διαφοραὶ τῶν πυρετῶν αἱ μὲν οἰκειόταται. Expl. f. 26ᵛ καὶ ἐκφεύξῃ θάνατον ἐκ κερασμάτων [?]).
52; s. XV. f. 1—22ᵛ (Θεόφ. καὶ Στέφ. ἔκ τε Ἱππ. καὶ Γαλ. π. τῆς τ. πυρ. διαφ. Expl. θερμασίας αὗται γίνονται).

[Diels II.106]

Excerpta varia.

Bologna: Bonon. 3632; s. XV. f. 262 (Inscr. Περὶ θεραπείας ψυχῆς; *vgl.* f. 16. Inc. Ἔλεγον οἱ πατέρες, ὅτι μόναχός τις ἐρχόμενός ἐστι. Expl. προσκύνει [?] τὸν δεσπότην Χριστόν).
London: Harleian. (Brit. Mus.) 6305; s. XVI. f. 161 (Θεραπεία μελαινῶν ἀλφῶν. Inc. Ὁ δὲ ἐν Ἀσίᾳ ὑπό τινος ἀγοραίου. Expl. πινόμενος μετὰ οἴνου ἀτοκίαν καὶ αὐτό ποιεῖ).
Modena: Mutinens. 61 (III B 9); s. XV. f. 31.
Paris:
Parisin.
2047; s. XV. f. 16ᵛ (Fragm. de phlebotomia).
2178; s. XV. f. 1 (Excerpta de pulsibus).
2228; s. XIV—XI. f. 59 (Exc. de excrementis).
2510; a. 1384. f. 108 (Praecepta medica et remedia varia).
Suppl. 629; s. XIX. f. 33 (Variae lectiones in Theophilum, e cod. Parisin. 2220).
Wien: Vindob. med. 28; s. XV. f. 2 (Ab init. mutil. Inc. Οἱ δὲ πελιοί. Expl. τὰ δὲ ἄλλα φυλάττουσιν κατὰ φ... + τέλος σὺν θεῷ ἁγίῳ τὸ περὶ σφυγμῶν ἀπὸ φωνῆς Θεοφίλου ἐκ τοῦ προγνωστικοῦ Γαληνοῦ).

Theophylactus Simocatta.

Versus in Galenum.

Inc. Σοὶ μέν, Γαληνέ.

Moskau: Mosquens. 464; s. XV. f. 301.

Περὶ διαφορᾶς φυσικῶν ἀπορημάτων καὶ ἐπιλύσεων αὐτῶν.
Quaestiones naturales.

Ed. Ideler, Phys. et Med. I p. 168—183.

Inc. Τὰς χελιδόνας ὑπὸ τῶν μητέρων ἀκήκοα.
Expl. τῶν δυσπορίστων λόγων τὴν ἐπιστήμην ἀπείληφα.

Modena: Mutinens. 135 (II E 2); s. XV. f. 123v.
Paris: Parisin. 993; s. XIV. f. 231v.

Theopompus.

Excerpta.

Bologna: Bonon. 1808; s. XV. f. 32v (Θυμίαμα μοσχάτον).

Theosebius.

Excerpta.

Bologna: Bonon. 3632; s. XV. f. 232v (Ὑποθέματα δυσεντερικὰ καὶ ἐπιθέματα).

Timocrates. [Diels II.107]

Excerpta.

Paris: Parisin. 2286; s. XIV. f. 89 (Remedia ad sedandos dentium dolores).

Timotheus Gazaeus.

Περὶ ζῴων τετραπόδων καὶ φυσικῶν αὐτῶν ἐνεργειῶν.
De animalibus quadrupedibus physicisque eorum facultatibus.

Partim ed. Cramer, Anecd. Oxon. IV p. 263, partim M. Haupt, Herm. III p. 5—30.
Vgl. Excerptor. Constantini de natura animilium libri II ed. Sp. Lambros, Suppl. Aristotel. I 1 praef. p. XII sq.

Inc. Περὶ καμίλων.
Expl. εἴδη ἐστὶν τῶν λύκων ...

Athos: Βιβλ. μον. Λαύρας (*Vgl.* Parisin. Suppl. 799. f. 18. Costomiris, Rev. des ét. gr. IV [1892] p. 99).
München: Monac. 514*; s. XIV. f. 239.
Oxford: Baroccian. 50; s. XI. f. 46.
Paris: Parisin. 2422*; s. XVI.

Vincentius Damodes.

[Περὶ φυσιολογίας.]
Physiologia.

Paris: Parisin. Suppl. 639; s. XVIII.

[Diels II.108]

Xenocrates.

Περὶ τῆς ἀπὸ τῶν ἐνύδρων τροφῆς.
De alimento ex aquatilibus.

Ed. Franz, Leipzig 1778.
D'Ancora, Neapel 1794.
Corais, Paris 1814.
Ideler, Phys. et Med. I p. 121—133.
Vgl. Daremberg Orib. I p. LVIII *und* 124.)

Inc. Πεποίηται μὲν ἡ νηχαλέα φύσις.
Expl. καὶ κοιλίας ὑπαγωγά.

Hamburg: nr.— (*Vgl.* Fabricius bibl. gr. IX. p. 454—474).
Leyden: Voss. misc. 22; s. XV (fine mutil.).
Paris: Parisin.
2290; s. XVIII. f. 1.
2291; s. XVI.
Rom: Vatic.? (*Vgl.* Daremb. 1. 1.).

Μετάφρασις περὶ θανάτου.
De morte. (Platonis Axiochus?)

Leyden: Voss. 8° 20; s. XVI. f. 1—58 (Initio mutil.).

Ioannes Zacharias Actuarius.

Opera varia.

Rom: Vatic. (*Vgl.* Costomiris, Rev. des ét. gr. X p. 435).
517.
1052.
1191.
1194
Verona: Veronens. 57 *bei* Montfaucon (*griechisch?*).

Περὶ ἐνεργειῶν καὶ παθῶν τοῦ ψυχικοῦ πνεύματος καὶ τῆς κατ' αὐτὸ διαίτης λόγοι Β'.
De spiritu animali libri II.

Ed. Ideler Phys. et Med. I 312—386.

Inc. (lib. 1) Ἐπειδή σου ταῖς ἔναγχός τε καὶ πρότριτα.
Expl. (lib. 2) μεταδιώκειν τἀμείνονα.

Berlin: Phillipps. 1582; s. XV. f. 111.
Brüssel: Bruxell. 11337—41; s. —. f. 1.
Dresden: Dresd.
Da 5; a. 1519. f. 2.
Da 67; s. — (Exempl. impress, a Ch. F. Matthaei c. cod. Da 5 collat.).
Escurial: Scorial. Φ. III. 12; s. XV. f. 130.
Florenz:
Laur. plut.
75, 9; s. XV. p. 114.
75, 11; s. XV. p. 82.
75, 16; s. XV. p. 105.
Riccard. 31 (K. II. 4); s. XIV. f. 275 (»Titulus hic prolatus ab usitato valde discrepat«).
Glasgow: Hunterian. V. 5. 11; s. XV. f. 1.
Leyden: Vossian. fol. 32; s. —.

London:

Arundel. (Brit. Mus.) 537; s. XV in. f. 156.

[Diels II.109] Medical Society H Hi 21. 22 = We 28. 29; s. XV. f. 1.

Mailand: Ambros. R 20 Sup.; s. —.

München: Monac. 69; s. XVI. f. 1.

Oxford:

Barocc. 2304; s. —.

Roe 15 (Bodl. 261); s. XV ex. f. 184.

Paris: Parisin.

2098; s. XIII. f. 119.

2153; s. XV. f. 435.

2232; s. XV. f. 63.

2234; s. XVI.

2256; s. XV. f. 240.

2304; s. XV. f. 114.

2305; a. 1418. f. 121.

2306; s. XV. f. 289.

2307; s. XVI. f. 453^{v}.

2308; s. XV. f. 204^{v}.

Rom: Vatic. 429; s. XV—XVI. f. 315 (*Nur* liber II?).

Venedig: Marcian.

298; s. XV.

529; s. XV.

Wien: Vindob. med. 21; s. —. f. 120—173.

Περὶ οὔρων λόγοι Ζ'.
De urinis libri VII.

Ed. Ideler Phys. et Med. II 3—192.

Inc. Πάλαι μὲν ἴσως φιλοτιμίας.
Expl. αὐτῶν δὲ τῶν λόγων ἀκριβής τις ἐπίσκεψις.

Berlin:

Phillipps.

1531; s. XVI. f. 98^{v}.

1582; s. XV. f. 1.

fol. 7 (247); s. XVI. f. 1.

Cambridge:

Caius Coll. 76; s. XV/XVI. f. 35.

Trinity Coll. 1386; s. XV. XVI. f. 9.
Dresden: Dresd. Da 5; a. 1519. f. 182.
Escurial: Scorial.
T. II. 14; s. XVI. f. 192.
Φ. III. 12; s. XV. f. 12.
Florenz: Laurent. plut.
74, 13; s. XV. p. 88.
75, 9; s. xv. p. 5.
75, 11; s. XV. p. 1 (Libri VI).
75, 16; s. XV. p. 4.
Leyden: Vossian. fol. 32; s. —.
London:
Arundel. (Brit. Mus.) 537; s. XV in. f. 1 (Inc. ποικίλης = Idel. II 4, 10).
Medical Society
H Hi 17 = We 30*; s. XV in. (Ex l. I. VI. VII).
H Hi 21. 22 = We 28. 29; s. XV. f. 44.
Wf 16; s. XVI ex.
Mailand: Ambros.
C 89 Sup.; s. —. f. 1 (»Deest magna pars libri I«).
R 20 Sup.; s. —.
München: Monac. 362; s. XVI. f. 112.
Oxford:
Miscell. 241.
Auct. T IV 3; s. XV. f. 8.
Roe 15 (Bodl. 261); s. XV ex. f. 105.
Paris:
Facult. med. (Anon. [fort. Actuar.] de urinis).
Coislin. 334; s. XV. f. 215.
Parisin.
2153; s. XV. f. 408.
2232; s. XV. f. 1 (L. I. II., ceterorum frgmta.).
2256; s. XV. f. 144^{v}.
2260; s. XVI. f. 42—120.
2270; s. XV—XIV. f. 231.
2304; s. XV. f. 1.
2305; a. 1418. f. 1.
2306; s. XV. f. 1.
2307; s. XVI. f. 1.
2308; s. xv. f. 55 (ab init. mutil.).
Rom: Vatic.
299; s. XV. f. 20^{v}.

2182*; s. XV. f. 81 (L. V prooem. 7—V 10, 13 = Idel. II 112—129) *und* f. 89 (L. VI pr. 6—VI 12, 10 = Idel. II 145—162).

Venedig:

Marcian.

296; s. XV.

510; s. XV (L. I).

App. cl. V 13; s. XIV—XVI. f. 25ᵛ.

Wien: Vindob. med.

3; s. —. f. 136—230.

21; s. —. f. 1—119.

26; s. XV. f. 1 (Ὀκταρίου).

44; s. XV—XVI. f. 136.

Ἰατρικὴ μέθοδος.
De methodo medendi libri VI.

L. I. II ed. Ideler Phys. et Med. II 353—463.

Inc. Ἐπειδή σοι εἰς τὴν ὑπὲρ τοῦ γένους ἡμῶν στελλομένῳ πρεσβείαν.
Expl. δοκῶμεν ἐκπεπονηκότες τὴν βίβλον.

Athos: Βιβλ. μον. Ἰβήρων 151; s. XV. f. — (Liber V).

Berlin:

Phillipps.

1528; s. XVI. f. 1 (Liber VI).

1582; s. XV. f. 159.

fol. 39 (275); s. — (»Abschr. von Buch 1. 2 von der Hand Schneiders«).

[Diels II.110] **Brüssel:** Bruxell. 11337—41; s. —. f. 138ᵛ. 239.

Dresden: Dresd. Da 5; a. 1519. *vor* f. 176ᵛ.

Escurial: Scorial.

Υ. III. 14*; s. XV. f. 6ᵛ.

Φ. 111. 12; s. XV. f. 175. 352ᵛ. 396. 411. 415.

Florenz: Laurent. plut.

75, 8; s. XV. p. 222.

75, 11; s. XV. p. 116b.

75, 16; s. XV. p. 192.

Leipzig: Lipsiens. 60; a. 1786. 87.

Leyden: Vossian. fol. 32; s. — (L. I—V).

London:

Arundel. (Brit. Mus.) 537; s. XV in. f. 196ᵛ (Expl. ἀποσιτίαι καὶ ἄλγη = Id. II 405, 28).

Medical Society
H Hi 21. 22 = We 28. 29; s. XV ex. f. 145—257v (*Abschrift der Bücher III—VI von Kalbfleisch, A. Meyer und H. Zimmer im Besitze der Berliner Akademie*).
NNa 11 = Wf 8; s. — (Inc. Ἡ μὲν παροιμία φησί, χελώνης. Expl. ἐνταῦθά πη συγκαταπαύειν).

Mailand: Ambros.
R 20 Sup.; s. — (L. I—V).
& 147 Sup.; s. XVI. f. 5v (Inscr. Βιβλίον ἰατρικὸν περιέχον πᾶσαν τέχνην ἐν ἐπιτόμῳ).

München: Monac. 69; s. XV. f. 46.

Oxford:
Laud. 62 (Bodl. 747); s. XVI. f. 1 (L. IV. V) *und* f. 95 (L. VIc. 8 ss. Inscr. Γαλ. Π. ἐμπλάστρων).
Roe 15 (Bodl. 261); s. XV ex. f. 218.

Paris:
Coislin. 334; s. XV. f. 1 *und* 19.
Parisin.
2153; s. XV. f. 290 (L. I—V).
2233; s. XVI (L. I—V et index l. VI).
2235; s. XVI. f. 1 (De medicamentorum compositione liber V) *und* f. 88 (De ratione medendi liber IV).
2256; s. XV. f. 280.
2304; s. XV. f. 191.
2305; a. 1418. f. 158.
2307; s. XVI. f. 122—451v.

Rom:
Palat. 370; s. XV. f. 151 (L. IV. V).
Reg. Suec. 181; a. 1364. f. 1 (L. I—V).
Vatic. 2182; s. XV. f. 97 (Inc. mutil. χείων ἡ ὑπόθεσις = Idel. I 355, 36) *und* f. 139v.

Venedig: Marcian. 298; s. XV.

Wien: Vindob. med.
21; s. —. f. 173—267v (L. I —III), f. 268–303 (L. VI cap. 1—31), f. 307—415v (L. IV. V).
22; s. —. f. 1—55 (L. IV. V).
23; s. —. f. 1 (Libri VI sub nomine Pyropuli[?]).
26; s. XV. f. 244—303 (L. III. VI) *und* f. 307—412 (Inc. *wie im* Londin. Medical Society NNa 11 = Wf 8).

Πραγματεία περὶ οὔρων βαρβάρων, μετενεχθεῖσα εἰς τὴν Ἑλλάδα παρὰ τοῦ ἰατρικωτάτου Χριστοδούλου, εἰς ῥυθμὸν δὲ καὶ τάξιν Ἑλληνικὴν ἐκτεθεῖσα παρὰ τοῦ σοφωτάτου καὶ ἰατρικωτάτου τοῦ ἀκτουαρίου κυροῦ Ιωάννου τοῦ Ζαχαρίου.
Tractatus de urinis, qui ex Avicenna translatus dicitur in graecam linguam a Christodulo, in ordinem redactus ab Actuario Zacharia.

Inc. Περὶ τοῦ ὑδατώδους οὔρου.

Athos: Βιβλ. Μον. Λαύρας Ω 69; s. —.
Madrid: Matrit. 9715; s. —.
Neapel: Neapol. 307 D III 23; s. XV. f. 139.
Palermo: Panorm. XIII. C. 3; s. —.
Paris: Parisin.
2260; s. XVI. f. 42.
2307; s. XVI.
Rom: Vatic. 299; s. XV. f. 17.
Turin: Taurin. 156b II 10; s. XVI. f. 154.
Venedig: Marcian. App. cl. V, 8; s. XIV. f. 110.

Περὶ ζῴων φθαρτικῶν.
De animalibus nocentibus.

Inc. Ζῷα τοίνυν φθαρτικά ἐστι.

Bologna: Bonon. 3632; s. XV. f. 380 (Ὀκταρίου).
Escurial: Scorial. Φ. III. 12; s. XV. f. 346.
Mailand: Ambros. R 20 Sup.; s. —.

[Diels II.111] Εἰς Γαληνοῦ περὶ θεραπευτικῆς μεθόδου.
In Galenum de methodo medendi.

Von Daremberg, Not. et Extr. I p. 23 *dem* Ioannes Archiatrus *zugeschrieben.*

Paris: Parisin. 2236; s. XV. f. 1 (Capp. 152).

Excerpta varia.

Dresden: Dresd. Da 5; a. 1519. f. 176v (Περὶ σταθμῶν καὶ χαρακτήριων αὐτῶν καὶ τῶν μέτρων).

Escurial: Scorial. Φ. III. 12; s. XV. f. 1 (Inc. Ξανθῆς χολῆς εἰς κένωσιν προκειμένης).
Paris: Parisin. 2144; s. XIV.

Zenarius.

Excerpta.

Paris: Parisin. 1991; s. XV. f. 29v (Excerpta de rebus medico-astrologicis).

Zosimus Panopolita.

Περὶ ἀρετῆς καὶ συνθέσεως ὑδάτων.
Liber de virtute et compositione aquarum.

Edd. Berthelot-Ruelle, Alchim. gr. II p. 107—113.

Inc. Θέσις ὑδάτων καὶ κίνησις.
Expl. τὸ μονόειδον ὡς πολύειδον.

Berlin: Phillipps. 1540 (ol. Meerm. 236); s. XVI. f. 69.
Paris: Parisin.
2249; s. XVI. f. 1.
2252; s. XVII. f. 265.
2327; a. 1478. f. 85.
Venedig: Marc. 299; s. XI. f. 92. 115.

Περὶ θείου ὕδατος. [Diels II.112]
Gemini commentarii de aqua divina.

Edd. Berthelot-Ruelle, Alchim. gr. II p. 141—145.

I. Inc. Λαβὼν ὠὰ ὅσα βούλει, ἔκζεσον.
Expl. οἷά πέρ εἰσιν. Ἔρρωσθε ἐν Χριστῷ τῷ Θεῷ Ἰησοῦ. Ἀμήν.

II. Inc. Τοῦτό ἐστι τὸ θεῖον καὶ μέγα μυστήριον.
Expl. ἀνάκειται δὲ τῷ ἐρωτύλῳ.

Berlin: Phillipps. 1540 (ol. Meerm. 236); s. XVI. f. 63.

Paris: Parisin.
2249; s. XVI. f. 96 (II).
2252; s. XVII. f. 219 (II).
2325; s. XIII. f. 86. 82 (I. II).
2327; a. 1478. f. 80. 83. 220 (II. I. II).
2329; s. XVI—XVII. f. 183ᵛ (I).
Venedig: Marcian. 299; s. XI. f. 113ᵛ. 188 (I. II).

Περὶ τῆς ἱερᾶς καί θείας τέχνης τῆς τοῦ χρυσοῦ καὶ ἀργύρου ποιήσεως.
De sacra divinaque arte auri et argenti faciendi.

Edd. Berthelot-Ruelle, Alchim. gr. II p. 145—148.

Inc. Λαβὼν ψυχὴν τοῦ χαλκοῦ.
Expl. κατείληφα τὴν τῶν φώτων ποσότητα.

Paris: Parisin.
2249; s. XVI. f. 18.
2251; s. XVII. f. 145.
2325; s. XIII. f. 118.
2327; a. 1478. f. 112.
2329; s. XVI—XVII. f. 41.

Περὶ ὀργάνων καὶ καμίνων.
De instrumentis et fornacibus.

Edd. Berthelot-Ruelle, Alchim. gr. II p. 244—227.

Inc. Ἡ τῆς ὁρωμένης καμίνου διαγραφή.
Expl. ἔστω ἀνεξάλειπτον. Ἔρρωσο.

Paris: Parisin. 2249; s. XVI. f. 94ᵛ.
Rom: Vatic. 1174; s. XIV—XV. f. 42.
Venedig: Marcian. 299; s. XI. f. 186.

Excerpta.

Berlin: Phillipps. 1540 (ol. Meerm. 236); s. XVI. f. 5 (Περὶ ἀσβέστου).

Addenda I.

S. 4 zu L. I 570—636, Laurent. 74, 1 *und* Marcian. 269: (*Collat. Kühleweins in dessen Besitz*). [Diels II.113]

S. 5 zu L. II 140—190, Laurent. 74, 1. 74, 11. 75,3 *und* Marcian. 269: (*Collat. Kühleweins in dessen Besitz*).

S. 6 zu Ambros. G 108 Inf.: (*Ediert von* Kühlewein, Hermes 25 p. 120 ff.).

S. 8 zu L. II 224—376, Marcian. 269: (*Collat. Kühleweins in dessen Besitz*).

S. 10 zu L. II 598—III 148, Laurent. 74, 1: (*Collat., Kühleweins in dessen Besitz*).

S. 11 zu L. III 272—336, Marcian. 269: (*Collat. Kühleweins in dessen Besitz*).

zu L. III 412—562, Marcian. 269: (*Collat., Kühleweins in dessen Besitz*).

zu L. IV 78—326, Parisin. 2142: (*Kalbfleischs Collat. von L. IV 78—109, 320—326 in Kühleweins Besitz*) *und zu* Marcian. 269 (*S. 12*): (*Kühleweins Collat. in dessen Besitz*).

S. 12 zu L. IV 340—394, Marcian. 269: (*Kühleweins Collat. in dessen Besitz*).

S. 14 zu L. IV 458—608, Marcian. 269: (*Kühleweins Collat. in dessen Besitz*) *und zu* Casinens. 97: (*Probe ediert von* Kühlewein, Hermes 17 p. 484 ff.).

S. *17 zu* L. IV 628—632, Laurent. 74, 1 *und* Marcian. 269: (*Kühleweins Collat. in dessen Besitz*).

S. 18 zu L. IV 638—643, Laurent. 74, 1 *und* Marcian. 269: (*Kühleweins Collat. in dessen Besitz*).

S. 19 zu L. V 72—468, Laurent. 74, 1 : (*Kühleweins Collat. von* B. Δ. *und 6 Seiten von* E *in dessen Besitz*), *zu* Vatic. 276: (*Tschiedels Collat. in Kühleweins Besitz*) *und zu* Marcian. 269: (*Kühleweins Collat. in dessen Besitz*).

S. 20 zu L. V 476—502, Marcian. 269: (*Kühleweins Collat. in dessen Besitz*).

zu L. V 588—732, Laurent. 74, 1: (*Kühleweins Collat. bis S. 277 Kühn in dessen Besitz*).

Füge hinzu: **Paris:** Parisin. 2253; s. XI. f. 1.

zu L. VI 2—26, Laurent. 74, 1 *und* Marcian. 269: (*Kühleweins Collat. in dessen Besitz*).

S. 21 zu L. VI 32—68, Marcian. 269: (*Kühleweins Collat. in dessen Besitz*).

S. 22 zu L. VI 72—86, Marcian. 269: (*Kühleweins Collat. in dessen Besitz*). *Die Schrift steht in den* Parisin. 2141. 2142. 2144. 2255 *als Anhang zu* περὶ φύσιος ἀνθρώπου; *danach ist das fol. zu bestimmen.*

S. 23 zu L. VI 140—204, Marcian. 269: (*Kühleweins Collat. in dessen Besitz*).

zu L. VI 208—270, Marcian. 269: (*Kühleweins Collat. in dessen Besitz*).

zu L. VI 276—348, Parisin. 2253: (*Kühleweins Collat. von* VI 294 L. — 340 ὑπεναντία γίνεται *in dessen Besitz. Von den genannten Worten ab fehlt der Schluß in der Handschrift*).

S. 24 zu L. VI 352—396, Marcian. 269: (*Kühleweins Collat. in dessen Besitz*).

S. 25 zu L. VI 466—524, Marcian. 269: (*Collat. Ilbergs und Kühleweins in Ilbergs Besitz*).

zu L. VI 526—636, Marcian. 269: (*Kühleweins Collat. in Ilbergs Besitz*).

[Diels II.114] *S. 26 zu* L. VI 640—662, Marcian. 269: (*Kühleweins Collat. in Ilbergs Besitz*).
zu L. VII 8—160, Marcian. 269: (*Kühleweins Collat. in dessen Besitz*).
S. 27 zu L. VII 166—302, Marcian. 269: (*Kühleweins Collat. in dessen Besitz*).
zu L. VII 312—430: *Die Schrift ist im Marcian, 269 nicht ganz vollständig erhalten.*
zu L. VII 436—452, Marcian. 269: (*Kühleweins Collat. in dessen Besitz*).
S. 28 zu L. VII 452—460, Marcian. 269: (*Kühleweins Collat. in dessen Besitz*).
zu L. VII 470—484, Marcian. 269: (*Kühleweins Collat. in dessen Besitz*).
S. 29 zu L. VII 486—542, Marcian. 269: (*Kühleweins Collat. in dessen Besitz*).
zu L. VII 542—614, Marcian. 269: (*Kühleweins Collat. in dessen Besitz*).
S. 30 zu L. VIII 10—232, Marcian. 269: (*Kühleweins Collat. in dessen Besitz*).
S. 31 zu L. VIII 476—508, Marcian. 269: (*Kühleweins Collat. in dessen Besitz*).
zu L. VIII 512 ff. I, Marcian. 269: (*Kühleweins Collat. in dessen Besitz*).
S. 33 zu L. IX 98—120, Marcian. 269: (*Kühleweins Collat. in dessen Besitz*).
S. 34 zu L. IX 152—160: Marcian. App. V 14 *ist* saec. XVI.
zu L. IX 168—196, Marcian. 269: (*Kühleweins Collat. in dessen Besitz*).
zu L. IX 226—244, Laurent. 74, 1 *und* Marcian. 269: (*Kühleweins Collat. in dessen Besitz*).
S. 35 zu L. IX 250—272, Laurent. 74, 1: (*Kühleweins Collat. in dessen Besitz*). *zu* Vatic. 277: (*Ilbergs Collat. in dessen Besitz*) *und zu* Marcian. 269: (*Nicht Ilberg, sondern Kühlewein besitzt eigenhändige Collation*).
zu L. IX 298—307, Marcian. 269: (*Kühleweins Collat. in dessen Besitz*). Marcian. App. V 14 *ist* saec. XVI.
S. 45 zu Hippocr. Προγνωστικά, latein. Übers.: *Vgl. den Abschnitt* Democritus Prognostica *in Teil* II *S.* 27.
S. 48 zu Ὅτι ὑπαρκτικαί εἰσιν αἱ τέχναι *und* Περὶ ὑπάρξεως ἰατρικῆς: *Diese Fragmente sind identisch mit einem Teile von* Περὶ τέχνης (= L. VI p. 2 sq. cap. 2).
S. 49 zu Πρόγνωσις περὶ τῶν δ' ὡρῶν: *Dies ist Excerpt eines Stückes von* Περὶ ἀέρων ὑδάτων τόπων (= L. II p. 42, 13—50, 12). *Füge hinzu* **Wien:** Vindob. gr. philos, et philol. 179; s. XV. f. 123ᵛ.
S. 58 zu Galen. *Opera varia:* **Dresden:** Dresdens. (»Galeni operum exemplar Aldinum ... hac re conspicuum, quod et in textu ipso nonnulla atramento sunt correcta et in margine librorum plurimorum adnotantur argumenta brevia, versiones latinae, variae denique lectiones haud paucae«. *Der III. Band fehlt. Vgl.* Ilberg, Philol. 48. N. F. II S. 57—66).
S. 76 zu K. VI 453—748, Titel: Lib. I c. 14—II c. 20 ed. G. Helmreich. Ansbach 1906.
S. 109 zu K. XIX 62—157, GRIECH. HDSS.: *Ilbergs Collation des* Laurent. plut. 74, 1 *und* 74, 3. *der* Parisini 2143. 2144. 2255, *des* Urbin. 68 *und des* Vatic. 277 *in dessen Besitz. Kühleweins Collation des* Marcian. 269 *und Karrers Collation des* Vatic. 277 *in Ilbergs Besitz. Vgl.* Ilberg *in den* Commentatt. in honor. Ribbeckii 1888 p. 327—354.

Addenda II.

Democritus. [Diels II.115]

Φυσικὰ καὶ μυστικά.
Physica et mystica.

Edd. Berthelot-Ruelle, Alchim. gr. I p. 41—53.

Inc. Βαλὼν εἰς λίτραν μίαν πορφύρας διοβόλου λίτραν.
Expl. ἐν ταῖς ἄλλαις μου γραφαῖς. Ἔρρωσθε ἐν ταύτῃ τῇ γραφῇ.

Paris:
Parisin.
2275; a. 1465. f. 7v.
2325; s. XIII. f. 8v.
2326; s. XVI. f. 1.
2327; a. 1478. f. 24v.
Suppl. 1022; s. XVII. f. 1.
Venedig: Marcian. 299; s. XI. f. 66v.

Βίβλος ε' προσφωνηθεῖσα Λευκίππῳ.
Liber V ad Leucippum.

Edd. Berthelot-Ruelle, Alchim. gr. I p. 53—56.

Inc. Ἰδοὺ μὲν ὃ ἦν, ὦ Λεύκιππε, περὶ τούτων τῶν τεχνῶν.
Expl. Κρύβε, ὦ Λεύκιππε, τὸ πᾶν· ἐφθόνησαν. Ἔρρωσο.

Florenz: Laurent. plut. 86, 16; a. 1492. sect. 35.
Paris: Parisin. 2327; a. 1478. f. 258.

Supplement I

Hippocrates

Under the title **Zeichenerklärung** (*Table of Symbols*), Diels' catalogue includes some abbreviations and *sigla*, the list of which appears on page 2 of the first issue of the catalogue (1905). Those abbreviations, utilized precisely in the present reproduction of Diels are the following with their respective explicitation:

*	=	die Hds. enthält nur Exzerpte.
[ ]	=	die Hds. ist nur aus Ackermann's *Hist. litteraria Hippocratis* (Kühn Med. Gr. Opp. XXI, 1 ff.) und *Hist. litt. Cl. Galeni* (Kühn M. G. O. I, XVII ff.) oder aus Littré (Œuvr. compl. d'Hippocr. Par. 1839—61. 10 Bde.) bekannt.
J.	=	Galenus, editio Iuntina 1528 (Exemplar der Vatikanischen Handbibliothek).
K.	=	Kühn.
L.	=	Littré.

*	=	the manuscript contains only extracts.
[ ]	=	the manuscript is known only through Ackermann's *Hist. litteraria Hippocratis* (Kühn Med. Gr. Opp. XXI, 1 sq.) and *Hist. litt. Cl. Galeni* (Kühn M. G. O. I, XVII ff.) or Littré (Œuvr. compl. d'Hippocr. Par. 1839—61. 10 vols).
J.	=	Galen, Iuntina 1528 edition (copy of the Vatican Library).
K.	=	Kühn.
L.	=	Littré.

Opera varia. [Diels N.25]
(Kat. I S. 3.)

Padua: S. Joann. in Viridario *usw.* = Holkham. 282 *nach Zuschrift von* Emil Jacobs (*Zu vgl.* R. Foerster, Philologus 42, 162).

Dazu: Constantinopol. Antonii Cantacuzeni (*bei* Foerster, De antiq. Cpolit. p. 24).

Προγνωστικόν.
(Kat. I S. 5.)

Mailand: Ambros.
P 90 Sup.; s. XV—XVI. f. 79v (»Dialecto communi scripta«).
Q 13 Sup.; s. XV—XVI *usw.*
Padua: S. Joann. in Viridario = Holkham. 282.
Rom: Palat. 199; s. XIII. f. 39 (*so*!). [M. W(ellmann).]

Ἀφορισμοί.
(Kat. I S. 12 ff.)

Athen: Βιβλ. τῆς Βουλῆς 68; s. XVIII. f. 299 (Expl. mut. sect. II τὰ πάντα εἶναι ἀσθενέστερα· περὶ δὲ ...).
Mailand: Ambros. T 19 Sup.; s. XV *usw.*
Padua: S. Joann. in Viridario = Holkham. 282.
Rom: Palat. 199; s. XIII. f. 44 (*so*!). [M. W.]

Περὶ φύσιος ἀνθρώπου. [Diels N.26]
(Kat. I S. 21.)

Padua: S. Joann. in Viridario = Holkham. 282.

Περὶ νούσων Α'.
(Kat. I S. 23.)

Athen: Βιβλ. τῆς Βουλῆς 39; s. XVIII. f. 1.

Περὶ παθῶν.
(Kat. I S. 23.)

Athen: Βιβλ. τῆς Βουλῆς 39; s. XVIII. f. 98v.

Περὶ ἱερῆς νούσου.
(Kat. I S. 24.)

Rom: Corsin. 1410 (36. E. 26); s. —; f. 348v (Inc. Μέλλοντας ἡμᾶς ἄρχεσθαι περὶ φύσεως ἀνθρώπου).

Περὶ νούσων Β' Γ'.
(Kat. I S. 26.)

Athen: Βιβλ. τῆς Βουλῆς 39; s. XVIII. f. 1 sqq.

Περὶ τῶν ἐντὸς παθῶν.
(Kat. I S. 27.)

Athen: Βιβλ. τῆς Βουλῆς 39; s. XVIII. f. 118v.

Περὶ φύσιος γυναικείης.
(Kat. I S. 27.)

Athen: Βιβλ. τῆς Βουλῆς 39; s. XVIII. f. 163 (Expl. καὶ ἣν ταῦτα φάγῃ ἢ πίῃ, ὡς πρὸς [sic] εἴπομεν, ὥστε ἀνάγκη ...).

Περὶ γονῆς.
(Kat. I S. 28.)

Padua: S. Joann. in Viridario = Holkham. 282.

Περὶ νούσων Δ'.
(Kat. I S. 29.)

Athen: Βιβλ. τῆς Βουλῆς 39; s. XVIII. f. 1 sqq.

Περὶ παρθενίων.
(Kat. I S. 30.)

Athen: Βιβλ. τῆς Βουλῆς 39; s. XVIII. f. 161^{v}.
Padua: S. Joann. in Viridario = Holkham. 282.

Περὶ ἑβδομάδων. [Diels N.27]
(Kat. I S. 32.)

Wien:
Colleg. S. J. Rossianus XI. 167; s. XVI. f. 12^{v} (Inc. ἰστέον ὡς ἱπποκράτης ἑπτὰ ἡλικίας. Expl. ibid. γέρων εἰς τὰς δεκατέσσαρας ἑβδομάδας).
Vindob. med. 41; s. XIV—XV. f. 83^{v} (*Wie im* Vindob. Rossian.).

Ἐπιστολαὶ κτέ.
(Kat. I S. 38.)

Wien: Vindob. Gollob Privatbesitz; s. XV—XVI. f.—. (Epp. 1—9. 25. 10—16. 18. 20. 19. 21. 17. 22—24).
Wolfenbüttel: Guelferb. 3132 (18. 1 Aug. 4°); s. XV. f. 115—116 (Epp. 1—3. 5).

Περὶ αἰσθήσεων.
(Kat. I S. 39.)

Ist Fragment der Ἐπιστολὴ πρὸς Πτολεμαῖον p. 287, 1—289, 6 Ermerins.

Περὶ ἀνατομῆς τῶν ζώντων.
(Kat. I S. 39.)

Dazu: Rhaedest. (*bei* Foerster, De antiq. Cpolit. p. 29).

Ἐπιστολὴ πρὸς Πτολεμαῖον περὶ κατασκευῆς ἀνθρώπου.
(Kat. I S. 40.)

Mailand: Ambros.
A 45 Sup.; s. XIII. f. 50 (Expl. συνάγεται ὁ ἐνιαυτὸς εἰς ἡμέρας τξε').

B 72 Sup.; s. XV. f. 116^{v} (Expl. ὑγιεῖ δ' ἔσονται).

F 23 Sup.; s. XV. f. 219^{v} (Inc. Ἀλλὰ μὴ ὑπολαμβάνῃς. Expl. ἐν τοῖς ἀριστεροῖς θύλῃ)

Wien:

Bibl. coll. S. J. Rossianus XI. 167; s. XVI. f. 9^{v} (Ἐκ τῶν τοῦ ἱπποκράτους περὶ τεσσάρων στοιχείων. Inc. συνέστηκεν ὁ κόσμος ἐκ. Expl. 11^{v} εἰσέρχεται εἰς τὴν κύστιν τὸ ὕδωρ = p. 279—285 Ermerins. Folgt f. 11^{v} περὶ αἰσθήσεων. Inc. αἰσθητήρια δὲ ἐστὶν. Expl. f. 12^{r} ὄνυχες δὲ ψυχρᾶς καὶ ξηρᾶς κράσεως εἰσὶν = p. 287, 1—289, 6 Ermerins).

Vindob. med. 41; s. XIV—XV. f. 82^{r}—83^{r}. 83^{r}—83^{v} (*Wie im* Vindob. Rossian.).

Ἐπιστολὴ πρὸς Πτολεμαῖον.
(Kat. I S. 41.)

Inc. Ἐπιμελούμενοι κτέ.

Mailand: Ambros. A 45 Sup.; s. XIII. f. 61^{v} (Expl. ἐκ τῆς προσθήκης τῶν ια' ἡμερῶν).

Περὶ ζωῆς καὶ θανάτου.
(Kat. I S. 41.)

Mailand: Ambros. H 2 Inf.; s. XVI. f. 240^{v}.

[Diels N.28] Ἰατροσόφιον.
(Kat. I S. 42.)

Dazu: Rhaedest. (*bei* Foerster, De antiq. Cpolit. p. 29).

Περὶ σώματος μορίων.
(Kat. I S. 43.)

Mailand: Ambros. H 2 Inf.; s. XVI. f. 268 (Inc. Βρέγμα τὸ λεγόμενον ἁπαλόν).

Περὶ οὔρων.
(Kat. I S. 44.)

Kommt in Betracht für Galenus Kühn XIX 609 ff.; vgl. Kat. I S. 113.

Περὶ παθῶν.
(Zu Kat. I S. 44.)

Athen: Atheniens. Βιβλ. τῆς Βουλῆς 68; s. XVIII. f. 220 (Exc. varia περὶ παθῶν ex Hipp., Gal., Paulo Nic., Paulo Aeg.).

Προγνωστικά.
(Kat. I S. 44.)

Athen: Βιβλ. τῆς Βουλῆς 68; s. XVIII. f. 109 (Προγν. μυστηριώδη).
Rom: Corsin. 1410 (36. E. 26); s. —. f. 343 (Inc. Εἱ δὲ κεφαλαλγίαν ἔχει ἢ οἴδημα).

Περὶ τῶν δ' στοιχειών καὶ χυμῶν, δι' ὧν συνίσταται ὁ ἄνθρωπος.
(Kat. I S. 46.)

Wien:
Bibl. coll. S. J. Rossianus XI. 167. s. XVI. f. 7v (Ἱπποκράτους περὶ τῶν δ' στοιχείων καὶ χυμῶν δι' ὧν συνίσταται ὁ ἄνθρωπος. Inc. Ἰστέον ὅτι ὁ ἄνθρωπος συνίσταται. Expl. 9v ὅσα δὲ γένηται ἐν χειμῶνι ἀπαλλάσσονται).
Vindob. med. 41. *usw.* f. 81r—82r (*Wie im* Vindob. Rossian.).

Φάρμακα.
(Kat. I S. 48.)

Rom: Corsin. 1410 (36. E. 26); s. —. f. 344 (Ἀλάτιον Ἱππ.).

Πρόγνωσις περὶ τῶν δ' ὡρῶν
(Kat. I S. 49.)

Ist = Aphor. III, 11–14, Littré IV, 490;
vgl. Boll *im* Catal. codd. astrol. VII p. 23 f.).

Excerpta varia. [Diels N.29]
(Kat. I S. 56.)

Mailand: Ambros. F 23 Sup.; s. XV. f. 131v (Διαίρεσις ἀνθρώπου. Inc. Διαιροῦμεν δὲ τὸν ἄνθρωπον. Expl. ἐξόχως ἐνταῦθα γενησόμενα), f. 222 (Inscr. Περὶ καταστάσεως ἀνθρώπου. Inc. Συνέστηκεν δὲ ὁ ἄνθρωπος ἐκ τινῶν, ἤγουν. Expl. φαντασία καὶ αἰσθήσεις).

Galen

Under the title **Zeichenerklärung** (*Table of Symbols*), Diels' catalogue includes some abbreviations and *sigla*, the list of which appears on page 2 of the first issue of the catalogue (1905). Those abbreviations, utilized precisely in the present reproduction of Diels are the following with their respective explicitation:

*	=	die Hds. enthält nur Exzerpte.
[ ]	=	die Hds. ist nur aus Ackermann's *Hist. litteraria Hippocratis* (Kühn Med. Gr. Opp. XXI, 1 ff.) und *Hist. litt. Cl. Galeni* (Kühn M. G. O. I, XVII ff.) oder aus Littré (Œuvr. compl. d'Hippocr. Par. 1839—61. 10 Bde.) bekannt.
J.	=	Galenus, editio Iuntina 1528 (Exemplar der Vatikanischen Handbibliothek).
K.	=	Kühn.
L.	=	Littré.

*	=	the manuscript contains only extracts.
[ ]	=	the manuscript is known only through Ackermann's *Hist. litteraria Hippocratis* (Kühn Med. Gr. Opp. XXI, 1 sq.) and *Hist. litt. Cl. Galeni* (Kühn M. G. O. I, XVII ff.) or Littré (Œuvr. compl. d'Hippocr. Par. 1839—61. 10 vols).
J.	=	Galen, Iuntina 1528 edition (copy of the Vatican Library).
K.	=	Kühn.
L.	=	Littré.

Saeculum einiger Ambrosiani. [Diels N.29]

C 4 Sup.; s. XV.
E 105 Sup.; s. XIII.
O 50 Sup.; s. XIII ex.
O 117 Sup.; s. XV—XVI.
Q 52 Sup.; s. XIV.
Q 87 Sup.; s. XV.
Q 94 Sup.; s. XV—XVI.
S 3 Sup.; s. XV—XVI.
T 19 Sup.; s. XV.
A 81 Inf.; s. XIII ex.
C 80 Inf.; s. XVI.

Opera varia.
(Kat. I S. 58.)

Leipzig: Institut f. Geschichte der Medizin: Basileensis (1538) des Galen mit Varianten und Korrekturen von der Hand des Leo Allatius.
Wolfenbüttel: Guelferbyt. Ebert 364 (7 und 8 Gud. lat.) *usw.*

Dazu: Constantinop. Antonii Cantacuzeni (*bei* Foerster, De antiq. Cpolit. p. 24).

Περὶ αἱρέσεων τοῖς εἰσαγομένοις.
(Kat. I S. 60.)

Moskau: Mosquens. 52 (*so!*) = 464 *und* 283 = 466.
Rom: Palat. 199; s. XIII. f. 4v (Expl. νῦν δὲ εἰσαγομένοις ἱκανὰ ταῦτα). [M. W.]

Πρὸς Πατρόφιλον περὶ συστάσεως ἰατρικῆς. [Diels N.30]
(Kat. I S. 60.)

Neapel: Borbon. III D 15*; s. XIV. f. 177v—178.

Τέχνη ἰατρική.
(Kat. I S. 63.)

Mailand: Ambros. C 102 Sup. (*nicht* Inf.); s. XV *usw.*

Venedig: Marcian. App. cl. V 9; s. XV. f. 179. [M. W.]

Περὶ φυσικῶν δυνάμεων.
(Kat. I S. 65.)

Rom: Vatic. 282; s. XVI. f. 50. [M. W.]

Περὶ ὀστῶν τοῖς εἰσαγομένοις.
(Kat. I S. 67.)

Mailand: Ambros.
Q 87 Sup.; s. XV *usw.*
S 3 Sup.; s. XV—XVI. *usw.*
Neapel: Borbon. III D 15; s. XIV. f. 184v—193v (mit Scholien).

Περὶ χρείας τῶν ἐν ἀνθρώπου σώματι μορίων.
(Kat. I S. 68 f.)

Wien: Colleg. S. J. Rossianus XI. 167; s. XVI. f. 1—310v.

Dazu: Constantinopol. Mich. Cantacuzeni (*bei* Foerster, De antiq. Cpolit. p. 27).

Περὶ ἀρίστης κατασκευῆς τοῦ σώματος ἡμῶν.
(Kat. I S. 71.)

Florenz: Laurent. 74, 10; s. XIV. f. 13v (Γαλ. περὶ κατασκ. τοῦ ἀνθρώπου. Inc. Οὐ μικρὸν μέν ἐστιν καταφρονῆσαι τὴν Πλάτωνος σοφίαν καὶ Ἀριστοτέλους καὶ Ἀσκληπιάδου καὶ Χείρωνος καὶ Ἱπποκράτους καὶ τοῦ Δημοκρίτου καὶ τοῦ μεγάλου Γαληνοῦ [sic]. Physiologischer Traktat in Frage und Antwort). [M. W.]
Rom: Palat. 199; s. XIII. f. 183v (Inscr. ρκδ' λόγος · ὧν [l. ὃν] ἐποίησαν Ἱπποκράτης καὶ ὁ μετ' αὐτοῦ [sic] Γαληνὸς καὶ περὶ φυσικῆς ἀκροάσεως. Inc. *wie im* Laurent. 74, 10). [M. W.]

[Diels N.31] Ὅτι ταῖς τοῦ σώματος κράσεσιν αἱ τῆς ψυχῆς δυνάμεις ἕπονται
(*so lautet die Überschrift in den Hss.*).
(Kat. I S. 72.)

Moskau: Mosquens. 292 *identisch mit* Mosq. 260.
München: Monac. 109 *usw.* f. 50—61. (*Ist vollständig. Photographische Proben im Besitz der Berl. Akademie.*)
Rom: Vatic. 154 = Reg. Suec. 154; *vgl.* J. v. Müller, Galeni Scripta minora II p. XXXIV.

Περὶ διαγνώσεως καὶ θεραπείας τῶν ἰδίων παθῶν.
(Kat. I S. 73.)

Wolfenbüttel: Guelferbyt. 837 (757 Helmst.) *usw.*

Περὶ τῶν Ἱπποκράτους καὶ Πλάτωνος δογμάτων.
(Kat. I S. 74.)

Neapel: Borbon. III D 15*; s. XIV. f. 175.

Περὶ τοῦ διὰ τῆς σμικρᾶς σφαίρας γυμνασίου.
(Kat. I S. 74.)

Ed. *nach Schoenes Collationen* Schäfer, Diss. Bonn. 1907.

Ὑγιεινῶν λόγοι.
(Kat. I S. 75.)

Dazu: Constantinopol. Mich. Cantacuzeni (*bei* Foerster, De antiq. Cpolit. p. 28).

Περὶ τροφῶν δυνάμεως.
(Kat. I S. 76 f.)

L. I c. 14—L. II c. 20 ed. G. Helmreich, Ansbach 1906. L. II c. 21—71 ed. G. Helmreich, Ansbach 1907.

Mailand: Ambros.
A 45 Sup.*; s. XIII. f. 43v.
B 108 Sup.; *usw.* f. 35.
München: Monac. 39* *usw.* f. 86 (*Photographien des Anfangs im Besitze der Berl. Akademie.* Expl. *des 1. Stücks* f. 121v περὶ ὠτίδων κτέ. ἐκ τοῦ περὶ ἐκείνου λόγου διαγνωσθήσεται) *und* f. 121v (Inscr. Σύνοψις τοῦ περὶ τροφῶν Γαλινοῦ. ὅτι τροφιμώτεροι οἶπε [sic]· περὶ πυρῶν ἤτοι ἄρτων. Inc. Ἠπιλημένοι [sic] καὶ τῷ οἴκῳ βαρύτεροι. Expl.

[Diels N.32] f. 126^{v} περὶ σκορόδων καὶ κρομύων καὶ πράσων κτέ. τοῖς γὰρ φλεγματώδεσι καὶ παχεῖς ἔχουσι χυμοὺς συμφέρει) *und* f. 126^{v} (Inscr. Ἐκ τοῦ τρίτου λόγου τοῦ περὶ τροφῶν. Inc. Περὶ τῆς ἀπὸ τῶν πεζῶν ζῴων τροφῆς κτέ. Αἱ σάρκες τῶν ζῴων αἵματος γεννητικαί. Expl. f. 130^{v} εἰς δὲ οὔρησιν χείρους τῶν λευκῶν).

Paris: Parisin. 1883. *usw.* (Expl. L. II c. 21).

Rom: Palat. 199 *usw.* (Expl. κἄπειτα προελθόντων ἡμῶν = K. VI 599, 6).

Wolfenbüttel: Guelferb. 4148 (64 Weißenb.) *usw.* (*Vgl.* K. Koch, Sitz.-Ber. d. Berl. Akad. 1907 p. 103—111).

Dazu: Constantinopol. Mich. Cantacuzeni (*bei* Foerster, De antiq. Cpolit. p. 28).

Περὶ εὐχυμίας καὶ κακοχυμίας τροφῶν.
(Kat. I S. 77.)

Florenz: Laurent. 74, 25; s. XIV (*Kalbfleischs Collation von VI 800, 6—809, 5 K. im Besitze von cand. phil. E. M. Arndt in Marburg).*

Περὶ τῶν ἐν τοῖς νοσήμασιν αἰτίων.
(Kat. I S. 78 f.)

Diese Schrift und die beiden folgenden bilden in lat. Übersetzung zusammen die 6 Bücher De accidenti et morbo, Kat. I S. 136.

Περὶ τῆς τῶν συμπτωμάτων διαφορᾶς.
(Kat. I S. 79.)

Mailand: Ambros. F 112 Sup.; s. XV. f. 1.

Περὶ αἰτίων συμπτωμάτων.
(Kat. I S. 79. 80.)

Mailand: Ambros. F 112 Sup.; s. XV. f. 15^{v} (In margine emendationes et variae lectiones).

Περὶ διαφορᾶς πυρετῶν.
(Kat. I S. 80 f.)

Rom: Palat. 199; s. XIII. f. 11. [M. W.]

Περὶ μαρασμοῦ.
(Kat. I S. 83.)

Paris: Parisin. Suppl. 635; s. XIII. f. 3 (*Nur der Schluß von p. 700, 4 an; Kalbfleischs Collation im Anhange zu den Abh. der Kgl. Pr. Akad. 1895 p. 4*[2]).

Περὶ σφυγμῶν τοῖς εἰσαγομένοις. [Diels N.33]
(Kat. I S. 86.)

Wolfenbüttel: Guelferb. Ebert 368 (11 Gud. gr.) *usw.*

Περὶ διαφορᾶς σφυγμῶν.
(Kat. I S. 87.)

Wolfenbüttel: Guelferb. Ebert 368 (11 Gud. gr.) *usw.*

Περὶ διαγνώσεως σφυγμῶν.
(Kat. I S. 87.)

Mailand: Ambros. O 50 Sup.; s. XIII ex. f. 129^v.

Σύνοψις περὶ σφυγμῶν.
(Kat. I S. 89).

Vgl. J. Gossen, De Gal. libro qui Σύν. π. σφ. inscribitur. Diss. inaug. Berol. 1907.

Περὶ κρίσεων.
(Kat. I S. 89.)

Rom: Vatic. 282 *usw.* (»Mit Lücken im 2. und 3. Buche.« M. W.).

Θεραπευτικῆς μεθόδου βιβλία.
(Kat. I S. 91 ff.)

Rom: Reg. Suec. 174; s. XIV (*Kalbfleischs Collation von X 830, 1—837, 15 K. im Besitze von cand. phil. E. M. Arndt, Marburg*).

Venedig: Marcian.
276 (*Mewaldts Probecollation im Besitze der Berl. Akademie. Collation von B. I und eines Teils von II im Besitze von Wellmann*).
284 (»stammt aus Marc. 276.« M. W.).
Wolfenbüttel: Guelferbyt. Ebert 369 (69 Gud. gr.) *usw.*

Dazu: Constantinopol. Mich. Cantacuzeni (*bei* Foerster, De antiq. Cpolit. p. 27). Rhaedest. (*bei* Foerster, De antiq. Cpolit. p. 30).

[Diels N.34] Τῶν πρὸς Γλαύκωνα θεραπευτικῶν βιβλία.
(Kat. I S. 93.)

München: Monac. 236 *usw.* (*Photographische Proben des Anfangs im Besitze der Berl. Akademie*).
Wolfenbüttel: Guelferb. Ebert 370 (69 Gud. gr.) *usw.*

Περὶ κράσεως καὶ δυνάμεως τῶν ἁπλῶν φαρμάκων.
(Kat. I S. 96.)

München: Monac. 469; s. XIV(?). f. 56—131. (*Andre Hand als vorher die von* Galenus εἰς Ἱπποκρ. π. διαίτης ὀξ. *und* π. τῶν ἐτησίων καιρῶν. — Inc. mut. τρύχνου τῆς ῥίζης ὁ φλοιός = K. XII 145, 18. Also Buch VIII Ende bis Buch XI Schluß des Werkes. *Photographie des Anfangs im Besitze der Berl. Akademie. Genaue Collation der ganzen Handschrift besitzt Helmreich*).
Rom: Vatic. 284; s. XI (Vorn unvollständig; enthält B. VI—XI mit Dioscurides περὶ ὕλης ἰατρικῆς verarbeitet). [M. W.]

Περὶ συνθέσεως φαρμάκων τῶν κατὰ τόπους.
(Kat. I S. 97 f.)

Venedig: Marcian. 288; s. XI (*Probecollation in Wellmanns Besitz*).

Περὶ εὐπορίστων.
(Kat. I S. 99 f.)

Mailand: Ambros.
C 102 Sup. (*nicht* Inf.); s. XV *usw.*
Q 94 Sup.; s. XV—XVI *usw.*

Εἰσαγωγὴ ἢ ἰατρός.
(Kat. I S. 100.)

München: Monac. 109. f. 22. (*Es fehlen* Kap. V *und* XI, *nicht* X. Lücken gelassen z. B. in Kap. XII, im Abschnitt περὶ ἰσχουρίας und öfter).
Venedig: Marcian. App. cl. V 9 (*Collationsprobe in Wellmanns Besitz*).

Εἰς τὸ Ἱπποκράτους περὶ φύσιος ἀνθρώπου.
(Kat. I S. 101.)

Mewaldts Collationen der beiden Laurentiani und Probecollation des Mutinensis im Besitze der Berl. Akademie. Expl. Mutin. 240: κεκραμένων (sic recte) γε. *Photographien des Reginens. im Besitze der Berl. Akademie.* Vindob. med. 34 = Parisin. Suppl. 447.

Εἰς τὸ Ἱπποκράτους περὶ διαίτης ὑγιεινῆς.
(Kat. I S. 101.)

Rom: Regin. (*Photographien im Besitze der Berl. Akademie*).

Εἰς τὸ Ἱπποκράτους περὶ διαίτης ὀξέων. [Diels N.35]
(Kat. I S. 102.)

Florenz: Laurent. 75, 5; s. XIV (*Kalbfleischs Collation von XV 626, 1—649, 18 K. im Besitze von cand. phil. E M. Arndt, Marburg*).
München: Monac. 469 *usw., nach alter Zählung* φυλλ. ιη'—ϙγ' *am rechten Rande (also vorher die ersten 17 Blätter verloren)*, f. 1—50^v^ *nach neuerer Zählung am untern Rande, die öfter mehrere Blätter überspringt.*

Εἰς τὸ Ἱπποκράτους περὶ χυμῶν.
(Kat. I S. 103.)

Mailand: Ambros. *muß heißen* C 119 Sup.; s. XVI.

Ἱπποκράτους ἐπιδημίαι καὶ Γαληνοῦ εἰς αὐτὰς ὑπομνήματα.
(Kat. I S. 104.)

Commentar zum 6. Buche griech. nicht vollständig erhalten, bricht ab bei Hip. Littré V 324.5. Volständige lat. Übers. sämtlicher 8 Bücher bei Jo. Bapt. Rasarius, Venedig 1562. *Vgl.* Rose, Hermes V p. 207 Anm. J. Ilberg, Rhein. Mus. 44 p. 236 ff.

München: Monac. 231; s. XVI. f. 1 (Inc. mut. μόνον προγνώσεται τὰς γινομένας νόσους = K. XVII A 5, 13. Expl. mut. τῶν ἔνδον τοῦ περιτοναίου μορίων, *also wie im* Marc. App. cl. V 15, = K. XVII A 791, 19. *Der Codex enthält* f. 1—106v Comm. I—III in Epid. A', f. 106v—228v Comm. I—III in Epid. Γ'. *Mewaldts Probecollation von* K. XVII A 5, 13—14, 14 *im Besitze der Berl. Akademie*).
Rom: Urbin. 64 (*Ist der Commentar des* Palladius; *vgl. Nachtrag zu diesem*).
Venedig: Marcian. App. cl. V 15 *usw.* (*Das* Expl. *ist vielmehr das von* Comm. III in Epid. Γ'; *vgl. oben* Monac. 231).

Ἱπποκράτους ἀφορισμοὶ καὶ Γαληνοῦ εἰς αὐτοὺς ὑπομνήματα.
(Kat. I S. 104 ff.)

Wien: Vindob. med. 34 *ist jetzt* Parisin. Suppl. 447.

Ἱπποκράτους προγνωστικὸν καὶ Γαληνοῦ εἰς αὐτὸ ὑπομνήματα.
(Kat. I S. 107 f.)

Rom:
Palat. 157; s. XIV. f. 2r. (*Teilweise Collation Heegs im Besitze der Berl. Akademie*).
Reg. Suec. 175; s. XIV. f. 2r. (*Probecollationen Heegs im Besitze der Berl. Akademie*).
Vatic. 1063; s. XIII. f. 1. (*Der Anfang des Commentars ist verloren gegangen. Anfang* = K. XVIII B 47. *Probecollationen Heegs im Besitze der Berl. Akademie*).
Wien: Vindob. 44; s. XV. XVI. f. 232 (*Probecollationen Heegs im Besitze der Berl. Akademie*).

[Diels N.36] Τῶν Ἱπποκράτους γλωσσῶν ἐξήγησις.
(Kat. I S. 109 f.)

München: Monac. 71 *usw.* (Sine auctoris nomine. Inscr. Κατὰ στοιχεῖον Ἱπποκράτους λεξικόν. Inc. Ἀγκρομήλη, ἄγκιστρον. Expl. f. 8v ὅτι καὶ ὥρα ἡ φροντὶς ... ἐνιαυτοῦ).

Εἰ ζῷον τὸ κατὰ γαστρός.
(Kat. I S. 110.)

Florenz: Laurent. 74, 3; s. XII. p. 105*b* (*Kalbfleischs Collation in dessen Besitz*).
Paris: (*Mit der Collation der Pariser Hdss. ist cand. prob. Hermann Wagner in Fulda beschäftigt*).

Ὅροι ἰατρικοί.
(Kat. I S. 111.)

Mailand: Ambros. T 19 Sup.; s. XV f. 22.
München: Monac.
109 *usw.* f. 1 (Inc. Τὴν τῶν ὅρων πραγματείαν κτέ. *Photographische Proben des Anfanges und Schlusses im Besitze der Berl. Akademie*).
469 *usw., nach alter Zählung am rechten Rande* φυλλ. ϙδ'–ϙη', *nach neuerer am unteren Rande* f. 51—55^{v} (Inscr. f. 51 mg. dextr. Γαληνοῦ βιβλίον Α' · τὰ ἐρωτήματα τῆς ἰατρικῆς τέχνης. Inc. Τί ἐστι τέχνη; τέχνη ἐστὶ σύστημα ἐγκαταλήψεως ἐγγεγυμνασμένη = K. XIX 350, 7. Expl. ποιεῖται τὴν κίνησιν ἔν τε κύκλῳ καὶ ἐπ' εὐθείας = K. XIX 377, 6. *Vielfach von Kühns Text im einzelnen abweichend. Photographien im Besitze der Berl. Akademie*).

Rom: Palat. 199*; s. XIII. f. 192 sq. (Inc. Γαληνοῦ [in mg.] περὶ μὲν τῶν νοσημάτων τῶν συμβαινόντων τοῖς ἀνθρώποις τὰ μέν ἐστι συνεχῆ, τὰ δὲ διαλείποντα = Gal. XIX 387 K.). [M. W.]
Venedig: Marcian. App. cl. V 9; s. XV. f. 500 (Ohne Namen. Περὶ ὅρων διαφόρων εἰδῶν· τί ἐστι διάφραγμα; διάφραγμά ἐστι νευρῶδες διεῖργον καὶ χωρίζον τά τε ἐν τῷ θώρακι = Gal. XIX 360 K. Expl. f. 507^{v} ἄφθα ἐστὶν ἕλκωσις ἐπιπόλαιος ἐν στόματι γινομένη· ἐπιπλάττει [sic] δὲ αὕτη ἡ ἕλκωσις μάλιστα παιδίοις = Gal. XIX 441 K.). [M. W.]

Ὅτι αἱ ποιότητες ἀσώματοι.
(Kat. I S. 111).

Ed. J. Westenberger, Galeni qui fertur de qualitatibus incorporeis libellus. Diss. inaug. Marp. Chatt. 1906.

Mailand: Ambros. *usw.* f. 202^{v}.

Περὶ κατακλίσεως νοσούντων προγνωστικά.
(Kat. I S. 112.)

Berlin: Phillipp. 1577 (Meerm. 287), s. XV. f. 87 (Inc. Συσχηματίζεται = K. XIX 532, 10—533, 6 γνωρίζεται).
Florenz: Laurent.
28, 13; s. XIV f. 224^{v} (Expl. ἀναιρεθήσονται γάρ. *Heegs Collationen im Besitze der Berl. Akademie*).
28, 14; s. XIV f. 154^{v} (*verloren gegangen; vgl.* Catal. cod. astrol. I p. 25).
28, 34; s. IX f. 5^{r} (*Heegs Abschrift im Besitze der Berl. Akademie*).
München: Monac. 105 *usw.* f. 218^{v} (Expl. mut. ἐὰν δὲ ἀγαθοποιὸς τὴν σελήνην θεωρήσῃ = K. XIX 545, 7. *Collationsprobe, K. XIX 529—532, besitzt W. Crönert. Mewaldts Probecollation K. XIX 529—531, 7 im Besitze der Berl. Akademie*).
Rom: Vatic. 1066; s. XVI f. 78^{r} (*Probecollation Heegs im Besitze der Berl. Akademie*).

[Diels N.37] Περὶ οὔρων.
(Kat. I S. 113.)

Paris: Parisin. 2308, *verbessere:* f. 15.

Περὶ οὔρων ἐκ τῶν Ἱπποκράτους κτλ.
(Kat. I S. 113).

Vgl. Hippokrates περὶ οὔρων Kat. I S. 44 *und unten* Gal. Περὶ οὔρων Kat. I S. 127.)

Florenz: Riccard. 41; s. XV f. 13. (*Teilweise Abschrift Heegs im Besitze der Berl. Akademie*).
Königsberg Pr.: Regim. bibl. urb. 16*b* 12; s. XIV—XV, *jüngere Hand.* f. 273^{v} (*Abschrift des Anfangs bis XIX 611, 7 K. von M. Odau im Besitze der Berl. Akademie*).
Paris: Parisin. 2308; s. XV. f. 12^{v}.

Περὶ σφυγμῶν πρὸς Ἀντώνιον.
(Kat. I S. 113.)

Florenz: Laurent. plut. 59, 14; s. XIII (*andere Hand; sonst* s. XV). f. 171^{v} (Inscr. Ποίημα μικρὸν φιλαρέτου περὶ σφυγμῶν πρὸς Ἀντώνιον φιλομαθῆ καὶ φίλον αὐτοῦ. *Also hier unter Philarets Namen!*).

Περὶ ἀντεμβαλλομένων.
(Kat. I S. 114.)

Mailand: Ambros. E 37 Sup.; s. XVI. f. 278.
Rom: Palat. 199; s. XIII. f. 15^{v} (Inc. Τὸ συνώνυμον ἀρχὴ τοῦ α' ἀντὶ ἀκανθίου σπέρματος λυχνίς. Expl. ἀντὶ ὠκιμοειδοῦς ἡδύοσμον ἄγριον). [M. W.]
Venedig: Marcian. 295; a. 1470 *usw.* [M. W.]

Περὶ τῆς ἀνατομῆς ἐπὶ τῶν ζώντων.
(Kat. I S. 116.)

Dazu: Constantinopol. Mich. Cantacuzeni (*bei* Foerster, De antiq. Cpolit. p. 27).

Περὶ διαίτης.
(Kat. I S. 118).

»Costomiris druckt nur einen Auszug der Foersterschen Kataloge ab.« Jacobs.

Περὶ διαίτης καὶ θεραπειῶν πρὸς ἀντικένσορα πατρίκιον.
(Kat. I S. 118.)

Paris: Parisin. *usw.* (*Abschrift besitzt E. O. Winstedt, Oxford*).

Περὶ τῶν ἐτησίων καιρῶν ὡς δεῖ διαιτᾶσθαι.
De temporibus etesiarum et quomodo iis utendum sit.
(Zu Kat. I S. 121.)

München: Monac. 469; s. XV. f. 55v, φυλλ. ϙη' *nach alter Zählung am rechten Rande.* (Inc. Ἀπὸ πλειάδων δύσεως ἕως τροπῶν χειμερινῶν. Expl. ζήσεις ἄνοσος τὸν ὑπόλοιπον τῆς ζωῆς σου χρόνον. *Mewaldts Abschrift und Photographie im Besitze der Berl. Akademie.*)

Ἰατροσόφια. [Diels N.38]
(Kat. I S. 123.)

München: Monac. 551; s. XV f. 334 (*Collation der Kapitelübersicht, der Vorrede und der ersten Abschnitte besitzt W. Crönert*).

Dazu:
Constantinopol. (*bei* Foerster. De antiq. Cpolit. p. 20 Inscr. Ἰατροσ. Γαληνοῦ καθ' Ἱπποκράτους).
Constantinopol. Mich. Cantacuzeni (*bei* Foerster p. 28 Inscr. ⟨Ἰατροσ.⟩ Γαλ. Καθ' Ἱπποκράτους).

Τοῦ Ἱπποκράτους εἰς τὰ ἀναλυτικά, ἐξηγεῖται αὐτὰ ὁ Γαληνός.
(Kat. I S. 124.)

Dazu: Constantinopol. (*bei* Foerster, De antiq. Cpolit. p. 23).
»Constantinopol. bei Verdier und Foerster identisch mit Vindob., nämlich der Hds. der Foersterschen Kataloge.« Emil Jacobs.

Περὶ κλοκίων.
De excrementis.
(Kat. I S. 125).

»Meine Vermutung über die Bedeutung des Titels bestätigt Thumb durch Hinweis auf Korais, Ἄτακτα I 338 und G. Meyer, Neugriech. Studien III 31.« Kalbfleisch.

Περὶ λίθων.
(Kat. I S. 126.)

Mailand: Ambros. A 45 Sup.; s. XIII. f. 31^{v}.

Περὶ σώματος μορίων.
(Kat. I S. 126.)

Mailand: Ambros. P 90 Sup.; s. XV—XVI. f. 68 (Inscr. Ὀνομασίαι τῶν ἐκτὸς τοῦ σώματος μορίων. Inc. Πρῶτον μὲν Ἀριστοτέλης. Expl. ἢ ἐκ τῆς κατὰ τὴν θέσιν τάξεως).

Περὶ νόσων.
(Kat. I S. 126.)

München: Monac. 39 *ist zu streichen.*

Περὶ οὔρων.
(Kat. I S. 128). [Diels N.39]

Kommt z. T. in Betracht für Galenus ed. Kühn XIX 609 ff.

Mailand: Ambros. Q 94 Sup.; s. XV—XVI. f. 332 (Inc. Οὖρον λευκὸν μὴ ἔχον ὑπόστασιν).
Rom: Corsin. 1410 (36. E. 26); s. —. f. 385 (Inc. *wie im* Scorial. Υ. III. 14. Expl. καὶ τῆς γενομένης προρρήσεως θεωρεῖν).
Wien: Vindob. phil. 178 *usw.* (Byzant. Werkchen. *Abschrift besitzt W. Crönert*).

Περὶ ποδάγρας.
(Kat. I S. 130).

Gehört dem Demetrius Pepagomenos ed. Bernard, Lugd. Bat. 1743; vgl. Krumbacher, Byz. Litt.-Gesch.² 615. 617.

München: Monac. 551; s. XV. f. 353ᵛ—359ᵛ (Inscr. Ἑρμηνεία περὶ τῆς ποδάγρας τοῦ σοφωτάτου Γαλ. Expl. μετὰ τοῦ p. 867 Bern. *Abschrift des Anfangs und Collation von Kap. 10 besitzt W. Crönert*).

Προγνωστικά
(Kat. I S. 130.)

München: Monac. 278 *ist zu streichen.*

Φάρμακα.
(Kat. I S. 132 ff.)

Rom: Corsin. 1410 (36. E. 26); s. —. f. 344 (Ἀλάτιον Γαλ.).
Wien:
Colleg. S. J. Rossianus XI 167; s. XV. f. 147ᵛ (Σκευασία τῆς ἱερᾶς Γαληνοῦ εἰς φλεγματικοὺς καὶ μελαγχολικούς. Inc. κολοκυνθίδος οὐγγίας δʹ. Expl. εἰς ἀποβροχὴν τῶν ὀπῶν).
Vindob. med.
31; s. XV. f. 149—150.
41; s. XIV—XV. f. 114—115.

Περὶ φλεβοτομίας.
(Kat. I S. 134. 135).

Vgl. Kühn XI 289, 15 ff.

Mailand: Ambros. C 4 Sup.; s. XV. f. 244^{v} (Inc. *wie im Londinens.*).
München: Monac. 39 *usw.* (*Photographien im Besitze der Berl. Akademie*).

[Περὶ φύσεως ἀνθρώπου].
(Kat. I S. 135.)

München: Monac. 39 *usw.* (*Ohne Überschrift. Photographien im Besitze der Berl. Akademie*).

[Diels N.41]

Excerpta varia.
(Kat. I S. 148 ff.)

Cairo: Patriarch. Alexandrin. 46 (*bei* Coxe, Mss. gr. of the Levant); s. XV. (Περὶ ὑποκρισέων [sic]).
Mailand: Ambros.
A 80 Sup.; s. XV ex. f. 261^{v}.
A 95 Sup.; s. XV. f. 78. 91.
E 6 Sup.; s. XIII. f. 235 (Inc. Τὴν γὰρ λογικὴν παρὰ τοῖς φιλοσόφοις. Expl. τῶν γε γραμμάτων μνημονεύειν δυνάμενον).
Q 87 Sup.; s. XV. f. 222 (Exc. de ossibus et musculis).
Neapel: Borbon. III D 15; s. XIV. f. 178^{v}—184^{v}.
Rom: Palat. 199; s. XIII. f. 186 (Περὶ πυρετῶν καὶ ἄλλων τινῶν· ἐκ τῶν Γαληνοῦ. 10 Kapitel. Inc. Μετὰ τὴν τῶν ὑγιεινῶν. Expl. τῆς ἀρίστης ἡλικίας τοῦ λείποντος ἡ δύναμις). [M. W.]
Venedig: Marcian. App. cl. V 9; s. XV. f. 469 (Γαλ. περὶ τόπων πεπονθότων. Inc. Διάγνωσις τῶν πεπονθότων τόπων γίνεται ἢ ἀπὸ συμπτωμάτων) *und* f. 471 (Γαλ. περὶ φυσικῶν δυνάμεων. Inc. Ἐν τούτῳ τῷ λόγῳ περὶ τῶν φυσικῶν μέλλει διδάξαι πλατύτερον). [M. W.]

The Other Physicians

Under the title **Zeichenerklärung** (*Table of Symbols*), Diels' catalogue includes some abbreviations and *sigla*, the list of which appears on page 2 of the first issue of the catalogue (1905). Those abbreviations, utilized precisely in the present reproduction of Diels are the following with their respective explicitation:

*	=	die Hds. enthält nur Exzerpte.
[ ]	=	die Hds. ist nur aus Ackermann's *Hist. litteraria Hippocratis* (Kühn Med. Gr. Opp. XXI, 1 ff.) und *Hist. litt. Cl. Galeni* (Kühn M. G. O. I, XVII ff.) oder aus Littré (Œuvr. compl. d'Hippocr. Par. 1839—61. 10 Bde.) bekannt.
J.	=	Galenus, editio Iuntina 1528 (Exemplar der Vatikanischen Handbibliothek).
K.	=	Kühn.
L.	=	Littré.

*	=	the manuscript contains only extracts.
[ ]	=	the manuscript is known only through Ackermann's *Hist. litteraria Hippocratis* (Kühn Med. Gr. Opp. XXI, 1 sq.) and *Hist. litt. Cl. Galeni* (Kühn M. G. O. I, XVII ff.) or Littré (Œuvr. compl. d'Hippocr. Par. 1839—61. 10 vols).
J.	=	Galen, Iuntina 1528 edition (copy of the Vatican Library).
K.	=	Kühn.
L.	=	Littré.

Abraham. [Diels N.42]

(Kat. II S. 3.)

»Gehört dem XI. Jahrhundert an; hat nur Recepte verfaßt«. Treu.

Adamantius.

Περὶ παλμῶν.
(Kat. II S. 3.)

»Sonst unter dem Namen des Melampus.« Mewaldt.

Aelius Promotus.

Δυναμερόν.
(Kat. II S. 4.)

Vgl. unten Ἰατρικά.

Mailand: Ambros. S 3 Sup.; s. XV—XVI. f. 21 (»Apogr. des Vatic.« M. W.).
Rom: Vatic. 299; s. XV. f. 451 (Inc. Τὰ λείποντα ἀπὸ τοῦ νη' κεφαλαίου ἐκ τοῦ βιβλίου τοῦ Προμώτου· ἄλλο βαπτικόν· κικίδα < δ'. »Diese Excerpte stammen aus cap. ρε' ff. des Δυναμερόν.« M. W. *Abschrift in Wellmanns Besitz*).
Venedig: Marc. 295; a. 1470 (*Vollständige Abschrift in Wellmanns Besitz*).

Φυσικὰ καὶ ἀντιπαθητικά.
(Kat. II S. 4.)

Inc. Πραγματείαν τεχνικὴν τοῖς πάθεσιν.
Expl. τὸ ἄκρον περίαπτε.

Mailand: Ambros. (*vgl.* f. 125^v).

Ἰατρικά.
(Kat. II S. 4.)

Im Titel lies: ἀπὸ τοῦ νη' κεφαλαίου usw.
»Ist Excerpt aus dem Δυναμερόν.« M. Wellmann.)

Περὶ ἰοβόλων καὶ δηλητηρίων φαρμάκων.
(Kat. II S. 4.)

Inc. Προεκθέσθαι βουλόμενος καὶ περὶ τῶν ἰοβόλων θηρίων.
Expl. ἢ μελίκρατον ὑδαρές.

Mailand: Ambros. S 3 Sup. (»Stammt aus Vatic. 299.« M. W.).
Rom: Vatic. 299 (*Abschrift besitzt E. O. Winstedt, Oxford*).

[Diels N.43]

Aëtius Amidenus.

Ἰατρικῶν λόγοι ΙΣΤ'.
(Kat. II S. 5 ff).

Liber XIII ed. Zervos, Athena XVIII 1906, p. 264—292; vgl. ebd. p. 240 ff.

Athos:
Βατοπεδ. A 29; s. XIV (Es fehlen B. V c. 137—143, VI und Schluß von XVI).
Λαύρ.
Ω 70; a. ,ϛϡμε' (= 1437).
Ω 72; s. XIV.
Berlin: Berol. fol.
37 *usw.* (*Nach Zervos Apogr. des Parisin. 2191*).
38; a. 1817 *usw.*
Neu-Ephesus: Ephes.; s. XIX. (L. IX—XVI).
Florenz:
»Laurent. 75, 5 + 75, 20 bilden Bd. I, 75, 18 + 75, 7 den II. Bd. derselben Aëtiushandschrift des XIV. Jahrhunderts.« M. W.
75, 10; s. XIV. f. 55—134. [M. W.]
Leipzig: Bibl. senat. 391 *usw.* (*Ist der Codex Boerhaaves. Apogr. des Vindob. med. 6 nach Zervos*).
Oxford: Canonic. 109 (*Nach Zervos Apogr. des Parisin. 2191*).
Padua: Bibl. S. Joann. in Viridario *usw.* = Holkham. nr. 283; *vgl.* R. Foerster, Philologus 42, 162.
Paris: Parisin.
1883 *usw.* (*Apogr. von Parisin. 2191*).
2192 *usw.* (*Apogr. von 2191*).
2196 (L. IX—XII 49 μαλάγματα διάφορα).
Patmos: Patmiac. (*Nach Zervos nur 2 Blätter, Buch I*).
Rom:
Palat. 199 (*Nach Zervos L. I—XI, ohne VII*).

Vatic.

297 *und* 298 (»enthalten Buch I—XVI.« M. W.).

1904 (»enthält nur B. I und einen Teil des Index.« M. W.).

1911; s. XIV (»B. I und B. II unvollständig, schließt mit cap. ρπγ'.« M. W.).

2202; s. XIV. f. 3—318 (»L. I—IV und Inhaltsverzeichnis von B. V z. T.« M. W.)

3062; s. XVI (*12 Blätter*).

3073; s. XVI.

Venedig: Marcian.

289 (»aus derselben Vorlage wie Weigelianus.« M. W.).

291; s. XVI (»B. I—XVI. Die letzte Seite, fol. 451, stammt aus einer andern Hds. und enthält Bruchstücke des Aëtius, B. VII cap. μζ' · περὶ ἀμβλυωπίας Γαληνοῦ κτλ. Inc. Χιτῶνας καὶ τὸ ὀπτικὸν πνεῦμα. Expl. ὑπαλίφειν ἐλαίῳ παλαιῷ μόνῳ.« M. W.).

596 (»L. I—VIII. Aus ihm stammt die Aldina.« M. W.).

Wien: Vindob. med. 12 *usw.* (L. IX init. mut. —XVI. *Apogr. des Parisin. 2191*).

Excerpta varia.

Florenz: Laurent. 75, 10; s. XIV. f. 51—52v (»Excerpte aus B. XIII.« M. W.) *und* f. 329 (Ἐκ τῶν Ἀετίου περὶ τῶν ἐν τοῖς σπλάγχνοις ἐρυσιπελάτων διαθέσεων κτλ. »Sind Excerpte aus B. XII«. M. W.).

Mailand: Ambros.

A 175 Sup. (*nicht* 157) *usw.*

I 166 Inf.; s. XVII. f. 62—73.

Rom: Vatic. 299 (»Ist B. I.« M. W.).

Africanus.

Ἐκ τῶν Ἀφρικανοῦ Κεστῶν κτλ.
(Kat. II S. 8.)

Rom: Vatic. 284; s. XI. f. 288v (Ἐκ τῶν Ἀ. κεστῶν περὶ τοῦ κιναμώμου. M. W.).

Περὶ σταθμῶν καὶ μέτρων. [Diels N.44]
(Kat. II S. 8).

Ed. P. de Lagarde, Symmicta I. Göttingen 1877 p. 167—173.)

Inc. Ἐπειδὴ πολλαχοῦ σταθμῶν τε καὶ μέτρων.
Expl. κατ' αὐτὴν τὸν σταθμὸν ἀεὶ ποιεῖν.

Paris: Parisin.
2720; s. XVI. f. 186v.
2731; s. XVI. f. 133v.
2830; a. 1515. f. 232.

Aglaias.

(Kat. II S. 8).

Vgl. M. Haupt, Opusc. III 609 f.

Mailand: Ambros. A 162 Sup.; s. XV. f. 69 (Expl. σύνθεσις ἥδε πέλει).

Alexander Aphrodisiensis.

Ἰατρικὰ ἀπορήματα καὶ φυσικὰ προβλήματα.
(Kat. II S. 9.)

Mailand: Ambros. M 41 Sup.; s. XV. f. 130.

Ἀπορίαι καὶ λύσεις διάφοροι.
(Kat. II S. 9.)

Mailand: Ambros. H 43 Sup.; s. XV—XVI. f. 110.

Alexander Rex.

Περὶ τῆς τῶν ἑπτὰ βοτανῶν δυνάμεως.
(Kat. II S. 10.)

Mailand: Ambrosian.
E 37 Sup.; s. XVI. f. 351.
H 2 Inf.; s. XVI. f. 250.

Alexander Trallianus.

[Diels N.45]

Περὶ ἑλμίνθων.
(Kat. II S. 12.)

Mailand: Ambros. R 111 Sup.; s. XVI. f. 264.

Andromachus.

Θηριακή.
(Kat. II S. 14.)

Rom: Palat. 48; s. XVI. f. 192.

Antonius Pyropulus.

(Kat. II S. 15.)

»Gehört dem 15. Jahrhundert an, ist also sicherlich zu streichen.« Treu.

Aretaeus.

(Kat. II S. 17 ff. Zu allen 4 Teilen des Werkes.)

Padua: »Bibl. Cathedr. P 129 ist zu streichen. Irrtum Kühns in seiner Ausgabe p. XV infolge von Montfaucon I p. 489, der einen Auszug aus Tomasinis Bibl. Patavinae gibt. P 129 bedeutet in Wahrheit: Tomasini p. 129, wo dieser seine eigne Hds. beschreibt.« E. Jacobs.

Dazu:
Rhaedest. (*bei* Foerster, De antiq. Cpolit. p. 29).
»Die Claromontani sind = den Phillipps. in Berlin.« Emil Jacobs.

Περὶ αἰτίων καὶ σημείων ὀξέων παθῶν.
(Kat. II S. 17.)

Neapel: Neapolit. III D 21 *usw.* (*Collationsprobe, K. p. 33—36, besitzt W. Crönert*).

[Diels N.46]

Asclepiades.

Ὑγιεινὰ παραγγέλματα.
(Kat. II S. 20.)

Athen: Βιβλ. τῆς Βουλῆς 68; s. XVIII. f. 212 (Asclep. et Dioscr. ὑγ. παραγγ. Inc. Μεταδιδόασθαι τὴν τροφὴν ἐξορμήσας).

S[anctus] Basilius.

Πρὸς Εὐστάθιον ἰατρόν.
(Kat. II S. 21.)

Vgl. Migne, Patrol. gr. 32 p. 684 ff. Ep. 189.

Inc. Ἔστι μὲν καὶ πᾶσιν ὑμῖν τοῖς τὴν ἰατρικὴν μετιοῦσι.
Expl. τὴν ἁγίαν Τριάδα διοριζόμεθα.

Bei Migne Vatic., Coislin., 2 Parisini regii.

Beniaminus.

Excerpta.
(Kat. II S. 22).

Nur Receptenmacher.

Berlin: Phillipps. 1583; s. XV. f. 105^v (Φάρμακα). [Treu.]
Mailand: Ambros. Q 94 Sup.; s. XV—XVI. f. 349—363.

Cassius Iatrosophista.

Ἰατρικαὶ ἀπορίαι κτέ.
(Kat. II S. 22.)

Mailand: Ambros. A 92 Sup.; s. XV—XVI. f. 45.

Chrysostomus (sic!).

Expl. διαφορεῖσθαι καὶ ἐξωθεῖσθαι πεποίηκεν.

Mailand: Ambros. Q 94 Sup.; s. XV—XVI *usw.*

Cleopatra.

[Diels N.47]

Περὶ μέτρων καὶ σταθμῶν.
(Kat. II S. 24.)

Mailand: Ambros.
A 57 Inf.; s. XVI. f. 98ᵛ.
A 193 Inf.; s. XVI. f. 100ᵛ.

Constantinus Melitiniota.

Ἀντίδοτοι.
(Kat. II S. 24.)

Berlin: Phillipps. 1562; s. XVI. f. 80 (Inscr. Αὗται αἱ ἀντίδοτοι ἐμετεγκομίσθησαν ἐκ τῶν Περσῶν εἰς τὴν Ἑλλάδα. Inc. Ἀντίδοτος διαφορητικὸν πνευμάτων παντὸς τοῦ σώματος. Remedia νγ').

Constantinus Taronites.

Siehe Nachtrag zu Taronitus.

Crateuas.

(Kat. II S. 25.)

Dazu:
Constantinop. (*bei* Foerster, De antiq. Cpolit. p. 20).
Constant. Antonii Cantacuzeni (*bei* Foerster p. 24).
Mich. Cantacuzeni (*bei* Foerster p. 27).

Cyrillus Alexandrinus.

Περὶ μέτρων καὶ σταθμῶν.
(Kat. II S. 25.)

Mailand: Ambros. C 69 Sup.; s. XV. XVI. f. 34 (Περὶ μετρικῶν ὀνομάτων). [Treu.]

Damnastes.

Περὶ κυουσῶν καὶ βρεφῶν θεραπείας.
(Kat. II S. 26.)

Florenz: *usw.* (*Abschrift besitzt auch W. Crönert*).

[Diels N.48]

Democritus.

Περὶ συμπαθειῶν καὶ ἀντιπαθειῶν.
(Kat. II S. 26.)

Mailand: Ambros. R 111 Sup.; s. XVI. f. 268.
Rom: Barberin. I 17; s. XV. f. 13^{v} (*Abschrift der ersten Hälfte besitzt W. Crönert*).

Excerpta varia.
(Kat. II S. 27.)

Rom: Vatic. 1174; s. XV. f. 1 (Ἐκ τῶν Δημοκρίτου *usw.* Inc. Ἡ φύσις τῇ φύσει τέρπεται) *und* f. 32^{v} (Ὁ δὲ Δημόκριτος ἐκ τούτων λαβὼν συνεγράψατο βιβλία δ' τῷ τῆς ἀφορμῆς ὀνόματι κτλ.) *und* f. 33^{v} (Ἐκ τῶν Δ. περὶ πορφύρας φυσικῆς. Inc. Βαλὼν εἰς λίτραν α' ποφρύρας). [M. W.]

Diocles.

Ἐπιστολὴ προφυλακτικὴ πρὸς Ἀντίγονον βασιλέα.
(Kat. II S. 27.)

München: Monac. 521; s. XV. f. 256^{v}.

Dioscurides.

Opera varia.
(Kat. II S. 29.)

Dazu: Rhaedest. (*bei* Foerster, De antiq. Cpolit. p. 30).

Περὶ ὕλης ἰατρικῆς.
(Kat. II S. 29 ff.)

Mailand: Ambros. L 119 Sup. (*nicht* C 119 Sup.) *usw.*
München: Monac. 236 *usw. ist zu streichen.*
Rom: Vatic. 284; s. XI. f. 1 (»Enthält eine illustrierte Compilation aus Gal. περὶ δυνάμεως φαρμάκων und D. περὶ ὕλης ἰατρικῆς, nach der galenischen Schrift geordnet; vorn unvollständig, umfaßt sie Gal. l. VI—XI. Inc. ρμ̅ περὶ δράβεως: — ⟨δράβη ἡ⟩ πόα. Expl. f. 251r Γαληνοῦ τῶν ἀπλῶν βιβλίον ια' ἐπληρώθη ἔχον ἀπὸ τοῦ Διοσκουρίδου ὅσα Γαληνῷ παραλέλειπται.« M. W. *Collationsprobe in Wellmanns Besitz*).

Dazu:
Constantinop. Antonii Cantacuzeni (*bei* Foerster, De antiq. Cpolit. p. 24).
Michael. Cantacuzeni (*bei* Foerster p. 27).
Rhaedest. (*bei* Foerster p. 30).

Περὶ δηλητηρίων φαρμάκων κτέ. [Diels N.49]
(Kat. II S. 31 f.)

Florenz: Laurent. 74, 23 (*Collation in Wellmanns Besitz*).
München: Monac. 236; s. XV. f. 83 (Πεδακίου Διοσκορίδου Ἀναζαρβέως λόγος ς' περὶ δηλητηρίων φαρμάκων καὶ τῆς αὐτῶν προφυλῶν [sic]. Expl. f. 100 τὰς ἀντιδότους ἀναγκαιότατα καὶ γενναιότατα).
Rom:
Palat. 48; s. XVI. f. 166v. [M. W.]
Vatic.
284; s. XI. f. 251v (*Abschrift in Wellmanns Besitz*).
289; s. XV. f. 98. [M. W.]

Venedig: Marcian.

271 (jetzt 727); s. XV (*Teilweise Collation in Wellmanns Besitz*).

272 (jetzt 728); s. XV (*Collation in Wellmanns Besitz*).

Περὶ ἰοβόλων κτἑ.

(Kat. II S. 32.)

Florenz: Laurent. 74, 23 (*Collation in Wellmanns Besitz*).

München: Monac. 236; s. XV. f. 100^{v}—123^{v} (Inscr. f. 100^{v} praemisso capitum indice: Βιβλίον ζ'^{ον} περὶ ἰοβόλων, ἐν ᾧ καὶ περὶ λυσσῶντος κυνός. Inc. Τὸν μὲν περὶ τῶν ἰοβόλων ζῴων. Expl. f. 112^{r} καὶ τελέως ἀβοήθητα παρασημειούμεθα. Subscr. f. 112^{v} Πεδ. Διοσκ. Ἀναζ. Κιλικίας βιβλίον ἔκδομον [leg. ἕβδομον]: προοίμιον περὶ ἰοβόλων καὶ περὶ σημειώσεως τῶν λυσσοδήκτων. *Photographische Proben im Besitze der Berl. Akademie.* — Inscr. f. 112^{v} Πεδ. Διοσκ. Ἀναζ. λόγος ὄγδοος περὶ σημειώσεως τῶν ὑπὸ ἰοβόλων δεδηκμένων [leg. δεδηγμένων]. Inc. Τοῖς δὲ ὑπὸ φαλαγγίων δεδηγμένοις. Expl. f. 118^{v} πρὸς ἕκαστον τῶν ἰοβόλων ἑξῆς ἴδωμεν. *Photographische Probe im Besitze der Berl. Akademie.* — Inscr. f. 119 Πεδ. Διοσκ. Ἀναζ. θεραπεῖαι τῶν ὑπὸ ἰοβόλων δεδηγμένων λόγος θ'^{ος} Inc. ⟨'Ε⟩ν τῇ σημει... περὶ σφικῶν. Expl. f. 123^{v} καὶ οὗτος ὁ θηριακὸς τρόπος. *Photographie des Anfangs im Besitze der Berl. Akademie. Die Bücher* Ζ' *bis* Θ' *bilden also zusammen die Schrift* Περὶ ἰοβόλων).

Rom:

Palat. 48; s. XVI. f. 177. [M. W.]

Vatic. 289; s. XV. f. 102. [M. W.]

Venedig: Marcian.

271 (jetzt 727); s. XV (*Teilweise Collation in Wellmanns Besitz*).

272 (jetzt 728); s. XV (*Collation in Wellmanns Besitz*).

Περὶ εὐπορίστων.

(Kat. II S. 32.)

Florenz:

Laurent.

74, 10 (*Collation in Wellmanns Besitz*).

74, 20 (*Teilweise Collation in Wellmanns Besitz*).

Riccard. 91 (*Collation in Wellmanns Besitz*).

Rom:

Palat. 400 »ist zu streichen«. M. W.

Vatic. 290 (»stammt aus Laurent. 74, 20.« M. W.).

Excerpta varia.
(Kat. II S. 34 f.)

Athen: Βιβλ. τῆς Βουλῆς 68; s. XVIII. f. 212 (Asclepiadis et Diosc. ὑγιεινὰ παραγγέλματα. Inc. Μεταδιδόασθαι τὴν τροφὴν ἐξορμήσας ἀταμιεύτας).
Mailand: Ambros.
Q 13 Sup.; s. XV—XVI. f. 258ᵛ.
Q 87 Sup.; s. XV f. 247ᵛ.
Rom:
Palat. 400; s. XV. f. 383 (»Βιβλίον Διοσκ. · αὕτη ἡ βίβλος περιέχει τέχνην πείρας ἰατρικῆς περὶ ἁπλῶν τε καὶ συνθέτων φαρμάκων κατὰ ἀλφάβητον ὑποτεταγμένων κτλ.« M. W.).
Vatic. 284 (»Was über ihn hier gesagt ist, kann jetzt wegfallen.« M. W.).

Dazu: Rhaedest. (*bei* Foerster, De antiq. Cpolit. p. 30. Inscr. Περὶ στεάτων).

Epiphanius.

[Diels N.50]

Φυσιολόγος.
(Kat. II S. 35.)

Dazu:
Cod. Jacobi τοῦ Μαρμαρέτου (*bei* Foerster, De antiq. Cpolit. p. 18).
Rhaedest. (*bei* Foerster p. 30).

Περὶ μέτρων καὶ σταθμῶν.
(Kat. II S. 36.)

I. (Ed. P. de Lagarde, Symmicta I. Göttingen 1877 p. 211—225.)

a) Inc. Κόρος σίτου μόδια λ'.
Expl. καθῶς εἶχον οἱ χρόνοι καὶ οἱ τόποι.
b) Inc. = a.
Expl. σίκλους ἑκατὸν εἴκοσι πέντε.

Oxford: Bodl. Misc.
211 (Auct. T II 11); s. XV f. 73—78ᵛ.
212 (Auct. T II 12); s. XVI f. 87—97ᵛ.
Paris: Parisin. 2665; s. XIV—XV f. 204—210.

II. (Ed. P. de Lagarde, Symmicta II. Göttingen 1880 p. 152—183.)

Inc. Εἴ τις θέλει τῶν ἐν ταῖς θείαις γραφαῖς.
Expl. ὃ ἑρμηνεύεται συνημμένον ἢ συνεστραμμένον.

Breslau: Rhedigeran.?; s. XIV—XV. f. 249.
Jena: Jenens.
London: Londin. Addit. (Brit. Mus.)
14620; s. IX.
17148; s. VII.
Paris: Parisin. 835; s. XVI. f. 206ᵛ.

Περὶ τῶν δώδεκα λίθων κτέ.
(Kat. II S. 36.)

Ed. Migne, Patrol. gr. 43 p. 305 ff.
Dindorf, Epiph. Opp. IV p. 233–236; vgl. p. 225–233.

Erotianus.

Der Imperialis Sambuci = einem der Vindobonenses, »= Vindob. 38ᶜ«. Jacobs.

Esdras Propheta.

Περὶ κρισίμων ἡμερῶν.
(Kat. II S. 37).

»Wird in vielen Iatrosophien als Receptenmacher angeführt.« Treu.)

Mailand: Ambros. O 117 Sup.; s. XV—XVI f. 91ᵛ (Inscr. Περὶ τῶν ἡμερῶν τῶν πεφωτισμένων καὶ ἀφωτίστων. Inc. Εἰσὶν αἱ ἡμέραι, ἃς ἐφανέρωσεν. Expl. ἃς δεῖ παρατηρεῖν).

[Diels N.51] Εἰς ὑδερικοὺς καὶ εἰς πάντα τὰ ψυχρὰ νοσήματα.
(Kat. II S. 37.)

Inc. *lies:* Μαμηρά, οὐγγίαν α'.

Wien:
Bibl. colleg. S. I. Rossianus XI. 167; s. XV. f. 156 (Inscr. καὶ ἡ τρίτη σκευασία τοῦ ἔσδρακος τοῦ σοφοῦ καὶ μεγάλου προφήτου εἰς — νοσήματα. Inc. μαμηρά, οὐγγίαν ᾱ. Expl. ἀπηφρισμένον τὸ ἀρκοῦν).

Vindob. med.
31; s. XV. f. 133—133v.
41; s. XIV—XV f. 92v—93v.

Euphemius Siculus.

Συνθέσεις.
(Kat. II S. 38.)

Paris: Parisin. 2194 *usw.* (Βιβλίον περιέχον συνθέσεις συναχθὲν καὶ πειραθὲν παρὰ Εὐφημίου Σικελοῦ τοῦ θαυμασιωτάτου καὶ Φιλίππου Ξηροῦ τοῦ Ῥιγινοῦ τῶν θαυμασίων ἰατρῶν. Inc. Σύνθεσιν σὺν θεῷ τροχίσκον). [Treu.]

Gregorius Nyssenus.

Περὶ καρασκευῆς ἀμθρώπου.
(Kat. II S. 40.)

Mailand: Ambros.
B 63 Sup.; s. XIV ex. f. 87 (Sine auct. nomine. Expl. c. 30 ἔστι δὲ καὶ ἄλλα τινά = Migne p. 241 A).
B 82 Sup.; s. XVI. f. 1 (Expl. c. 22 τὴν τοῦ ἀδὰμ κλῆσιν).
C 88 Sup.; s. X in. f. 54 (Expl. ἐπιτεχνηθέντος τῇ ὕλῃ = Migne p. 253 C).
F 107 Sup.; s. X f. 75 (Fragmenta).
H 11 Sup.; s. XIII. XIV. f. 265.
Q 14 Sup.; s. XV f. 97v (91v).
E 10 Inf.; s. XI f. 91 (Inc. ⟨γεγονό⟩των διέλαθεν = Migne p. 144 cap. 8).
Patmos: Patmiac. ΚΓ' (*bei* Migne, Patrol. gr. 149 p. 1049).

Gregorius Theologus.

Ἀλάτιον.
(Kat. II S. 41.)

München: Monac.
105 *usw.* f. 333v (*Abschrift besitzt W. Crönert*).
287; s. XIV f. 1 (*Abschrift in Crönerts Besitz*).

Harpocration.

Excerpta varia.
(Kat. II S. 41.)

Berlin: Philipp. 1577 (Meerm. 287); s. XV f. 186—198.

[Diels N.52]

Heliodorus.

Πρὸς Θεοδόσιον περὶ τῆς τῶν φιλοσόφων μυστικῆς τέχνης.
(Kat. II S. 41).

»Ed. Fabricius, Bibl. Graeca VI[1] p. 774—781. Gehört einem Alchemisten Heliodorus.« Treu.

Inc. Σκῆπτρα γαίης μέδοντες, ὡς πανέμφρονες.
Expl. εἰς κυκλικοὺς αἰῶνας αἰώνων, ἀμήν.

Mailand: Ambros.
A 57 Inf.; s. XVI. f.37.
A 193 Inf.; s. XVI. f. 35v.

Χειρουργούμενα.
Chirurgia.
(Vgl. Kat. II S. 42.)

Papyrus im Besitze von Ad. Cattaui, Cairo; s. III(?). Zwei Spalten (Inc. ἐὰν δὲ ⟨ἐπὶ πλεῖον ᾗ⟩ ἐψειλωμέν⟨ον τ⟩ὸ κρα⟨νίο⟩ν ἐμποδίζον τὴν συνσάρκωσιν. Expl. μᾶλλον ἔχονται τοῦ ἀποτελέσματος ἔμπροσθεν.

Herausgegeben von I. Nicole, kommentiert und dem 2. Buche der Χειρουργούμενα des H. zugewiesen von J. Ilberg in: Wilckens Archiv für Papyrusforschung IV S. 269—283).

Hermes Trismegistus.

Opera varia.
(Kat. II S. 43).

Vgl. Kyranus.

Dazu:
Constantinop. Antonii Cantacuzeni (*bei* Foerster, De antiq. Cpolit. p. 25).
Michaelis Cantacuzeni (*bei* Foerster p. 27).
Rhaedest. (*bei* Foerster, De antiq. Cpolit. p. 30. Ἑρμ. τρισμ. βιβλία τρία ἰατρομαθηματικά).

Μέθοδος εἰς πᾶσαν καταρχήν ἐπιτήδειος.
(Kat. II S. 43.)

Inc. Πρὸ πάντων δεῖ.
Expl. μηδὲν κτώμενον.

Florenz: Laurent. 28, 14; s. XIV ex. f. 241.
Rom: Vatic. *usw.*; s. XV. f. 18v.
Venedig: Marc. 334; s. XIV f. 49.

Κυρανίδες.
(Kat. II S. 43).

Vgl. Ernst Meyer. Geschichte der Botanik. II. Königsberg 1855 p. 348—366. H. Haupt, Philol. 48 [1889] p. 371 ff. P. Tannery, Revue des étud. gr. XVII [1904] p. 335 ff.)

Berlin: Phillipp. 1577 (Meerm. 287)*; s. XV. f. 186—198.

Ἰατρομαθηματικὰ πρὸς Ἄμμωνα. [Diels N.53]
(Kat. II S. 44.)

Erlangen: Erlangens. bibl. univ. 89; s. XV. f. 177v (Inc. Ἐν τῇ καταβολῇ τοῦ ἀνθρωπίνου σπέρματος).
Florenz: Laurent.
28, 13; s. XIV. f. 221.

28, 34; s. XI. f. 1 (»Ab editione Ideleriana paululum differt«).
München: Monac. 401; s. XVI. f. 318 (Inc. mut. κινδυνεῦσας [sic] εἰς χρόνον = Idel. I 431, 36. Expl. mut. κατακλιθῇ τις Κρόνου συνόντος = Id. I 438, 10. »Multis locis discrepat scriptura huius codicis ab editione Ideleri sive Hoeschelii«).
Turin: Taurin. C VI 21 (b VI 18); s. XVI. f. 66 (Ἐκ τῶν ἰατρομαθηματικῶν Ἑρμοῦ καὶ Πετοσιριος καὶ τῶν συναγωγῶν Πρωταγόρου).

Περὶ κατακλίσεως νοσούντων.
(Kat. II S. 44.)

Florenz: Laurent. 28, 33; a. 1542. f. 246ᵛ (Inscr. Ἑρμοῦ π. κατακλίσεως. Inc. Ψήφισον τὸ ὄνομα. Expl. ὑγιαίνει).

Περὶ βοτανῶν χυλώσεως.
(Kat. II S. 44.)

Venedig: Marcian. App. V 13; s. XIV—XV. f. 157.

Πρὸς τὸν Ἀσκληπιὸν λόγος καθολικός.
(Kat. II S. 44).

Füge hinzu beim Titel: Ad Aesculapium liber universalis.

Περὶ βοτανῶν τῶν ιβ' ζῳδίων.
(Kat. II S. 45).

Ed. Pitra, Analecta sacra V p. 291.

Inc. Κριοῦ ἐλελίσφακον.
Expl. φυσικὴν ἀποτέλεσιν.

Erlangen: Erlangens. bibl. univ. 89; s. XV. f. 175ᵛ.
Paris: Parisin. 2243; a. 1339. f. 654ᵛ (Anonym.).

Περὶ τῆς τῶν ιβ' τόπων ὀνομασίας (so!) καὶ δυνάμεως.
(Kat. II S. 45).

Nicht medizinisch, rein astrologisch.

Inc. Ὁ α'ος τόπος ὁ καὶ ὡροσκόπος καλεῖται.
Expl. ἢ καταδίκη περιτρέψει.

Erlangen: Erlangens. bibl. univ. 89; s. XV. f. 159.
Paris: Parisin. 2506; s. XIII. f. 1.
Venedig: Marc. 335; s. XV. f. 28.

Περὶ βοτανῶν τῶν ζ' πλανήτων.
(Kat. II S. 45).

Ed. Fr. Boll, Catal. codd. astrol. VII append.

Inc. Βότανον Ἡλίου πολύγονον.
Expl. κόκκον σίτου ἢ κριθῆς.

Erlangen: Erlangens. bibl. univ. 89; s. XV. f. 175v.
Paris: Parisin. 2243; a. 1339. f. 654v (Anonym.).

Excerpta varia. [Diels N.54]
(Kat. II S. 47.)

Rom: Urbin. 67; s. XIV—XV. f. 186v (»Ἀντίδοτος πρὸς ποδαλγικοὺς πάνυ πεπειραμένη αἰγυπτιακὴ τρισμέγιστος, φοβερὰ δόκιμος γεναμένη εἰς ὑγείαν πολλῶν ἀνθρώπων.« M. W.).

Herophilus.

Περὶ πυρεσσόντων.
(Kat. II S. 48).

»Rührt von Hierophilus Sophista her.« M. Wellmann.

Hierophilus Sophista.

Περὶ πυρεσσόντων.
(Zu Kat. II S. 49).

Vgl. Nachtrag zu Herophilus περὶ πυρεσσόντων.

Ioannes Archiatrus.

(Kat. II S. 52.)

München: Monac. 288 *usw. ist im Titel folgendes zu verbessern:* εὐίατα γενέσθαι ὠφέλειαν καὶ ἴασιν. (*Abschrift besitzt W. Crönert*).

Ioannes Chrysostomus.

Vgl. Nachtrag über Chrysostomus.

Ioannes Dioecetas.

(Kat. II S. 53.)

»Doch wohl διοικητής.« Treu.

Τῆς τελείας τῆς ἰατρικῆς βιβλία. (*So lautet der Titel nach Treu.*)

[Diels N.55]

Ioannes Episcopus Prisdrianensis.

Παρεκβολαὶ περὶ διαχωρημάτων.
(Kat. II S. 54.)

Paris: Parisin. 2286 *usw.* (Expl. τοὺς ἐν βάθει πάσχοντας ἀφανεῖν τόπους). [Treu.]

Συγγραφὴ περὶ οὔρων.
(Kat. II S. 55.)

Paris: Parisin. 2286 *usw.* (Inscr. Περὶ οὔρων διάγνωσις καὶ πραγματεία ἀρίστη. Inc. Τὴν περὶ τῆς τῶν οὔρων διαφορᾶς πραγματείαν). [Treu.]

Ἐκ τῆς Παλλαδίου, Ἀρχελάου, Στεφάνου Ἀλεξανδρέως
καὶ διαφόρων παλαιῶν ἰατρῶν περὶ ἐντέρων.
(Treu. Kat. II S. 55.)

Inc. Τὸ τοῦ ἀνθρώπου.

Ioannes Staphidaces.

(Kat. II S. 55.)

Rom: Vatic. 282 *usw.* (»Σύνθεσις ἀκριβὴς διαφόρων πράξεων ἐκβληθεῖσα καὶ συντεθεῖσα ὡς ἀναγκαῖον [in mg. ἰωάννου τοῦ σταφιδάκη]. Inc. Κουφότερον καθαρτικόν· ἐπιθύμου ςΓ δ'· μυροβάλατα ςΓ η'. Expl. f. 444ᵛ ἔχον τὴν σαμίαν αἰγυπτίαν ῥόδα.« M. W.).

Iustus. [Diels N.56]

(»Häufig Receptenmeister in den Iatrosophien.« Treu.)

Leo.

Σύνοψις ἰατρικῆς.
(Kat. II S. 57.)

Paris: Parisin. *usw.* (*Abschrift besitzt E. O. Winstedt, Oxford*).

Logadius.

Excerpta.
(Kat. II S. 58).

»Häufig als Receptenmeister in den Iatrosophien genannt.« Treu.

Rom: Angelic. *usw.*: εἰς ξανθοχολ. *usw. gehört zur Überschrift.*
Wien:
Bibl. colleg. S. J. Rossian. XI. 167; s. XV. f. 139v (σκευασία τῆς ἱερᾶς λογαδίου εἰς ξανθο(χο)λικοὺς καὶ μελαγχολικοὺς καὶ φλεγματικούς. Inc. θύμου οὐγγίαν α'. Expl. 139v ἀφρονίτρου οὐγγίας β').
Vindob. med.
31; s. XV. f. 133v—136v.
41; s. XIV—XV. f. 93v—96.

Lucas.

Σκευασία ἁλατίου.
(Kat. II S. 58.)

»Recht häufig in den Iatrosophien.« Treu. »Stammt aus des Manuel Comnenos Δυναμερόν.« M. Wellmann.

München: Monac. 551; s. xv. f. 303 (*Abschrift besitzt W. Crönert*).
Rom: Vatic. 299; s. XV. f. 148 (»Ἁλάτιον σκευασθὲν ὑπὸ τοῦ ἁγίου ἀποστόλου Λουκᾶ ἔχον ἐνεργείας τῶν ὑποτεταγμένων κεφαλαίων. Expl. ἐν αὐτῷ τὰς τροφὰς πάσας.« M. W.).
Wien:
colleg. S. J. Rossianus XI. 167; s. XV. f. 137v. (Inc. ἔχων ἐνεργείας. Expl. ἐν αὐτῷ τὰς τροφὰς πάσας).
Vindob. med.
31; s. XV. f. 130v—131.
41; s. XIV—XV. f. 88—89.

Excerpta varia.
(Kat. II S. 58.)

Berlin: Phillipps. 1583; s. XV. f. 31.

Dazu: Constantinop. Michaelis Cantacuzeni (*bei* Foerster, De antiq. Cpolit. p. 27).

Macarius Maximus,

d. i. Μακάριος (beatus) Maximus, scil. Confessor.

Περὶ ψυχῆς.
(Kat. II S. 59)

Ed. Migne, Patrol. gr. 91 p. 353—361.

Magnus Emesenus.

[Diels N.57]

Περὶ οὔρων.
(Kat. II S. 59. 60.)

Dazu:
Constantinop. Mich. Cantacuzeni (*bei* Foerster p. 27).
Rhaedest. (*bei* Foerster, De antiq. Cpolit. p. 30).

Manuel Comnenus.

Δυναμερόν.
De compositione medicamentorum.
(Zu Kat. II S. 60.)

Rom: Vatic. 299; s. XV. f. 131 (»Τῶν σκευασιῶν ἡ βίβλος αὕτη πέλει καὶ δυναμερὸν σὺν θεῷ λεγομένη. Ἀρχὴ καὶ πρώτη σκευασία τῆς θηριακῆς. Es folgt Index von ος' Kapiteln und Index der σκευασίαι τῶν ἐμπλάστρων mit οθ' Kapiteln. Text beginnt f. 132 mit Überschrift: π' σκευασία τοῦ ζουλαπίου κυρίου Μανουὴλ Κομνηνοῦ· σκευασία τῆς θηριακῆς. Aus dieser Schrift stammt des Lucas σκευασία ἁλατίου.« M. W.).

Marcellinus.

Περὶ σφυγμῶν.
(Kat. II S. 60.)

Ed. H. Schoene, Festschrift zur 49. Philologenversammlung in Basel 1907 p. 455—471.

Bologna: Bonon. *usw.* (Inc. Σφυγμὸν θήγειν καὶ περὶ σφυγμῶν ὅσα χρὴ μαθήν = Zeile 2 Schoene. Expl. τὴν ἐπιπλοκὴν ἔχων = Zeile 485 Sch.).

Wien: Vindob. med.
15; s. XV. *usw.*
16; s. XIV. *usw.*

Marianus.

(Fällt fort; s. u.)

Excerpta.
(Kat. II S. 62.)

Rom: Barberin. *usw.* (Εὑρισκόμενα *usw., also aus dem Besitze des Mariano Tucci*).

Maximus (Planudes?)

»Schwerlich von Planudes.« Treu. *Vgl. Nachtrag zu* Meletius *Excerpta varia.*

[Diels N.58]

Melampus Ἱερογραμματεύς.

Περὶ παλμῶν μαντικὴ πρὸς Πτολεμαῖον βασειλέα.
Ex palpitatione divinatio ad regem Ptolemaeum.
(Kat. II S. 62.)

Ed. Fr. Sylburg, Aristotelis var. opusc. Frankfurt 1589 p. 223—235.
Darnach J. G. F. Franzius, Scriptores Physiognomiae vett. Altenburg 1780 p. 451—500.
Vgl. R. Foerster,
Herm. 10 p. 465.
De Polemonis physiognomicis, Progr. Kiel 1886 p. 20f.
Philologus 46 p. 259.
und Adamantius περὶ παλμῶν Kat. II S. 3.
Neuausgabe von H. Diels erscheint in diesen »Abhandlungen« 1907.)

München: Monac. 583 (olim Uffenbachianus); a. 1656 (Apogr. der Editio Romana).
Paris: Parisin.
2037; s. XVI. f. 41 (desgl.).
2118; s. XVI. f. 56 (*W. Nachstädts Collation im Besitze der Berl. Akademie*).
2154; s. XIV. f. 280 (*Abschrift besitzt R. Foerster. Abschrift des Anfangs von W. Nachstädt und Photographien des Ganzen im Besitze der Berl. Akademie*).

Περὶ ἐλαιῶν τοῦ σώματος.
De naevis corporis.

Ed. Sylburg p. 235 ff. J. G. F. Franzius p. 501—508.

Inc. Ἐάν ἐστι εἰς τὸ πρόσωπον.
Expl. καὶ πτωχοὶ ἔσονται.

Berlin: Phillips. 1576 (Meerm. 286); s. XVI. f. 23ᵛ.
Paris: Parisin. 2037; s. XVI. f. 54.

Meletius Monachus.

Περὶ ψυχῆς.
(Kat. II S. 62.)

Vgl. unten Nachtrag zu περὶ φύσεως ἀνθρώπου *aus* Monac. 39.

Περὶ φύσεως ἀνθρώπου.
(Kat. II S. 63.)

Athen: Βιβλ. τῆς Βουλῆς 43; s. XIII. f. 122.
Mailand: Ambros. P 90 Sup.; s. XV—XVI. f. 4.
München: Monac. 39 *usw.* (Inscr. Πόνημα ἐν συνόψει περὶ φύσεως ἀνθρώπου ἐξερανισθὲν καὶ συντεθὲν παρὰ Μελετίου μοναχοῦ ἐκ τῶν τῆς ἐκκλησίας ἐνδόξων καὶ τῶν ἔξω λογάδων καὶ φιλοσόφων. Inc. Τὰ περὶ τῆς τοῦ ἀνθρώπου κατασκευῆς καὶ ἐξ ὅσων ἐστὶ φύσεων. Expl. f. 71 ἐκ τῶν λαμβανομένων τροφῶν. *Darauf folgt, wie zu dem Werke des Meletius gehörig,* περὶ ψυχῆς πρόλογος. Inc. Ὁ περὶ ψυχῆς ὧδε [sic] λόγος οὐ τὸ τί ἐστιν ἡ ψυχή, *vgl.* Med.-Kat. II S. 62. Expl. f. 72ᵛ προαίρεσις — ἐπιθυμία, λογικαί — ἄλογοι. *Dahinter wiederum ohne Abtrennung von dem frühern* f. 72ᵛ: Περὶ ψυχῆς λόγος δεύτερος. Inc. Ἐπειδὴ δὲ ἐκ ψυχῆς καὶ σώματος συνέστη ὁ ἄνθρωπος. Expl. f. 79ᵛ σῶμα δὲ τὴν φράσιν. δόξαν χριστῷ τῷ θεῷ usw. ἀμήν).

[Diels N.59]

Dazu:
Constantinopol. (*bei* Foerster, p. 20. Inscr. Περὶ τῆς τοῦ ἀνθρώπου κατασεκυῆς).
Cpolit. Antonii Cantacuzeni (*bei* Foerster p. 24).
Michaelis Cantacuzeni (*bei* Foerster p. 27. Inscr. Περὶ τῆς τοῦ ἀνθρ. κατασκ.).
Rhaedest. (*bei* Foerster, De antiq. Cpolit. p. 30).

Excerpta varia.
(Kat. II S. 64.)

Paris: Parisin. 2240 *usw.* (»Die Verse sind nicht politische, sondern ein Kanon in der Form eines Kirchenliedes [τῶν οὐρανίων ταγμάτων; cf. Christ und Paranikas Anthol. Gr. carminum Christianorum, Lips. 1871 p. 64 ff.]. In den genannten Pariser Mss. wird er Meletius zugeschrieben, in anderen Mss. anderen: z. B. Nicophorus Blemmydes in Vindob. med. Graec. 32; s. XV—XVI. f. 35. Parisin. 2303; s. XV. Parisin. suppl. 629; s. XIX, besonders aber, und wohl mit Recht, dem Maximus Planudes; z. B. Parisin. 2286; f. 101. Vindob. theol. Gr. 295; s. XV—XVI. f. 312. Unter Maximus Planudes' Namen ist dieser Kanon ediert von Ideler, Phys. et med. Gr. II 318—322. Ideler hatte natürlich keine Ahnung, daß er Verse herausgab.« Treu.)

Mercurius Monachus.

Περὶ σφυγμῶν.
(Kat. II S. 64. 65.)

Mailand: Ambros. D 33 Sup.; s. XV. f. 66 (Expl. μίαν καὶ δύο = Ideler p. 255, 27).
Paris: Parisin. 2315; s. xv. f. 1 (»Περὶ σφυγμῶν κάλλιστον καλλίστου ἀνδρὸς μοναχοῦ μερκουρίου. Inc. Τὸ σῶμα τοῦ ἀνθρώπου. Expl. κατὰ τὴν ἡμετέραν δύναμιν ἐξεθέμεθα.« Treu.)
Rom: Vatic. 299 *usw.* (»Inc. Τὸ σῶμα τοῦ ἀνθρώπου συνέστηκεν ἐκ δ' στοιχείων. Expl. f. 101v κατὰ λέξιν τοιόνδε.« M. W. *Abschrift besitzt E. O. Winstedt, Oxford*).

Methodius Patriarchus,

d.i. »Patriarch«, *nämlich von* Konstantinopel,
»also zu schreiben Patriarcha«. Treu.

(Kat. II S. 65.)

Nemesius Emesenus.

Περὶ φύσεως ἀνθρώπου.
(Kat. II S. 66. 67.)

Mailand: Ambros. P 32 Sup.; a. 1564. f. 1 (Sub nomine Pachomii).

München: Monac. 419 *usw.* (Inc. Τὸν ἄνθρωπον ἐκ ψυχῆς νοερᾶς καὶ σώματος ἄριστα κατεσκευάσθαι. Expl. f. 32ᵛ τὰ γὰρ φύσει τὰ αὐτὰ παρὰ πᾶσιν. *Photographie des Anfangs und Schlusses im Besitze der Berl. Akademie*).
Patmos: Patmiac. monast. St. Ioann. Evang. 11 (*bei* Coxe, Mss. gr. of the Levant); s. X in. (*vgl.* nr. Λ' *bei* Migne, Patrol. gr. 149, 1049).

Neophytus Prodromenus. [Diels N.60]

Συλλογὴ περὶ βοτανῶν.
(Kat. II S. 68.)

Paris: Parisin. 2286 *usw.* (»Fol. 105 ist ursprünglich das 1. Fol. des Codex. Der ganze Codex 2286 ist von Neophytus' Hand; f. 168ʳ folgende Verse: πίναξ ἀκριβὴς τῆς παρούσης πυκτίδος πᾶσιν ἐναργῶς ἴασιν δωρουμένης θεοῦ τὸ δῶρον καὶ πόνος νεοφύτου τῆς προδρομικῆς etc. — ἡ βίβλος ἥδε τῆς φιλανθρώπου τέχνης. Die Blätter des Codex sehr durcheinander. Der Index aber sehr vollständig.« Treu).
Rom: Palat. 199; S. XIII. f. 17 (Λέξις βοτανῶν κατὰ στοιχεῖον ἀλφαβήτου. Inc. Ἄρκευστον ἢ καντζάρου ἢ κέδρος. *Aufgenommen und hierher gestellt von* M. Wellmann).

Nepualius.

Περὶ τῶν κατὰ συμπάθειαν καὶ ἀντιπάθειαν.
(Kat. II S. 68.)

Mailand: Ambros. R 111 Sup.; s. XVI. f. 266ᵛ.
Neapel: Borbon. I 17; s. XV. f. 9 (Inscr. Τῶν κατὰ ἀντιπάθ. καὶ συμπ. *Abschrift des Anfangs besitzt W. Crönert*).

Nicolaus Myrepsus.

Δυναμερόν.
(Kat. II S. 69).

»In 48 Abteilungen in alphabetischer Ordnung.« Treu.

Athen: Atheniens. 1478 (*vgl.* Krumbacher, Byz. Litt.^{2} 617f.).
Berlin: »Phillipps. 1583 hat mit diesem Werke nichts zu tun, muß also fort;
Paris: ebenso muß fort Parisin. 2315; f. 276.

Da steht nur ἑρμενία νικολάου, περὶ ἐμπλάστρου πάνυ ὠφέλιμον. Hinzuzufügen wäre noch [nach Foerster p. 31] aus der Rhädestosbibliothek: νικολάου τοῦ μυρεψικοῦ ἰατρικόν. Und endlich ist zu erwähnen, daß es eine lateinische Übersetzung des Werkes gibt, Ingolst. 1549, vom Tübinger Leonhard Fuchs. Die Handschrift, die er benutzt hat, scheint verloren. Die Übersetzung ist bei Stephanus und sonst öfter wieder gedruckt.« Treu.

Dazu: Constantinop. Michaelis Cantacuzeni (*bei* Foerster, De antiq. Cpolit. p. 27).

Oribasius.

Opera varia.
(Kat. II S. 70.)

Dazu: Rhaedest. (*bei* Foerster, De antiq. Cpolit. p. 29).

[Diels N.61] Σύνοψις πρὸς Εὐστάθιον.
(Kat. II S. 71.)

Venedig: Marcian. 295*; a. 1470. f. 177ᵛ (»Ohne Überschrift«. Wellmann).

Excerpta varia.
(Kat. II S. 73.)

Mailand: Ambros. G 69 Sup.; s. XV. f. 341.
Rom: Palat. 199; s. XIII. f. 16ᵛ (Περὶ μέτρων καὶ σταθμῶν ἰατρικῶν. Inc. Ὁ μέδιμνος ἔχει) *und* f. 149ᵛ sq. (folgende Capitel, die = Orib. I 436 ff.: περὶ κατακλίσεως, ἐκ τῶν Ἀντύλλου καὶ Γαληνοῦ ἐκ τῶν ποιουμένων βοηθημάτων, περὶ ἡσυχίας ἐκ τοῦ αὐτοῦ λόγου, περὶ ἀσιτίας ἐκ τοῦ αὐτοῦ λόγου, περὶ ὕπνου καὶ ἐγρηγόρεως Γαληνοῦ, περὶ τῆς ἐξ ὕπνου ὠφελείας Ἀντύλλου, περὶ ἐγρηγόρεως τοῦ αὐτοῦ, περὶ λαλιᾶς τοῦ αὐτοῦ. Dann περὶ τῶν μέσων ἐδεσμάτων τῶν αὐτῶν Γαληνοῦ = Orib. I 173. Dann folgen die weitern Capitel Orib. I 174. 177. 182. 178) *und* f. 168ᵛ (Περὶ λουτρῶν σαφὲς = Orib. II 369) *und* f. 181ᵛ (Περὶ τῶν ἐν τοῖς συμπτώμασιν αἰτίων = Orib. III 208. Daran schließen sich weitere Excerpte bis fol. 183ᵛ). [M. W.]

Palladius.

Περὶ πυρετῶν.
(Kat. II S. 75.)

Florenz: Laurent. 74, 11 (*Bianchis Collation in dessen Besitz*).

Περὶ βρώσεως καὶ πόσεως.
(Kat. II S. 75.)

Florenz: Laurent. 74, 2 (*Bianchis Collation in dessen Besitz*).

Εἰς τὸ περὶ ἀγμῶν Ἱπποκράτους.
(Kat. II S. 76.)

Florenz: Laurent. *usw.* (*Bianchis Collation in dessen Besitz. Buddenhagens Collation in Schoenes Besitz*).

Σχόλια τῆς ἕκτης ἐπιδημίας.
(Kat. II S. 76.)

Berlin: Phillipps. 1525 (*Mewaldts Collation des I. Buches in Bianchis Besitz*).
Florenz: Laurent.
75, 21 (*Collationen Bianchis in dessen Besitz*)
und
75, 22 (*Collationen Bianchis in dessen Besitz*).
Rom: Urbin. 64; s. X—XI. f. 48ᵛ (*Unter dem Namen des* Galen).

Pamphilus. [Diels N.62]

»Nur in Receptensammlungen.« Treu.

Pancharius.

Περὶ κατακλίσεως νοσούντων.
(Kat. II S. 76).

Ed. A. Olivieri, Catal. codd. astrol. I p. 118—122.

Inc. ⟨Ἐν Κριῷ⟩. Σελήνη πρὸς Ἄρην.
Expl. ἀπαραβάτως καὶ [εἰς] χρόνια πάθη.

Florenz: Laurent. 28, 34; s. XI. f. 16.

Paulus Aegineta.

Ἐπιτομὴ ἰατρική.
(Kat. II S. 77. 78.)

Paris:
Coislin.
8; f. 1. s. X (= ed. Aldina Venetiis 1528, fol. 26ᵛ lin. 4 — fol. 27ʳ l. 12) *und* f. 283. s. X (= ed. Ald. fol. 29ʳ l. 10 — fol. 29ᵛ l. 36).
123; f. A (*vor* f. 1) s. X (= ed. Ald. fol. 79ʳ l. 38 — fol. 80ʳ l. 18).
Suppl. gr. 1156; f. 23. s. X (= ed. Ald. fol. 77ᵛ l. 26 — fol. 78ᵛ l. 9) *und* f. 24. s. X (= ed. Ald. fol. 87ᵛ l. 11 — fol. 88 l. 13) *und* f. 25. s. X (= ed. Ald. fol. 95ᵛ l. 12 — fol. 96ʳ l. 13).
Patmos: Monast. St. Ioann. Evang. *usw.* (nr. 71 *bei* Coxe, Mss. gr. of the Levant); s. XIII. (»imperf.«).
Venedig: Marcian. 292 (*Collationsprobe von B. IV, V, VII in Wellmanns Besitz*).
Wien: Vindob. med. 12; s. XIV—XV. f. 92—142 (Liber VI).
Wolfenbüttel: Guelferb. Ebert 2 (47 Gud. gr.) *usw.*

Dazu: Rhaedest. (*bei* Foerster, De antiq. Cpolit. p. 31).

Περὶ ἀντεμβαλλομένων.
(Kat. II S. 78.)

Rom: Vatic. 299; s. XV. f. 153ᵛ. [M. W.]

Περὶ μέτρων καὶ σταθμῶν.
(Kat. II S. 79.)

Venedig: Marcian. 295; a. 1470. f. 176ᵛ (Inc. Τὸ ἰταλικὸν κεράμιον. Expl. τὸ μικρὸν μύστρον Γ^{ρ} κ' < ς' < θ'). [M. W.]

Excerpta varia.
(Kat. II S. 79.)

Athen: Βιβλ. τῆς Βουλῆς 68; s. XVIII. f. 220 (Exc. π. παθῶν ex Hipp., Gal., Paulo Nic., Paulo Aeg.).
Mailand: Ambros. B 113 Sup.; s. XIV in. f. 229ᵛ (Π. δυνάμεως τοῦ πηγάνου. Inc. Πηγάνου ἐν ταῖς βοτάναις πάσαις).

Paulus Nicaeensis.

(Kat. II S. 81.) [Diels N.63]

Vgl. Skeuos G. Zervos, Janus, Arch. intern. pour l'histoire de la médecine etc. 1901 p. 487 ff.

Inc. Πολλῶν τε καὶ ποικίλων γενομένων νοσημάτων.

Athen: Βιβλ. τῆς Βουλῆς 68*; s. XVIII. f. 220 (Exc. περὶ παθῶν ex Hipp., Gal., Paulo Nic., Paulo Aeg.).
Wien: Bibl. colleg. S. J. Vindob. Rossianus XI. 167; s. XV. f. 1. (Pinax Inc. α' · περὶ ἐπισκέψεως. Expl. 2ᵛ ρλ' · περὶ παρονυχίας. f. 12ᵛ de cognitione et curatione variorum morborum. Inc. f. 12ᵛ πολλῶν τε καὶ ποικίλων. Expl. f. 135ᵛ τὴν σάρκα πανταχόθεν ἀπὸ τοῦ ὄνυχος).

Dazu: Constantinop. (*bei* Foerster, De antiq. Cpolit. p. 20. Inscr. Ἰατροσόφιον Π. Νικαίου, μαθητοῦ τοῦ Ἱπποκράτους). Cpolit. Michaelis Cantacuzeni (*bei* Foerster p. 27).

Petosiris.

Ἐπιστολὴ πρὸς Νεχεψώ.
(Kat. II S. 82.)

Mailand: Ambros. H 2 Inf.; s. XVI. f. 228ᵛ (Inc. Περὶ ἑνὸς ἑκάστου. Expl. ὁ κίνδυνος ἢ οὔ).

Philaretus.

Περὶ σφυγμῶν.
(Kat. II S. 83 f.)

Florenz: Laurent. 59, 14: *dieses Werk von einer Hand des XIII.* (*!*) *Saec.*

Philippus Xerus.

Συνθέσεις.
Compositiones medicamentorum.
(Zu Kat. II S. 85.)

Paris: Parisin. 2194; s. XV. f. 454 (Βιβλίον περιέχον συνθέσεις συναχθὲν καὶ πειραθὲν παρὰ Εὐφημίου Σικελοῦ τοῦ θαυμασιωτάτου καὶ Φιλίππου Ξηροῦ τοῦ Ῥιγινοῦ τῶν θαυμασίων ἰατρῶν. Inc. Σύνθεσιν σὺν θεῷ τροχίσκον). [Treu.]

Philo.

Excerpta varia.
(Kat. II S. 85.)

Wien:
Colleg. S. J. Rossianus XI. 167; s. XV. f. 156r (Φίλωνος · φιλῶ τὴν σκευασίαν πάνυ εἰς φλεγματικοὺς καὶ πνευματικούς. Inc. κρόκου οὐγγίας β'. Expl. καὶ μέλιτος τὸ ἀρκοῦν).
Vindob. med.
31; s. XV. f. 163.
41; s. XIV—XV. f. 132.

[Diels N.64]

Philumenus.

Περὶ ἰοβόλων ζῴων καὶ τῶν ἐν αὐτοῖς βοηθημάτων.
(Kat. II S. 85.)

Rom: Vatic. 284 (*Abschrift in Wellmanns Besitz, der den Tractat im Corpus Med. veröffentlichen wird*).

Ptolemaeus.

Centiloquium.
(Kat. II S. 87.)

»n'aurait pas dû être mentionné.« Cumont.

Pythagoras.

Ψῆφοι.
(Kat. II S. 87.)

Mailand: Ambros.
A 45 Sup.; s. XIII. f. 55.
H 2 Inf.; s. XVI. f. 247.

Rufus.

Opera varia.
(Kat. II S. 88.)

Dazu: Rhaedest. (*bei* Foerster, De antiq. Cpolit. p. 29).

Περὶ τῶν ἐν νεφροῖς καὶ κύστει παθῶν.
(Kat. II S. 88.)

München: Monac. 469 *usw.* (*Vielfach zerstört.* Inc. f. 148r. Expl. f. 160v mut. νίτρῳ μετὰ ὄξους ἀνατρίβειν = Dbg. p. 61, 4. *Fortsetzung auf* f. 164r, *bis zum Schlusse des Werkes. Photographien im Besitze der Berl. Akademie. Collation besitzt Helmreich*).
Rom:
Barberin. 382 (I 91)
und
Vatic. 291 (*Collation von beiden besitzt Helmreich*).

Περὶ σατυριασμοῦ καὶ γονορροίας.
(Kat. II S. 88.)

München: Monac. 469 *usw.* (*Vielfach zerstört.* Inc. f. 164[v] Τοῦ αὐτοῦ, scil. Ῥούφου, περὶ ... flg. Z. ᾧ τὸ αἰδοῖον *vgl. Anfang des Werkes,* Dbg. p. 64, 1. f. 164[v] expl. εἰ πρὸς τοῦτο ... = Dbg. p. 67, 1. *Fortsetzung auf* f. 161[r] ⟨ε⟩ὑρίσκεται· πῶς οὖν = Dbg. p. 67, 2, *und so fort* f. 161. 162 *bis* 163[v], *dann* f. 165. Subscr. f. 165[v] περὶ σατυριασμοῦ ἢ [sic] γονοροί⟨ας⟩. *Photographien im Besitze der Berl. Akademie. Collation besitzt Helmreich*).

[Diels N.65] Περὶ ὀνομασίας τῶν τοῦ ἀνθρώπου μορίων.
(Kat. II S. 89.)

Mailand: Ambros.
H 22 Sup.*; s. XV. f. 11 *und* 12[v].
& 141 Sup.; s. XVI. f. 1.

Σύνοψις περὶ σφυγμῶν.
(Kat. II S. 90.)

Paris: Parisin. 2193 *usw.* f. 400—401 (Sonst dem Galen zugeschriebenes Werk).

Περὶ φαρμάκων καθαρτικῶν.
(Kat. II S. 90.)

München: Monac. 469 *usw.* f. 137—147[v] (*Von derselben Hand vorher* Galenus π. κράσ. κ. δυν. τῶν ἁπλ. φαρμ. *und* Galenus Τίνας δεῖ καθαίρειν καὶ ποίοις καθαρτηρίοις καὶ πότε. *Letzteres Buch hat folg. Subscr.:* ἐνταῦθα τέλος Γαληνοῦ μονοβίβλου, *dann auf derselben Zeile:* ἡ ἀρχὴ Ῥούφου μονοβίβλου. Inc. οὔτε πάντας τοὺς ὁπωσοῦν διακειμένους καθαρτέον. Expl. στήθους καὶ πνεύμονος. *Photographien im Besitze der Berl. Akademie*).
Rom: Palat. 199; s. XIII. f. 181[v] (Περὶ καθάρσεως τῆς κατὰ κοιλίαν πρόγνωσις Ῥούφου Ἐφεσίου = Orib. II 94f.). [M. W.]

Excerpta varia.
(Kat. II S. 91.)

Mailand: Ambros. Q 94 Sup.; s. XV—XVI. f. 347 (Inc. Κολοκυνθίδος ἐντεριώνης. Expl. εἶτα καὶ τὴν ἀντίδοτον).

Wien:

Colleg. S. J. Rossianus XI. 167; s. XV. f. 148r (σκευασία ἱερᾶς τοῦ ῥούφου τοῦ ἐφεσίου εἰς δυσπνοιικοὺς καὶ δυσουριῶντας καὶ παχυφλεγματικούς. Inc. Χαμανδρίνου οὐγγίας ι'. Expl. μέλιτος ἀπηφρισμένον τὸ ἀρκοῦν).

Vindob. med.

31; s. XV. f. 150r—150v.

41; s. XIV—XV. f. 115v—116v.

Severianus. (Wohl der Bischof der Galater.)

Περὶ τῆς προσηγορίας τοῦ ἀνθρώπου.
(Kat. II S. 91.)

Vgl. Migne, Patrol. gr. 56, 473 C f.

Soranus.

Περὶ ἐπιδέσμων.
(Kat. II S. 92.)

Florenz: Laurent. 74, 7 *usw.* (*27 Blätter. H. Schoenes Collation der Schrift und Films der Illustrationen in Ilbergs Besitz*).

Ἱπποκράτους γένος.
(Kat. II S. 93.)

Mailand: Ambros. L 110 Sup.; s. XV. f. 233.

[Diels N.66]

Stephanus Alexandrinus.

Περὶ χρυσοῦ ποιήσεως.
(Kat. II S. 95.)

Mailand: Ambros.
E 37 Sup.; s. XVI. f. 308ᵛ.
A 57 Inf.; s. XVI f. 1.
A 193 Inf.; s. XVI. f. 1.

Περὶ τῆς ἱερᾶς καὶ μεγάλης ἐπιστήμης κτλ.
(Kat. II S. 96.)

»In der Überschrift zu verbessern τῆς χρυσοποιίας (☉ποιίας hat die Handschrift).« M. Wellmann.

Stephanus Atheniensis.

(Kat. II S. 97.)

Saecula der Ambrosiani:
Q 94 Sup.; s. XV—XVI.
S 19 Sup.; a. 1349.

Περὶ διαφορᾶς πυρετῶν.
(Kat. II S. 97 ff.)

Florenz: Laurent. 86, 20 (*Bianchis Collation in dessen Besitz*).

Stephanus Ἀρχιατρὸς τῶν Μαγγάννων.

(Kat. II S. 98.)

»Das Mangana-Hospital ist erst Mitte des 11. Jahrhunderts gegründet worden.« Treu.

Syncellus.

Excerpta.
(Kat. II S. 99).

»Das ist Michael syncellus oder syngelus (kirchliches Amt). Von ihm nur Recepte in Iatrosophien.« Treu.

Rom: Urbin. 67; s. XIV—XV. f. 187 (Ἀντίδοτος τοῦ Συγκέλλου). [M. W.]
Wien:
Colleg. S. I. Rossianus XI. 167; s. XV. f. 153ᵛ (σκευασία συγκέλλου τοῦ πανολβίου. Inc. πεπέρεως κοινοῦ. Expl. μέλιτος τὸ ἀρκοῦν).
Vindob. med.
31; s. XV. f. 159ʳ—159ᵛ.
41; s. XIV—XV. f. 127—127ᵛ.

Synesius.

Περὶ πυρετῶν.
De febribus.
(Kat. II S. 99).

Ed. Jo. St. Bernard, Amstelod. 1749.
Vgl. Daremberg, Not. et Extr. des Ms. p. 78.

Inc. Διελθόντες τῇ χάριτι τοῦ Θεοῦ ἐν τοῖς προλαβοῦσι λόγοις.
Expl. ὀλίγον κρόκου καὶ ῥοδοστάγματος.

Leyden: Vossian. fol. 65; s. XV (*benutzt von* Bernard).

[Diels N.67]

Περὶ ἐνυπνίων
(προθεωρία *ist im Titel zu streichen.*)

Ed. Migne, Patrol. gr. 66 p. 1281—1320.

Inc. Ἀρχαῖον ὄμμα καὶ λίαν Πλατωνικόν.
Expl. ὅταν κατὰ Θεόν τι πιστεύηται.

Πρὸς Διόσκορον.
(Kat. II S. 100.)

Mailand: Ambros.
E 37 Sup.; s. XVI. f. 301.
A 57 Inf.; s. XVI. f. 65ᵛ.
A 193 Inf.; s. XVI. f. 64.

Ἐπιστολὴ ὑπὲρ τοῦ σιλφίου.
(Kat. II S. 100).

Ed. Migne, Patrol. gr. 66 p. 1490. Ep. 106.

Mailand: Ambros.
B 72 Sup.; s. XV. f. 1 ff.
L 44 Sup.; s. XIV ex. f. 1 ff.

Taronitus.

(Kat. II S. 100.)

»D. i. Constantinus Taronites«; vgl. Berol. Phillipps. 1583. f. 104. Treu.

Berlin: Phillipps. 1583; s. XV. f. 104 (Ἀντίδοτος λίθων θρυπτικὴ καὶ διουρητικὴ συντεθεῖσα παρὰ κυροῦ Κωνσταντίνου τοῦ Ταρωνείτου). [Treu.]

Theodoretus.

»Die Angabe im cod. Phillipps. (ich habe sie noch nicht angesehen) ist mindestens zweifelhaft: es gibt z. B. eine Antidotus Theodoretus ex anacordiis, z. B. bei Aetius ed. H. Stephanus, Medicae artis principes, col. 661d; vgl. auch Nicol. Myrepsus bei Stephanus l. l. I col. 406. 442. 449. Theodoretus ist also gar kein Name, sondern bedeutet dasselbe wie z. B. Antidotus Theodotus. Viele Stellen im Index zu Stephanus' 2. Bande der Principes s. v. Theodoretos. — Mit der Stelle im Barocc. steht's schwerlich anders.« Treu. *Also* Theodoretus *wohl zu streichen; ebenso zu tilgen das Citat aus Stephanus.*

Theodorus.

»Ein Receptenfabrikant des XI. saec.; der Theodorus im Ottobon. ist wohl ein anderer. Auch Nicol. Myrepsus kennt Theodori. — In Sathas Μεσσαιωνικὴ βιβλιοθ. I p. 274: θεοδώρου τοῦ παναρέτου στίχοι ἰαμβικοὶ, ‚γϡ', περὶ ἰατρικῶν ὑποθέσεων.« Treu.

Theophilus. [Diels N.68]

Περὶ διαχωρημάτων.
(Kat. II S. 102.)

Cairo: Patriarch. Alexandrin. 46 (*bei* Coxe, Mss. gr. of the Levant); s. XV.

Ἐκ τῶν Ἱπποκράτους καὶ Γαληνοῦ περὶ ἰατρικῆς ἐπιστήμης.
(Kat. II S. 105.)

Rom: Palat. 199; s. XIII. f. 190 (Expl. ἀποτελεῖται ἀπὸ τῆς μήτρας). [M. W.]

Excerpta varia.
(Kat. II S. 106.)

Paris: Parisin. 2286; s. XIV. f. 121v (Περὶ χρωμάτων).

Theophylactus Simocatta.

Περὶ διαφορᾶς φυσικῶν ἀπορημάτων.
(Kat. II S. 106.)

Wien: Vindob. phil. 178; s. XV. f. 305v (Anonym; Ideler p. 174, 13—183, 22. *Collation besitzt W. Crönert*).

Vincentius Damodes

»Zu streichen. Autor des XVII.—XVIII. Jahrhunderts« Treu.

Xenocrates.

Περὶ τῆς ἀπὸ τῶν ἐνύδρων τροφῆς.
(Kat. II S. 108.)

Hamburg: Hamburgens. 200 (*in den* Philologica Hamburgensia, Hambg. 1905) = philol. 313; s. XVII. f. 21—27 (*Abschrift des Werkes von der Hand* H. Lindenbrogs).

[Diels N.69]

Ioannes Zacharias Actuarius.

Ἰατρικὴ μέθοδος.
(Kat. II S. 109.)

Berlin: *Abschrift der Berliner Hdss. besitzt M. Treu.*
Mailand: Ambros.
O 123 Sup.; s. XVI. f. 1 (L. V. VI).
R 20 Sup.; s. XV. f. 20.

Περὶ ζῴων φθαρτικῶν.
(Kat. II S. 110.)

»Ist nicht von Ioannes Zacharias.« Treu.

Mailand: Ambros. R 20 Sup. »enthält die Schrift nicht«. Treu. *Also zu streichen.*

Excerpta varia.

Dresden: Dresd. Da 5 »zu streichen; ist nicht von Zacharias, denn vor περὶ σταθμῶν usw. steht nicht τοῦ αὐτοῦ.« Treu.

Zenarius.

Καταρχαί.
Exordia.
(Kat. II S. 111).

Ed. A. Olivieri, Catal. codd. astrol. I p. 128—129.

Inc. Ἐκκείσθω δὲ καὶ κατὰ Ζηνάριον πῶς τινες πηγνύουσι τὰς καταρχάς.
Expl. ὁ δὲ Ἑρμῆς Ὑδροχόῳ.

Florenz: Laurent. 28, 34; s. XI. f. 22v.
Paris: Parisin. 1991; s. XV. f. 49.

Zosimus Panopolita.

Περὶ ἀρετῆς καὶ συνθέσεως ὑδάτων.
(Kat. II S. 111.)

Mailand: Ambros.
E 37 Sup.; s. XVI. f. 290v.
A 57 Inf.; s. XVI. f. 104v.
A 193 Inf.; s. XVI. f. 106v.

Excerpta varia.
(Kat. II S. 112.)

Mailand: Ambros.
A 57 Inf.; s. XVI.
A 193 Inf.; s. XVI.

www.ingramcontent.com/pod-product-compliance
Ingram Content Group UK Ltd.
Pitfield, Milton Keynes, MK11 3LW, UK
UKHW051029041026
15470UKWH00016B/1820

9 783110 600643